Straight A's
in
Anatomy &
Physiology

Straight A's

in

Anatomy & Physiology

Lippincott Williams & Wilkins
a Wolters Kluwer business
Philadelphia · Baltimore · New York · London
Buenos Aires · Hong Kong · Sydney · Tokyo

STAFF

Executive Publisher
Judith A. Schilling McCann, RN, MSN

Editorial Director
David Moreau

Clinical Director
Joan M. Robinson, RN, MSN

Art Director
Mary Ludwicki

Senior Managing Editor
Jaime Stockslager Buss, ELS

Editorial Project Manager
Coleen M.F. Stern

Clinical Project Manager
Beverly Ann Tscheschlog, RN, BS

Editors
Margaret Eckman, Diane M. Labus,
Gale Thompson

Clinical Editor
Marcy S. Caplin, RN, MSN

Copy Editors
Kimberly Bilotta (supervisor),
Tom DeZego, Amy Furman,
Shana Harrington, Lisa Stockslager,
Pamela Wingrod

Designer
Matie Anne Patterson

Digital Composition Services
Diane Paluba (manager),
Joyce Rossi Biletz, Donna S. Morris

Associate Manufacturing Manager
Beth J. Welsh

Editorial Assistants
Megan L. Aldinger, Karen J. Kirk,
Linda K. Ruhf

Indexer
Karen C. Comerford

STRA&P011106

**Library of Congress
Cataloging-in-Publication Data**

Straight A's in anatomy and physiology.
    p. ; cm.
  Includes bibliographical references and index.
  1. Human physiology—Outlines, syllabi, etc. 2. Human anatomy—Outlines, syllabi, etc. 3. Human physiology—Examinations, questions, etc. 4. Human anatomy—Examinations, questions, etc. 5. Nurses—Licenses—United States—Examinations—Study guides. I. Lippincott Williams & Wilkins.
  [DNLM: 1. Anatomy—Examination Questions. 2. Anatomy—Nurses' Instruction. 3. Physiology—Examination Questions. 4. Physiology—Nurses' Instruction. QS 18.2 S896 2007]
  QP41.S895 2007
  612—dc22
ISBN13 978-1-58255-562-1
ISBN10 1-58255-562-1 (alk. paper)   2006024927

Contents

Advisory board

Ivy Alexander, PhD, CANP
Assistant Professor, Yale University
New Haven, Conn.

Susan E. Appling, RN, MS, CRNP
Assistant Professor, Johns Hopkins University School of Nursing
Baltimore

Paul M. Arnstein, PhD, APRN-BC, FNP-C
Assistant Professor, Boston College

Bobbie Berkowitz, PhD, CNAA, FAAN
Chair & Professor, Psychosocial & Community Health
University of Washington
Seattle

Karla Jones, RN, MSN
Nursing Faculty, Treasure Valley Community College
Ontario, Ore.

Manon Lemonde, RN, PhD
Associate Professor, University of Ontario (Oshawa) Institute of Technology

Sheila Sparks Ralph, RN, DNSC, FAAN
Director & Professor, Division of Nursing & Respiratory Care
Shenandoah University
Winchester, Va.

Kristine Anne Scordo, RN, PhD, CS, ACNP
Director, Acute Care Nurse Practitioner Program
Wright State University
Dayton, Ohio

Robin Wilkerson, RN, BC, PhD
Associate Professor, University of Mississippi
Jackson

Contributors and consultants

Rita Bates, RN, MSN
Team Leader, Fundamentals of Nursing, ADN
University of Arkansas
Fort Smith

Lynn Cherry, RN, MSN
Education Specialist
Henry Ford Hospital
Detroit

Kim Cooper, RN, MSN
Nursing Department Program Chairperson
Ivy Tech Community College
Terre Haute, Ind.

Lillian Craig, RN, MSN, FNP-C
Adjunct Faculty
Oklahoma Panhandle State University
Goodwell

Diane J. Lane, RN, MSN
Instructor, Vocational Nursing
Silva Health Magnet High School
El Paso, Tex.

Virginia Lester, RN, MSN
Assistant Professor in Nursing
Angelo State University
San Angelo, Tex.

Linda Ludwig, RN, BS, MEd
Practical Nursing Instructor
Canadian Valley Technology Center
El Reno, Okla.

William J. Pawlyshyn, RN, BSN, MS, MN, M.DIV, APRN-BC, ANP-C
Nurse Practitioner
Cape Cod Ear, Nose & Throat Specialists
Hyannis, Mass.

Maria Elsa Rodriguez, RN
Clinical Educator
Kindred Hospital
San Diego

Janis Simpson, RN, BSN, MA, EdS
Practical Nursing Coordinator
Tennessee Technology Center
Athens

Betty E. Sims, RN, MSN
Nurse Consultant
Board of Nurse Examiners
Austin, Tex.

Kimberly Such-Smith, RN, BSN, LNC
President, Healthcare Advocate
Nursing Analysis & Review, LLC
Byron, Minn.

Allison J. Terry, RN, MSN, PhD
Nurse Consultant
Alabama Board of Nursing
Montgomery

How to use this book

Straight A's is a multivolume study guide series developed especially for nursing students. Each volume provides essential course material in a unique two-column design. The easy-to-read interior outline format offers a succinct review of key facts as presented in leading textbooks on the subject. The bulleted exterior columns provide only the most crucial information, allowing for quick, efficient review right before an important quiz or test.

Special features appear in every chapter to make information accessible and easy to remember. **Learning objectives** encourage the student to evaluate knowledge before and after study. The **Chapter overview** highlights major concepts. The NCLEX®-style questions found in the **NCLEX checks** at the end of each chapter offer additional opportunities to review material and assess knowledge gained before moving on to new information.

Other features appear throughout the book to facilitate learning. **Clinical alerts** appear in color to bring the reader's attention to important, potentially life-threatening considerations that could affect patient care. **Time-out for teaching** highlights key areas to address when teaching patients. **Go with the flow** charts promote critical thinking. Last, a Windows-based software program (see CD-ROM on inside back cover) poses more than 250 multiple-choice and alternate-format NCLEX-style questions in random order to assess your knowledge.

The *Straight A's* volumes are designed as learning tools, not as primary information sources. When read conscientiously as a supplement to class attendance and textbook reading, *Straight A's* can enhance understanding and help improve test scores and final grades.

Foreword

As an experienced family nurse practitioner who has taught prelicensure registered nursing students and graduate nursing students, I'm always appreciative of texts that provide a straightforward review of complex material. Students often don't keep their textbooks from anatomy and physiology and, therefore, have no basis on which to conduct a review. In addition, texts are scarce that contain anatomy and physiology material that's succinct yet detailed and, most importantly, that are reader friendly. That's why *Straight A's in Anatomy & Physiology* is a must have for your reference shelf.

This review text not only presents the basic concepts of anatomy and physiology but also reviews each body system in an innovative format that makes the learning process easy. Each chapter begins with clearly stated learning objectives and a chapter overview that summarizes the topics featured within. The book's unique two-column design presents a simple-to-follow outline in the main text along with an outer column highlighting key points, so students can retrieve important facts lightning fast and study more efficiently for an exam.

Perhaps most important to prelicensure registered nursing students are the NCLEX-style questions, including alternate-format types, at the end of each chapter, which provide the correct answers and rationales for correct and incorrect answer choices. In addition to the 200 end-of-chapter questions, students can continue to test themselves with the more than 250 NCLEX-style questions on the CD-ROM in the back of the book.

Straight A's in Anatomy & Physiology isn't just for prelicensure registered nursing students, it's also useful for any registered nurse or advanced practice nurse who wishes to review anatomy and physiology. Even more-experienced clinicians will find that the clear diagrams and succinct, bulleted information are a quick-and-easy way to brush up on their knowledge of anatomy and physiology. And once you learn the *Straight A's* way, you'll reach for other books in the series when it's time to study!

Nancy M. George, PhD, APRN, BC
Assistant Professor (Clinical)
Wayne State University
College of Nursing
Detroit

1

Overview of anatomy and physiology

LEARNING OBJECTIVES

After studying this chapter, you should be able to:

- Define anatomy and physiology.
- Describe common terms used in anatomy and physiology.
- Identify directional terms used to describe the location of body structures.
- Identify body reference planes.
- Name the major body cavities and the organs found in each.
- Describe how the human body achieves homeostasis.

CHAPTER OVERVIEW

Every nurse needs a basic understanding of anatomy and physiology, including knowledge of how the body is organized, how its parts function together, and how disease and other factors may affect its structures and functions. This chapter reviews basic anatomy and physiology terms, body reference planes, body cavities and their contents, body regions, and the principles of homeostasis.

Types of anatomy

- Gross: studies structures visible to the eye
- Regional: studies limited regions of the body
- Developmental: studies structural changes occurring over time
- Microanatomy: studies structures using a microscope
- Applied: applies anatomic findings to medical diagnosis and treatment
- Pathologic: studies diseased or injured tissue

Types of physiology

- Cell: studies cell functions
- Systems: studies operation of organ systems
- Pathophysiology: studies changes caused by disease or aging
- Exercise: studies cell and organ function during activity
- Neurophysiology: studies nerve cell functions
- Endocrinology: studies effects of hormones on body functions
- Immunology: studies body's defense mechanisms

DEFINITIONS

● **Anatomy**
- Anatomy: study of the body's structure and the relationship of its parts
- Includes several subdivisions that address specific aspects of structure
  - *Gross anatomy* (macroscopic anatomy) is the study of anatomic structures visible to the unaided eye
  - *Regional anatomy* is the study of limited portions or regions of the body, such as the head and neck
  - *Developmental anatomy* is the study of structural changes from conception through old age
  - *Microanatomy* (microscopic anatomy) is the study of anatomic structures using a microscope
  - *Applied anatomy* is the application of anatomic findings to the diagnosis and treatment of medical disorders
  - *Pathologic anatomy* (morbid anatomy) is the study of abnormal, diseased, or injured tissue

● **Physiology**
- Physiology: study of how body parts function, including their chemical and physical processes
- Includes several subdivisions that address specific aspects of function
  - *Cell physiology* is the study of cell functions
  - *Systems physiology* is the study of organ system operation
  - *Pathophysiology* is the study of functional changes caused by disease and aging
  - *Exercise physiology* is the study of cell and organ functions during skeletal muscle activity
  - *Neurophysiology* is the study of nerve cell functions
  - *Endocrinology* is the study of the effects of hormones on body functions
  - *Immunology* is the study of the body's defense mechanisms
- Can also be subdivided according to the function of specific structures
  - *Cardiovascular physiology* is the study of the heart and blood vessels
  - *Respiratory physiology* is the study of air passageways and lungs
  - *Renal physiology* is the study of kidneys
  - *Reproductive physiology* is the study of reproductive structures
- Also covers *complementarity,* or how the functions of a body part reflect (complement) its structure; for example, the structure of the heart valves controls the direction of blood flow through the heart

Anatomic and directional terms
- Used by clinicians and throughout health science fields to describe exact location of body structures; terms are derived mainly from Greek or Latin
- *Anatomical position:* position of the body when erect and facing forward, with arms at the sides and palms turned forward
- *Superior (cranial):* toward the head
- *Inferior (caudal):* toward the tail or lower part of the body
- *Anterior (ventral):* toward the front of the body
- *Posterior (dorsal):* toward the back of the body
- *Medial:* toward the midline of the body
- *Lateral:* away from the midline of the body
- *Proximal:* closest to the trunk, point of origin of a part, or center of the body
- *Distal:* farthest from the trunk, point of origin of a part, or center of the body
- *Superficial:* toward or at the body surface
- *Deep:* farthest from the body surface

Body reference planes
- Imaginary lines that divide the body and its organs into sections
- Used to describe the body's structural plan and the anatomic relationship of its parts
- Includes three major body reference planes — sagittal, frontal, and transverse — which lie at right angles to one another (see *Body reference planes,* page 4)
  - *Sagittal plane* runs longitudinally (lengthwise), dividing the body into right and left regions
    - Called the median sagittal plane or midsagittal plane when exactly midline
    - Called the parasagittal plane when not exactly midline
  - *Frontal plane* (coronal plane) runs longitudinally but at a right angle to the sagittal plane, dividing the body into anterior and posterior regions
  - *Transverse plane* runs horizontally at a right angle to the vertical axis, dividing the body into superior and inferior regions
- Also includes the *oblique plane,* which is slanted and lies between horizontal and longitudinal planes

BODY ORGANIZATION AND FUNCTION

Structural organization
- Characteristic of the body and all its parts
- Each higher level is increasingly more complex than the previous level

Body reference planes

Body reference planes are directional terms used to locate body structures. This illustration shows the median sagittal, frontal, and transverse planes, which lie at right angles to one another.

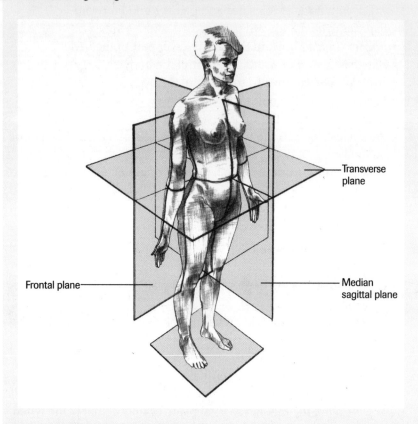

Transverse plane

Frontal plane

Median sagittal plane

Key facts about structural organization

- Chemical level: most basic level; consists of atoms and molecules
- Cellular level: basic structures and functions; consists of cells
- Tissue level: cells and surrounding substances work together
- Organ level: different tissues perform a function
- Systems level: different organs perform complex functions
- Organismic level: highest level

– *Chemical level* includes the atoms and molecules needed to maintain life
– Cellular level consists of cells—the body's basic structural and functional unit
– Tissue level combines similar cells and surrounding substances into groups that work together
– Organ level organizes different kinds of tissues—usually in recognizable shapes—to perform a special function
– Systems level consists of different kinds of organs arranged to perform complex functions
– Organismic level (highest level) brings together all lower level structures into a functioning, living being
• Changes gradually
– Structures typically grow and develop until young adulthood
– After young adulthood, body structures typically age and atrophy

Body cavities

This illustration shows the body's two major cavities—dorsal and ventral. The dorsal cavity, located posteriorly, is subdivided into the cranial and vertebral cavities. The ventral cavity, located anteriorly, is subdivided into the thoracic and abdominopelvic cavities.

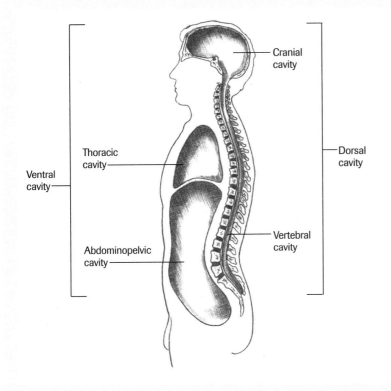

Key body cavities

- Dorsal: posterior region; cranial and vertebral cavities
- Ventral: anterior region; thoracic and abdominopelvic cavities
- Oral (mouth)
- Nasal (nose)
- Orbital (eyes)
- Tympanic (middle ear bones)
- Synovial (movable joints)

● Body cavities
- Spaces within the body that house the internal organs
- Include two major closed cavities—dorsal and ventral—containing the internal organs (see *Body cavities*)
  - Dorsal cavity is located in the posterior region of the body; it's divided into cranial and vertebral cavities
    - *Cranial cavity* (skull) encases the brain
    - *Vertebral cavity,* also called the *spinal cavity* or *vertebral canal,* is formed by the series of bones (vertebrae) that enclose the spinal cord
  - Ventral cavity is located in the anterior region of the trunk
    - Walls and outer surface of its organs are covered by a thin membrane called the *serosa*
      - *Parietal serosa* lines the cavity wall
      - *Visceral serosa* covers the organs

• Divided into thoracic and abdominopelvic cavities
  – Thoracic cavity is superior to the abdominopelvic cavity (separated by the diaphragm, a large dome-shaped muscle), surrounded by the ribs and chest muscles, and divided into the pleural cavities and mediastinum
    • Two lateral *pleural cavities* each contain a lung (serosa in these cavities is called the *pleura*)
    • *Mediastinum* contains the heart (enclosed in a membranous serosal sac called the *pericardium,* which forms the pericardial cavity), large vessels of the heart, trachea, esophagus, thymus, lymph nodes, and portions of other vessels and nerves
  – *Abdominopelvic cavity* is subdivided into the superior portion (abdominal cavity) and inferior portion (pelvic cavity), which aren't separated by muscle or membrane (serosa in these cavities is called the *peritoneum*)
    • *Abdominal cavity* contains the stomach, spleen, liver, small intestine, most of the large intestine, and other organs
    • *Pelvic cavity* contains the bladder, some of the large intestine, some reproductive organs, and the rectum
• Also includes other cavities: oral, nasal, orbital, tympanic, and synovial
  – *Oral cavity* (mouth) contains the teeth and tongue and is continuous with other GI structures
  – *Nasal cavity* (nose) is divided medially and is continuous with the respiratory tract
  – *Orbital cavities* house the eyes
  – *Tympanic cavities* (temporal bone) contain the auditory ossicles (small bones of the middle ear)
  – *Synovial cavities* are enclosed within fibrous capsules that surround freely movable joints

● **Body regions**
• Specific areas of the body with a particular nerve, vascular supply, or special function
• Used to describe the anatomic locations of body structures
• Abdominal regions are most widely used body region terms (see *Abdominal regions*)
  – *Umbilical region* (navel) surrounds the umbilicus; prominent structures include sections of the small and large intestines, inferior vena cava, and abdominal aorta
  – *Epigastric region* (stomach) is superior to the umbilical region; prominent structures include the pancreas and portions of the stomach, liver, inferior vena cava, abdominal aorta, and duodenum

Abdominal regions

This illustration shows an anterior view of the abdominal regions.

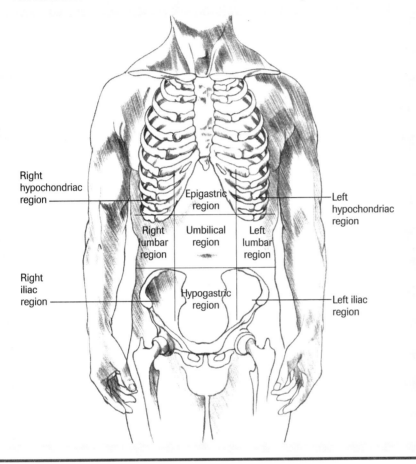

Right
hypochondriac
region

Epigastric
region

Left
hypochondriac
region

Right
lumbar
region

Umbilical
region

Left
lumbar
region

Right
iliac
region

Hypogastric
region

Left iliac
region

Key structures of the hypogastric region

- Portions of the sigmoid colon
- Urinary bladder
- Ureters
- Small intestine

- *Hypogastric region* (pubic region) is inferior to the umbilical region; prominent structures include portions of the sigmoid colon, urinary bladder, ureters, and small intestine
- Right and left *inguinal regions* (iliac regions) are lateral to the hypogastric region; prominent structures include portions of the small and large intestines
- Right and left *lumbar regions* (loin regions) are lateral to the umbilical region; prominent structures include portions of the small and large intestines and portions of the right and left kidneys
- Right and left *hypochondriac regions* are lateral to the epigastric region; both contain portions of the diaphragm and kidneys
  · Right region contains the right side of the liver and portions of the diaphragm and kidneys

Key structures of the right and left hypochondriac regions

Right

- Right side of the liver
- Portion of the diaphragm
- Portion of the kidneys

Left

- Spleen
- Portion of the diaphragm
- Portion of the kidneys

· Left region contains the spleen and portions of the diaphragm and kidneys

● **Homeostasis**
- Condition of relative constancy in the body's internal environment
- Occurs only when the body's internal environment meets certain criteria
  - Water, gases, and ions are all in the proper concentration
  - Normal temperature is maintained
  - Sufficient fluid volume is available to maintain cellular health
- Maintained and restored by nervous and endocrine systems through homeostatic mechanisms
  - Homeostatic mechanisms operate by negative feedback
  - Change in one direction feeds back to cause a change in the opposite direction

NCLEX CHECKS

It's never too soon to begin your NCLEX preparation. Now that you've reviewed this chapter, carefully read each of the following questions and choose the best answer. Then compare your responses with the correct answers.

1. The nurse is assessing a 1-year-old boy and discussing with his parents the changes they can expect to see in their child over the next year. In this discussion, the nurse uses knowledge of which subdivision of anatomy?
- ☐ **1.** Gross
- ☐ **2.** Developmental
- ☐ **3.** Microanatomy
- ☐ **4.** Pathologic

2. While teaching a client with newly diagnosed diabetes mellitus, the nurse explains that the client needs to see a specialist in which area?
- ☐ **1.** Endocrinology
- ☐ **2.** Exercise physiology
- ☐ **3.** Neurophysiology
- ☐ **4.** Immunology

3. The nurse auscultates the client's heart sounds with a stethoscope. Which structural level is the nurse assessing?
- ☐ **1.** Chemical
- ☐ **2.** Cellular
- ☐ **3.** Tissue
- ☐ **4.** Organ

4. The nurse places the stethoscope over the upper left side of the client's chest to listen to his lungs. The nurse documents that breath sounds were auscultated in which location?

- ☐ **1.** Inferior chest
- ☐ **2.** Anterior chest
- ☐ **3.** Posterior chest
- ☐ **4.** Medial chest

5. The nurse is assessing a client's rash and comparing lesions on the right side of his body with lesions on the left side. Which reference plane does the nurse use to divide the body lengthwise into right and left regions?

- ☐ **1.** Frontal
- ☐ **2.** Sagittal
- ☐ **3.** Transverse
- ☐ **4.** Oblique

6. The nurse is caring for a client who has a chest tube placed through the chest wall into the space surrounding his right lung. The nurse explains to the client that the end of the chest tube is located in which cavity?

- ☐ **1.** Cranial
- ☐ **2.** Abdominal
- ☐ **3.** Thoracic
- ☐ **4.** Vertebral

7. A client complains of abdominal pain and points to the epigastric region when the nurse asks him to point to the area where the pain is located. Identify the area on the illustration where the client feels pain.

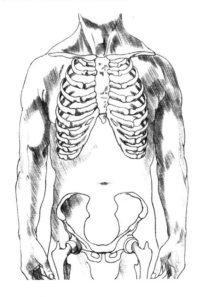

8. A client has sustained injuries to his mediastinum following a motor vehicle accident. Which structure would the nurse anticipate is injured?

☐ **1.** Small intestine
☐ **2.** Heart
☐ **3.** Bladder
☐ **4.** Brain

9. The nurse knows that which condition must be met for a client's body to be in a state of homeostasis?

☐ **1.** Water, gases, and ions must be in proper concentration.
☐ **2.** The body must maintain an above normal temperature.
☐ **3.** The nervous and cardiovascular systems must operate by negative feedback.
☐ **4.** The nervous and endocrine systems must operate by positive feedback.

10. When teaching a class on heart disease to high-risk clients, the nurse discusses the structure of the body and the relationship of its parts. Which term is the nurse discussing?

☐ **1.** Anatomy
☐ **2.** Physiology
☐ **3.** Complementarity
☐ **4.** Homeostasis

ANSWERS AND RATIONALES

1. CORRECT ANSWER: 2
Developmental anatomy is the study of structural changes from conception through old age. The nurse uses knowledge of developmental anatomy to explain to the parents the changes that will occur in their child over the next year. Gross, or macroscopic, anatomy is the study of anatomic structures visible to the unaided eye. Microanatomy (microscopic anatomy) is the study of anatomic structures that can be seen only by using a microscope. Pathologic, or morbid, anatomy is the study of diseased or injured tissue.

2. CORRECT ANSWER: 1
Diabetes mellitus is an endocrine disorder; thus, the client will need to see a specialist in endocrinology (the study of the effects of hormones on the body). A specialist in exercise physiology focuses on the study of cell and organ function during skeletal muscle activity. A specialist in neurophysiology specializes in the study of nerve cell functions. A specialist in immunology studies the body's defense mechanisms.

3. CORRECT ANSWER: 4
The heart is an organ; therefore, the nurse is assessing the client at the organ structural level. The chemical level consists of the atoms and mol-

ecules that maintain life. The cellular level consists of the cells that are the body's basic structural and functional units. The tissue level combines similar cells and surrounding substances that work together.

4. CORRECT ANSWER: 2

The nurse placed the stethoscope over the client's upper left chest, which is the anterior (ventral) position or toward the front of the body, left of midline. Documenting the inferior chest would indicate that the nurse placed the stethoscope over the lower portion of the chest. Noting the posterior (dorsal) position would indicate that the nurse placed the stethoscope over the client's back. Documenting the medial position would indicate that the nurse placed the stethoscope toward or over the body's midline.

5. CORRECT ANSWER: 2

The nurse uses the sagittal plane, which runs lengthwise through the body, to divide the body into right and left regions. The frontal (coronal) plane also runs lengthwise but at a right angle to the sagittal plane, dividing the body into anterior and posterior regions. The transverse plane runs horizontally through the body at a right angle to the vertical axis, dividing the body into superior and inferior regions. The slanted oblique plane lies between the horizontal and longitudinal planes.

6. CORRECT ANSWER: 3

The lungs are located in the thoracic cavity. The cranial cavity (skull) contains the brain. The abdominal cavity contains the stomach, intestines, spleen, liver, and other organs. The vertebral cavity surrounds the spinal cord.

7. CORRECT ANSWER:

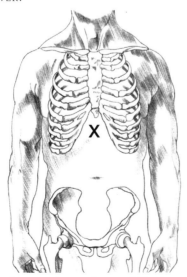

The epigastric region is superior to the umbilical region and contains most of the pancreas as well as portions of the stomach, liver, inferior vena cava, abdominal aorta, and duodenum.

8. CORRECT ANSWER: 2

The mediastinum, located in the ventral cavity, contains the heart, large vessels of the heart, trachea, esophagus, thymus, lymph nodes, and portions of other vessels and nerves. The small intestine is located in the abdominal cavity, which also contains the stomach, spleen, liver, most of the large intestine, and other organs. The bladder is located in the pelvic cavity, which also contains some of the large intestine, some reproductive organs, and the rectum. The cranial cavity contains the brain.

9. CORRECT ANSWER: 1

Homeostasis requires the proper concentrations of water, gases, and ions within the body as well as a normal temperature. The nervous and endocrine systems maintain homeostasis through negative feedback. The cardiovascular system isn't part of the homeostatic mechanism.

10. CORRECT ANSWER: 1

Anatomy is the study of the body's structures and the relationship of its parts. Physiology is the study of how body parts function, including their chemical and physical processes. Complementarity refers to the way that the functions of a body part reflect its structure. Homeostasis is a condition of relative constancy in the body's internal environment.

2

Chemical organization

LEARNING OBJECTIVES

After studying this chapter, you should be able to:

● Describe the basic chemical principles.
● Understand the chemical composition of the body.
● Identify the structure of an atom.
● Describe chemical bonds and reactions.
● Explain the differences between inorganic and organic compounds.

CHAPTER OVERVIEW

The chemical level is the simplest level of structural organization, yet it's the most important. Without the proper chemicals in the proper amounts, the cells—and eventually the body—will die. Not only is the body composed of chemicals, but all of its activities are chemical in nature as well. This chapter reviews the basic principles of chemistry, such as atomic structure and chemical bonds and reaction, and the inorganic and organic compounds in the body.

BASIC PRINCIPLES

● **Matter and energy**
  • Matter: anything that has mass and occupies space

– Matter may be a solid, liquid, or gas
– All forms of matter are composed of chemical elements
• Energy: the capacity to do work (put mass into motion)
– Two basic types are *potential* (stored) and *kinetic* (energy of motion)
– Forms of energy include chemical, electrical, and radiant
• Matter and energy can't be created or destroyed; however, matter can be converted to energy

● **Chemical elements**
• Element: a form of matter that can't be broken down into simpler substances by normal chemical reactions
• When two or more elements combine, they're called a *compound* (see *Understanding elements and compounds*)
• Periodic table of elements lists 109 chemical elements, each with its own chemical symbol

Key facts about matter

• Anything that has mass and occupies space
• Can be solid, liquid, or gas
• Can be converted to energy
• Can't be created or destroyed

Key facts about energy

• The capacity to do work
• Two types: potential and kinetic
• Forms: chemical, electrical, and radiant
• Can't be created or destroyed

Key facts about elements and compounds

• Element: form of matter that can't be broken down further
• Periodic table has 109 chemical elements
• Two or more elements combine to form a compound

Understanding elements and compounds

The best way to remember the difference between elements and compounds is to understand how atoms combine to form each.

ATOMS ALONE
A single atom constitutes an element; for example, an atom of hydrogen is also the element hydrogen. However, an element can also be composed of more than one atom—a molecule.

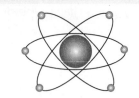

MOLECULES: TWO (OR MORE) OF THE SAME
A molecule is a combination of two or more atoms. If these atoms are all the same element (such as all hydrogen atoms), they're considered a *molecule* of that element (a molecule of hydrogen).

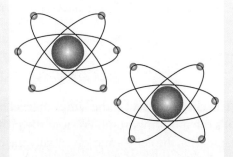

COMPOUNDS: WHERE THE DIFFERENT COME TOGETHER
If the atoms combined are different elements (such as a carbon atom and an oxygen atom), the molecule formed is a *compound* (such as CO, or carbon monoxide).

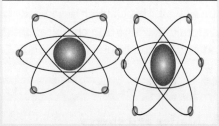

What's a body made of?

This chart shows the chemical elements of the human body from most to least plentiful.

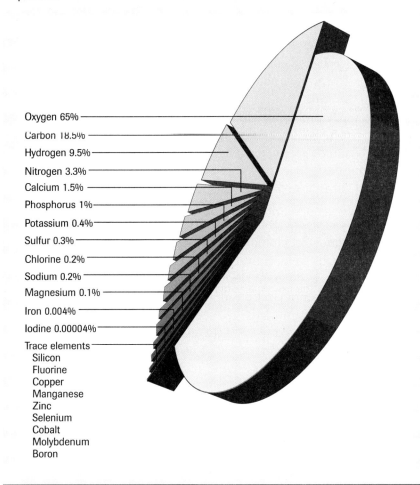

Oxygen 65%
Carbon 18.5%
Hydrogen 9.5%
Nitrogen 3.3%
Calcium 1.5%
Phosphorus 1%
Potassium 0.4%
Sulfur 0.3%
Chlorine 0.2%
Sodium 0.2%
Magnesium 0.1%
Iron 0.004%
Iodine 0.00004%
Trace elements
  Silicon
  Fluorine
  Copper
  Manganese
  Zinc
  Selenium
  Cobalt
  Molybdenum
  Boron

Key elements in the human body

- Oxygen: 65%
- Carbon: 18.5%
- Hydrogen: 9.5%
- Nitrogen: 3.3%
- Calcium: 1.5%
- Phosphorus: 1%

- Oxygen, carbon, hydrogen, and nitrogen make up 96% of total body weight (see *What's a body made of?*)
- Calcium and phosphorus compose another 2.5% of total body weight
- An imbalance of chemicals in the body can cause cell death

● **Atoms**
- *Atom:* smallest unit of matter that can take part in a chemical reaction (an element is composed of atoms of a single type such as carbon)
- When two or more atoms combine, they're called a *molecule*
- When one atom combines with or breaks apart from another atom, a *chemical reaction* occurs

Key facts about atoms

- Smallest unit of matter that can take part in a chemical reaction
- Electrically neutral
- Two or more combine to form a molecule
- Each consists of a nucleus and one or more electron shells
- Nucleus contains protons and neutrons
- Atomic weight: the total mass of protons, neutrons, and electrons
- Mass number: the sum of the mass of protons and neutrons

Types of subatomic particles

- Protons: positive, in nucleus
- Neutrons: neutral, in nucleus
- Electrons: negative, in outer shell, number of electrons = number of protons in the nucleus

- Each atom consists of a nucleus (dense central core) and one or more electron shells (surrounding energy layers)
- Three basic subatomic particles: protons, neutrons, and electrons
  – Protons (p+) are positively charged particles in the atom's nucleus
    · Each element has a unique number of protons
    · Number of protons determines the element's *atomic number* (each element has a unique atomic number)
    · The positive charge of a nucleus equals the number of its protons
    · One proton weighs the same as one neutron, which is equal to 1,836 times the weight of one electron
  – Neutrons are uncharged (neutral) particles in the atom's nucleus
    · All atoms of an element don't necessarily have the same number of neutrons
    · *Isotopes* are atoms that have a different number of neutrons from most atoms of an element
  – Electrons are negatively charged particles that orbit around the nucleus in different electron shells
    · Number of electrons in an atom equals the number of protons in its nucleus
    · Negative charges of electrons cancel out the positive charges of protons; because of this cancellation, atoms are electrically neutral
    · Each electron shell surrounding the nucleus can accommodate a maximum number of electrons (the innermost shell can hold no more than two electrons; the outermost shells can hold many more)
    · Electrons play a key role in chemical bonds and reactions
      - An atom with single (unpaired) electrons in its outer electron shell can participate in chemical reactions
      - An atom's *valence* (combining capacity) equals the number of unpaired electrons in its outer shell
- Atomic weight (atomic mass) equals the total mass of an atom's protons, neutrons, and electrons (p + n + e)
- Mass number is the sum of the mass of an atom's protons and neutrons (p + n); because electrons have little mass, an atom's mass number may nearly equal its atomic weight

● **Chemical bonds**
- Chemical bonds: forces of attraction that hold together the atoms of a molecule
- Formation usually requires energy (chemical bond breakage usually releases energy)

Key facts about chemical bonds

- Forces of attraction that hold together the atoms of a molecule
- Require energy to form
- Release energy when broken

Picturing ionic and covalent bonds

A chemical bond is a force of attraction that binds the atoms of a molecule to-gether. These illustrations show how ionic and covalent bonds form.

IONIC BONDS

In an ionic bond, an electron is transferred from one atom to another. For ex-ample, this is what happens when an electron is transferred by forces of attrac-tion from a sodium (Na) atom to a chlorine (Cl) atom. The result is a molecule of sodium chloride (NaCl).

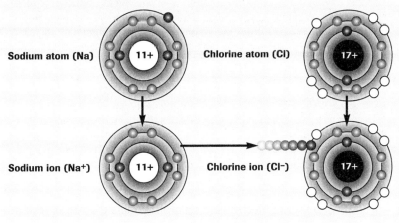

COVALENT BONDS

In a covalent bond, atoms share a pair of electrons. This is what happens when two hydrogen (H) atoms form a covalent bond.

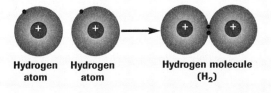

- Types of chemical bonds: ionic, covalent, and hydrogen
  - Ionic bonds form when valence electrons are transferred from one atom to another
  - Covalent bonds form when atoms share pairs of valence elec-trons (see Picturing ionic and covalent bonds)
  - Hydrogen bonds form when two atoms associate with a hydro-gen atom (oxygen and nitrogen commonly form hydrogen bonds)
- **Chemical reactions**
  - Depend on energy as well as particle concentration, speed, and orientation

Types of chemical bonds

- Ionic: when valence electrons are transferred from one atom to another
- Covalent: when atoms share pairs of valence electrons
- Hydrogen: when two atoms associate with a hydrogen atom

Types of chemical reactions

- Synthesis: two or more substances combine to form a new, more complex substance
- Decomposition: a substance breaks down into two or more simpler substances
- Exchange: combination of decomposition and synthesis reactions
- Reversible: the product of a chemical reaction reverts to its original reactants or vice versa

---

Comparing chemical reactions

When chemical reactions occur, they involve unpaired electrons in the outer shells of atoms. Here are the four basic types of chemical reactions.

SYNTHESIS REACTION (ANABOLISM)
A synthesis reaction combines two or more substances (reactants) to form a new, more complex substance (product). This results in a chemical bond.

$$A + B \rightarrow AB$$

EXCHANGE REACTION
An exchange reaction is a combination of a decomposition and a synthesis reaction. This reaction occurs when two complex substances decompose into simpler substances. The simple substances then join (through synthesis) with different simple substances to form new complex substances.

$$AB + CD \rightarrow A + B + C + D \rightarrow AD + BC$$

DECOMPOSITION REACTION (CATABOLISM)
In a decomposition reaction, a substance decomposes (breaks down) into two or more simpler substances, leading to the breakdown of a chemical bond.

$$AB \rightarrow A + B$$

REVERSIBLE REACTION
In a reversible reaction, the product reverts to its original reactants and vice versa. Reversible reactions may require special conditions, such as heat or light.

$$A + B \leftrightarrow AB$$

- Four basic types: synthetic, decomposition, exchange, and reversible (see *Comparing chemical reactions*)
  - *Synthesis reactions* involve the combination of two or more substances (reactants) to form a new, more complex substance (product)
    - Chemical bonds form
    - Collectively, synthesis reactions in the body are called *anabolism*
  - *Decomposition reactions* involve the breakdown of a substance into two or more simpler substances
    - Chemical bonds break
    - Collectively, decomposition reactions in the body are called *catabolism*
  - *Exchange reactions* combine decomposition and synthesis reactions
    - Two complex substances undergo decomposition into simpler substances
    - Through synthesis, the simple substances combine with different simple substances to form new complex substances
  - *Reversible reactions* allow the product to revert to its original reactants and vice versa; these reactions may require special conditions to take place (such as heat or light)

INORGANIC COMPOUNDS

● **Key concepts**
  - Usually small compounds lacking carbon that are formed from biomolecules (most biomolecules form organic compounds)
  - Major inorganic compounds: water and inorganic acids, bases, and salts

● **Water**
  - Body's most abundant substance
  - Excellent solvent and suspension medium; it easily forms polar covalent bonds
  - Acts as a lubricant in mucus and other body fluids
  - Enters into chemical reactions (such as nutrient breakdown during digestion)
  - Absorbs and releases heat slowly, which helps the body maintain homeostasis
  - Needs a great deal of heat to convert from a liquid to a gas (this function keeps the body cool through perspiration)

● **Inorganic acids, bases, and salts**
  - When molecules of inorganic acids, bases, and salts are in water, they undergo *ionization* (separation of ions)
    – *Acids* ionize into hydrogen ions (H^+) and anions (negatively charged ions); for example, HCl dissociates into H^+ and the anion Cl^-
    – *Bases* ionize into hydroxide ions (OH^-) and cations (positively charged ions); for example, KOH dissociates into OH^- and the cation K^+
    – *Salts* ionize into cations and anions but not H^+ or OH^- ions; for example, KCl dissociates into the cation K^+ and the anion Cl^-
  - When acids and bases react together, they form salts
  - To maintain homeostasis, body fluids must achieve *acid-base balance*
    – The greater the number of H^+ in a solution, the more acidic it is
    – The greater the number of OH^- in a solution, the more basic (alkaline) it is
    – The pH scale measures acidity or alkalinity of body fluids
      · *Neutral solutions* have a pH of 7.0 and contain equal amounts of H^+ and OH^-
      · *Acidic solutions* have a pH below 7.0 and contain more H^+ than OH^-
      · *Basic (alkaline) solutions* have a pH above 7.0 and contain more OH^- than H^+
    – In the body, pH is maintained by various buffer systems (see chapter 17, Fluid, electrolyte, and acid-base balance)

Key facts about inorganic compounds
- Small compounds lacking carbon formed from biomolecules
- Includes water and inorganic acids, bases, and salts

Key characteristics of water
- Acts as solvent and suspension medium
- Acts as lubricant
- Absorbs and releases heat slowly, helping maintain homeostasis

Key characteristics of inorganic acids, bases, and salts
- Undergo ionization in water
- Form salts when they react together
- To maintain homeostasis, body fluids must achieve acid-base balance
- The greater the number of H^+ in a solution, the more acidic it is
- The greater the number of OH^- in a solution, the more basic (alkaline) it is

Key facts about organic compounds

- Contain carbon and hydrogen formed from biomolecules
- Use covalent bonds
- Major organic compounds: carbohydrates, lipids, proteins, and nucleic acids

Key characteristics of carbohydrates

- Store and release energy
- Grouped by size as monosaccharides, disaccharides, and polysaccharides

Key characteristics of lipids

- Group of water-insoluble biomolecules
- Triglycerides: most plentiful; protect, insulate, and provide and store energy
- Phospholipids: major component of cell membranes
- Steroids: cholesterol (required to form other steroids), bile salts (aid in digestion and absorption of vitamins), male and female sex hormones (reproduction and sexual characteristics), and vitamin D (regulates body's calcium concentration)
- Lipoproteins: help transport lipids to various parts of the body
- Eicosanoids: prostaglandins (which serve diverse functions) and leukotrienes (which mediate inflammatory and allergic responses)

ORGANIC COMPOUNDS

● **Key concepts**
- Compounds containing carbon and hydrogen that form from biomolecules and use covalent bonds
- Major organic compounds: carbohydrates, lipids, proteins, and nucleic acids

● **Carbohydrates**
- Include sugars and starches as well as glycogen and cellulose
- Serve mainly to store and release energy
- Grouped by size as monosaccharides, disaccharides, and polysaccharides
  - *Monosaccharides* have three to seven carbon atoms and combine to form disaccharides or polysaccharides through dehydration synthesis; this process yields the more complex saccharide and water
  - *Disaccharides* are a combination of two monosaccharides; examples include sucrose (table sugar) and lactose (milk sugar)
  - *Polysaccharides* are large carbohydrates made from many monosaccharides (glycogen is the major polysaccharide)
  - Disaccharides and polysaccharides break down into monosaccharides by hydrolysis; adding water to larger molecules yields smaller molecules

● **Lipids**
- Diverse group of water-insoluble biomolecules
- Major lipids: triglycerides, phospholipids, steroids, lipoproteins, and eicosanoids
  - *Triglycerides* (neutral fats) are the most plentiful lipids in the diet and the body
    - Protect, insulate, and provide and store energy
    - Have three molecules of a fatty acid and one molecule of glycerol
  - *Phospholipids* function as the major component of cell membranes
    - Have one molecule of glycerol, two molecules of a fatty acid, and a phosphate group
    - Phosphatidylcholine (lecithin) is a common phospholipid
  - *Steroids* (cholesterol, bile salts, male and female sex hormones, and vitamin D) have different functions
    - *Cholesterol,* a part of cell membranes, is required to form all other steroids
    - *Bile salts* emulsify fats during digestion and promote the absorption of vitamins A, D, E, and K

- *Male and female sex hormones* are responsible for reproduction function and sexual characteristics
- *Vitamin D* helps regulate the body's calcium concentration
– *Lipoproteins* help transport lipids to various parts of the body
– *Eicosanoids* include prostaglandins and leukotrienes
  - *Prostaglandins* serve diverse functions, such as modifying hormone responses, promoting the inflammatory response, and opening airways
  - *Leukotrienes* mediate the inflammatory and allergic responses

● **Proteins**
- Polypeptides composed of *amino acids* (the building block of proteins)
- Sequence of amino acids in a protein's polypeptide chain determines its conformation (shape), which determines its functions
- Typical functions include providing structure and protection, regulating biological processes, promoting muscle contraction, transporting substances, and serving as enzymes
- *Enzymes,* the largest group of proteins, act as catalysts for vital chemical reactions

● **Nucleic acids**
- Include deoxyribonucleic acid (DNA) and ribonucleic acid (RNA)
- DNA is the primary hereditary molecule composed of nitrogenous bases, sugars, and phosphate groups
  – Includes two long chains of deoxyribonucleotides coiled into a double-helix shape
  – Deoxyribose and phosphate units alternate in the backbone of the chains
  – Base pairs of adenine-thymine and guanine-cytosine hold the two chains together
  – Each human DNA molecule contains a specific sequence of more than 100 million base pairs; this sequence is the same in all the DNA in one individual and different from the DNA of all other individuals
- RNA guides protein synthesis from amino acids
  – Unlike DNA, RNA has a single-chain structure
  – Contains ribose instead of deoxyribose, and substitutes uracil for the base thymine

Key characteristics of proteins

- Polypeptides composed of amino acids
- Provide structure and protection
- Regulate biological processes
- Promote muscle contraction
- Transport substances
- Enzymes (largest group) act as catalysts for vital chemical reactions

Key characteristics of nucleic acids

- DNA is the primary hereditary molecule
- RNA guides protein synthesis from amino acids

TOP 10

Items to study for your next test on chemical organization

1. Comparison of matter and energy
2. Chemical elements
3. Structures of the atom
4. Types of chemical bonds
5. Four types of chemical reactions
6. Differences between organic and inorganic compounds
7. Acid-base balance
8. Role of water in the body
9. Characteristics of carbohydrates, lipids, and proteins
10. Differences between RNA and DNA

NCLEX CHECKS

It's never too soon to begin your NCLEX preparation. Now that you've reviewed this chapter, carefully read each of the following questions and choose the best answer. Then compare your responses with the correct answers.

1. When planning a client's care, the nurse needs to keep in mind that which three chemical elements are the most abundant?
☐ **1.** Phosphorus, hydrogen, and oxygen
☐ **2.** Carbon, oxygen, and calcium
☐ **3.** Oxygen, carbon, and hydrogen
☐ **4.** Oxygen, carbon, and phosphorus

2. The nurse knows that a proton has which charge?
☐ **1.** Positive charge
☐ **2.** Negative charge
☐ **3.** Neutral charge
☐ **4.** Mixed charge

3. The nurse is teaching a client about proper nutrition. In answer to the client's question, which example of an organic compound does the nurse provide?
☐ **1.** Water
☐ **2.** An electrolyte
☐ **3.** A protein
☐ **4.** An acid

4. The nurse is teaching a class on nutrition to clients with newly diagnosed diabetes mellitus and correctly explains that which substance is a carbohydrate?
☐ **1.** Monosaccharide
☐ **2.** Amino acid
☐ **3.** Lipid
☐ **4.** Enzyme

5. When assessing a client's nutritional status, the nurse must keep in mind that protein has which primary function in the body?
☐ **1.** Maintains fluid and electrolyte balance
☐ **2.** Transports lipids
☐ **3.** Provides structure and protection
☐ **4.** Maintains normal pH

6. In the illustration below, identify the electron in the sodium atom that will be transferred to a chlorine atom to form a sodium chloride molecule by ionic bonding.

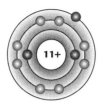

7. The nurse knows that which reaction involves the breakdown of a substance into two or more simpler substances?
- ☐ **1.** Synthesis
- ☐ **2.** Exchange
- ☐ **3.** Reversible
- ☐ **4.** Decomposition

8. The nurse is assessing the drainage from a client's nasogastric tube. Which finding would indicate acidic stomach contents?
- ☐ **1.** pH of 3.0
- ☐ **2.** pH of 7.0
- ☐ **3.** pH of 9.0
- ☐ **4.** pH of 11.0

9. When assessing a client's fluid and electrolyte balance, the nurse understands that water has which characteristic?
- ☐ **1.** It requires little heat to change from a liquid to a gas.
- ☐ **2.** It absorbs and releases heat quickly.
- ☐ **3.** It readily forms ionic bonds.
- ☐ **4.** It's a solvent and suspension medium.

10. The nurse knows that DNA contains which base pair?
- ☐ **1.** Adenine-uracil
- ☐ **2.** Adenine-thymine
- ☐ **3.** Guanine-ribose
- ☐ **4.** Cytosine-uracil

ANSWERS AND RATIONALES

1. CORRECT ANSWER: 3
Oxygen, carbon, hydrogen, and nitrogen—the most abundant elements of the human body, respectively—make up 96% of total body weight. Calcium and phosphorus compose another 2.5% of total body weight.

2. CORRECT ANSWER: 1

Protons are positively charged particles in the atom's nucleus. Electrons are negatively charged particles that orbit around the nucleus in different electron shells. Neutrons are uncharged (neutral) particles in the atom's nucleus.

3. CORRECT ANSWER: 3

Organic compounds all contain carbon. Examples include carbohydrates, lipids, proteins, and nucleic acids. Water, electrolytes, and acids are inorganic compounds.

4. CORRECT ANSWER: 1

Monosaccharides are carbohydrates with three to seven carbon atoms. They combine to form disaccharides or polysaccharides. Amino acids are the building blocks of proteins. Lipids are water-insoluble biomolecules that consist of triglycerides, phospholipids, steroids, lipoproteins, and eicosanoids. Enzymes are proteins that act as catalysts for vital chemical reactions.

5. CORRECT ANSWER: 3

Proteins provide structure and protection. They also regulate biological processes, promote muscle contraction, transport substances, and serve as enzymes.

6. CORRECT ANSWER:

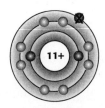

The electron that will be transferred is the outermost unpaired electron in the outer shell. An ionic bond is formed when valence electrons are transferred from one atom to another.

7. CORRECT ANSWER: 4

A decomposition reaction involves the breakdown of a substance into two or more simpler substances. In a synthesis reaction, two or more substances (reactants) combine to form a new, more complex substance (product). An exchange reaction combines both decomposition and synthesis reactions. In a reversible reaction, products revert to their original reactants and vice versa. A reversible reaction may need a special condition, such as heat or light.

8. CORRECT ANSWER: 1

An acidic solution has a pH of less than 7.0. A neutral solution has a pH of 7.0, and a basic solution has a pH greater than 7.0.

9. CORRECT ANSWER: 4

Water is the body's most abundant substance and acts as an excellent solvent and suspension medium. Because it absorbs and releases heat slowly, water helps the body remain in a homeostatic state. A large quantity of heat is required to convert water from a liquid to a gas, which allows water to cool the body through perspiration. Water readily forms polar covalent bonds.

10. CORRECT ANSWER: 2

In DNA, two long chains of deoxyribonucleotides coil into a double-helix shape. Base pairs of adenine-thymine and guanine-cytosine hold the two chains together. RNA substitutes uracil for the base thymine.

3

Cell organization

LEARNING OBJECTIVES

After studying this chapter, you should be able to:
- Describe cell structures and their functions.
- Discuss cellular energy production.
- Identify how substances move across a cell membrane.
- Describe cell division.
- Understand the phases of mitosis and meiosis.

CHAPTER OVERVIEW

Although the cellular level is the second level of structural organization, it's the first level for living matter. Learning about cell organization and function can help the nurse better understand certain disease processes, drug actions, and laboratory tests. This chapter reviews cellular components and energy production. It also explains substance movement across the cell membrane as well as cell division, including the phases of mitosis and meiosis.

CELLULAR COMPONENTS

● **Key concepts**
- Cells are structural and functional units of all living matter
- Smallest body structures that can perform all the fundamental activities of life (such as movement, ingestion, excretion, and reproduction)
- Consist of three major components: protoplasm, a cell membrane, and a nucleus (see *Inside the cell,* page 28)

● **Protoplasm**
- Viscous, translucent material containing a large percentage of water, inorganic ions (such as potassium, calcium, magnesium, and sodium), and naturally occurring organic compounds (such as proteins, lipids, and carbohydrates)
- *Nucleoplasm* is the protoplasm of the cell's nucleus; it plays a role in reproduction
- *Cytoplasm* is the protoplasm of the cell body that surrounds the nucleus (all the cell's contents from the cell membrane to the nucleus); it contains cytosol, organelles, and inclusions
  - *Cytosol* is the semifluid medium in the cytoplasm that makes up intracellular fluid; it contains proteins, enzymes, nutrients, and ions
  - *Organelles* are metabolic units that perform a specific function to maintain the life of the cell; they include mitochondria, ribosomes, the endoplasmic reticulum, Golgi apparatus (or complex), lysosomes, centrosomes, peroxisomes, and cytoskeletal elements
    · *Mitochondria* are the energy-producing cellular structures containing enzymes that oxidize food nutrients; this oxidation produces *adenosine triphosphate* (ATP), which provides energy for many cellular activities
    · *Ribosomes* are nucleoprotein particles attached to the endoplasmic reticulum and the site of protein synthesis
    · *Endoplasmic reticulum,* a system of interconnecting, fluid-filled, tubular channels, connects all parts of the cytoplasm
      - Rough (granular) endoplasmic reticulum is covered with ribosomes
      - Smooth endoplasmic reticulum contains enzymes to synthesize lipids
    · *Golgi apparatus* synthesizes carbohydrate molecules, which combine with protein produced by rough endoplasmic reticulum to form secretory products (such as lipoproteins)

Key facts about protoplasm
- Viscous, translucent material containing water, inorganic ions, and organic compounds
- Nucleoplasm: protoplasm of the cell's nucleus
- Cytoplasm: protoplasm of the cell body; contains cytosol, organelles, and inclusions

Types of organelles
- Mitochondria: produce energy through the production of ATP
- Ribosomes: site of protein synthesis
- Endoplasmic reticulum: channels connecting all parts of the cytoplasm
- Golgi apparatus: synthesize carbohydrate molecules
- Lysosomes: responsible for digestion within the cell
- Centrosomes: contain centrioles, which move to opposite poles of a cell during division
- Peroxisomes: contain oxidases, which reduce oxygen to hydrogen peroxide and hydrogen peroxide to water
- Cytoskeletal elements: form protein structure network

Key components of a cell

- Cytoplasm
- Lysosome
- Cell membrane
- Mitochondrion
- Golgi apparatus
- Nucleus
- Ribosome
- Endoplasmic reticulum

Inside the cell

This cross section shows the components and structures of a cell.

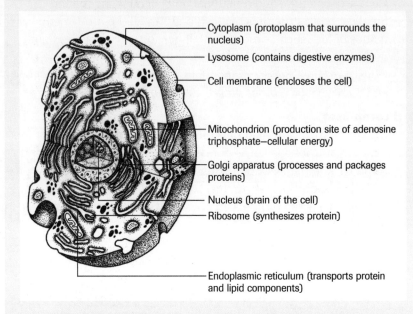

- Cytoplasm (protoplasm that surrounds the nucleus)
- Lysosome (contains digestive enzymes)
- Cell membrane (encloses the cell)
- Mitochondrion (production site of adenosine triphosphate—cellular energy)
- Golgi apparatus (processes and packages proteins)
- Nucleus (brain of the cell)
- Ribosome (synthesizes protein)
- Endoplasmic reticulum (transports protein and lipid components)

· *Lysosomes* are digestive bodies that break down damaged or foreign material in the cells (see *Lysosomes at work*)

· Centrosomes contain *centrioles,* short cylinders adjacent to the nucleus; during cell division, they move to opposite poles of the cell and form the mitotic spindle

· Peroxisomes contain *oxidases*, enzymes capable of reducing oxygen to hydrogen peroxide and hydrogen peroxide to water

· Cytoskeletal elements form a network of protein structures

– *Inclusions* are chemicals produced by the cell (such as melanin, glycogen, and triglycerides) that aren't contained by a membrane but some have particular shape

● Cell (plasma) membrane
- Semipermeable structure that surrounds the cell
- Regulates passage of certain materials in and out of the cell
- Separates the cell's internal environment from its external one

● Nucleus
- Control center of the cell that directs the activities of the cytoplasmic structures
- Contains genetic material of the cell
- Also contains one or more *nucleoli,* spherical structures that synthesize ribonucleic acid (RNA)

Key facts about the nucleus

- Control center of the cell
- Contains genetic material
- Contains one or more nucleoli
- Nuclear membrane separates the nucleus from the cytoplasm

Lysosomes at work

Lysosomes are the organelles responsible for digestion within a cell. Phago-cytes assist in this process. Here's how lysosomes work.

FUNCTION OF LYSOSOMES

Lysosomes are digestive bodies that break down foreign or damaged material in cells. A membrane surrounds each lysosome and separates its digestive enzymes from the rest of the cytoplasm.

BREAKING IT DOWN

The lysosomal enzymes digest matter brought into the cell by *phagocytes*, special cells that surround and engulf matter outside the cell and then transport it through the cell membrane. The membrane of the lysosome fuses with the membrane of the cytoplasmic spaces surrounding the phagocytized material; this fusion allows the lysosomal enzymes to digest the engulfed material.

• Has a *nuclear membrane,* which separates the nucleus from the cytoplasm; pores in this membrane allow certain substances to pass through

CELLULAR ENERGY PRODUCTION

● **Key concepts**
• Cellular activities require energy
• Mitochondria are the cellular power stations
  – Contain enzymes that oxidize food nutrients
  – Oxidation produces *ATP,* a chemical fuel for cellular processes
    • ATP is composed of a nitrogen-containing compound (adenine) joined to a five-carbon sugar (ribose) to form adenosine
      - Adenosine is joined to three phosphate groups
      - Chemical bonds between the first and second and the second and third phosphate groups contain a large amount of energy
    • ATP must be converted to adenosine diphosphate (ADP) to produce energy (remember the three R's)
      - *Rupture*—when the terminal high-energy phosphate bond ruptures, ATP is converted to ADP
      - *Release*—liberation of the third phosphate releases the energy stored in the chemical bond
      - *Recycle*—mitochondrial enzymes use the energy obtained by oxidizing food nutrients to reconvert ADP and the liberated phosphate back into ATP (the ATP is then available again for energy production)

Key processes of lysosomes

• Enzymes digest matter brought into the cell by phagocytes
• Lysosome membrane fuses with the membrane of the cytoplasmic spaces (surrounds phagocytized material)
• Fusion allows enzymes to digest the engulfed matter

Key facts about cellular energy production

• Mitochondria are the cellular power stations
• Mitochondria contain enzymes that oxidize food nutrients
• Oxidation produces ATP
• Energy is produced when ATP is converted to ADP

Key ATP processes

• Rupture: ATP is converted to ADP
• Release: Energy stored in the chemical bond is released
• Recycle: ADP is reconverted to ATP for further energy production

SUBSTANCE MOVEMENT ACROSS THE CELL MEMBRANE

● **Key concepts**
- Each cell interacts with body fluids through the interchange of substances across the cell membrane
- Substances move between cells and body fluids by one of four main mechanisms: diffusion, osmosis, active transport, or endocytosis
- Transport of fluids and dissolved substances across capillaries into *interstitial fluid* (fluid surrounding the cells) is facilitated by filtration

● **Diffusion**
- Passive transport method that doesn't require cellular energy
- Dissolved particles (solute) move from an area of higher concentration to one of lower concentration
- Several factors influence the diffusion rate
  - *Concentration gradient* (difference in particle concentration on either side of the plasma membrane) affects diffusion (the greater the concentration gradient, the faster diffusion occurs)
  - Small particles diffuse more rapidly than large particles
  - Lipid-soluble particles diffuse more rapidly than other particles through the lipid layers of the cell membrane
  - *Electrical charge* of particles can speed or slow diffusion
    - If electrically charged particles (ions) on either side of the cell membrane have opposite charges, diffusion occurs more rapidly (ions with opposite charges attract each other)
    - If ions on either side of the membrane have the same charge, diffusion occurs more slowly (ions with the same charge repel each other)
- *Facilitated diffusion* occurs when a carrier molecule in the cell membrane picks up the diffusing substance on one side of the membrane and deposits it on the other side

● **Osmosis**
- Passive transport method that involves molecule movement from a solution of higher concentration to one of lower concentration (see *Understanding osmosis*)
- Movement of water (solvent) molecules across the cell membrane differentiates osmosis from diffusion; water moves from a dilute solution (with a higher concentration of water molecules) to a concentrated solution (with a lower concentration of water molecules)
- Mechanism depends on the *osmotic pressure* of a solution
  - Osmotic pressure measures the "water-attracting" property of a solution (determined by the number of dissolved particles in a

Key facts about diffusion

- Passive transport method that doesn't require energy
- Dissolved particles move from an area of higher to lower concentration
- Concentration gradient, particle size, and particle type affect diffusion rate
- Facilitated diffusion: the diffusing substance is picked up on one side of the membrane and deposited on the other side

Key facts about osmosis

- Passive transport method in which molecules move from a solution of higher to lower concentration
- Water molecules move from an area of dilute solution (with a higher concentration of water molecules) to concentrated solution (with a lower concentration of water molecules)
- Depends on osmotic pressure

Understanding osmosis

This illustration shows the movement of fluid from an area of lower solute concentration to an area of higher solute concentration until the concentration is equal in both areas. This movement is known as *osmosis*.

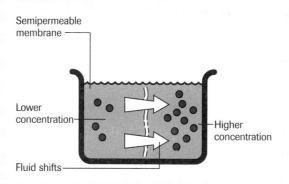

Semipermeable membrane

Lower concentration

Higher concentration

Fluid shifts

Key facts about osmotic pressure

- Measures the "water-attracting" property of a solution (determined by the number of dissolved particles in a solution)
- Osmotic pressure differences between intracellular and extracellular fluids cause osmosis
- A change in the osmotic pressure of body fluids triggers a water shift between cells and extracellular fluids

given volume of solution, not by their size or electrical charge); for example, a calcium chloride molecule ($CaCl_2$) dissociates (ionizes) in solution into three particles: a calcium ion and two chloride ions (its osmotic pressure is higher than that of a larger glucose molecule, which doesn't dissociate into ions when dissolved in solution)

– Water movement in and out of cells by osmosis depends on the osmotic pressure differences between intracellular and extracellular fluids (normally, intracellular osmotic pressure equals extracellular osmotic pressure; consequently, water content of cells doesn't change)

– Osmotic pressure changes in body fluids cause water to shift between cells and extracellular fluids, impairing or disrupting cell functions
  - When osmotic pressure of extracellular fluid is lower than that of intracellular fluid, water enters cells, causing them to swell and, possibly, rupture
  - Conversely, when osmotic pressure of extracellular fluid is higher than that of intracellular fluid, water moves into extracellular fluid, causing cells to shrink

● **Active transport**
- Transport method that moves a substance across the cell membrane (a *carrier molecule* in the cell membrane combines with the substance, transports it through the membrane, and deposits it on the other side of the membrane)
  – Usually, a substance moves from an area of lower concentration to an area of higher concentration (against the concentration gradient)
  – A substance may move from an area of higher concentration to an area of lower concentration (with the concentration gradient)

Key facts about active transport

- Moves a substance across the cell membrane using a carrier molecule
- Usually moves from an area of lower to higher concentration
- Requires energy from ATP breakdown

Key facts about endocytosis

- Active transport method in which a substance is engulfed by the cell
- Divided into phagocytosis and pinocytosis
- Phagocytosis: the cell ingests particles too large to pass through the cell membrane
- Pinocytosis: the cell engulfs substances in solution

Key facts about filtration

- Pressure forces fluid and dissolved particles through a membrane
- Amount of pressure determines the filtration rate

Key facts about cell division

- Chromosomes duplicate before a cell divides
- In duplication, DNA chains separate
- Uncontrolled cell division can cause excess tissue formation
- Cells normally divide by mitosis or meiosis

Key facts about mitosis

- Form of cell division for all cells except gametes
- Parent cell divides to produce two identical daughter cells
- Occurs in one inactive phase and four active phases

- Requires energy from ATP breakdown to transport a substance across a cell membrane

● **Endocytosis**
- Active transport method in which a substance is engulfed by the cell rather than passing through the cell membrane
  - Cell surrounds the substance with part of its membrane
  - Part of the membrane separates, forming a vacuole that moves to the cell interior
- Divided into phagocytosis and pinocytosis
  - In *phagocytosis*, the cell engulfs and ingests particles too large to pass through the cell membrane
  - In *pinocytosis*, the cell engulfs substances in solution or very small particles in suspension

● **Filtration**
- Pressure applied to a solution on one side of the cell membrane forces fluid and dissolved particles through the membrane; the filtration rate depends on the amount of pressure
- Filtration serves two main purposes
  - It promotes transfer of fluids and dissolved materials from blood across capillaries into interstitial fluid (pressure of capillary blood provides filtration force)
  - Filtration from blood flowing through capillaries in the kidneys results in urine formation

CELL DIVISION

● **Key concepts**
- Each cell must replicate itself for life to continue
- Before a cell divides, its chromosomes duplicate
- In duplication, deoxyribonucleic acid (DNA) chains separate
  - Double helix separates into two DNA chains (serves as the template for constructing a new chain)
  - Individual DNA nucleotides link into new strands, with bases complementary to those in the originals
  - Two identical double helices (duplicates of the original DNA chain) form, each containing one of the original strands and a newly formed complementary strand (see *DNA duplication*)
- Uncontrolled cell division may cause excess tissue to form (may develop into a tumor, growth, or neoplasm)
- Continuous cell division occurs in phases
- Cells normally divide by mitosis or meiosis

● **Mitosis**
- Form of cell division that all cells undergo (except gametes)
  - Parent cell with 46 chromosomes (diploid) undergoes division and gives rise to two daughter cells

DNA duplication

The basic structural unit of deoxyribonucleic acid (DNA) is the nucleotide, which is composed of a phosphate group, deoxyribose, and a nitrogen base made of adenine (A), guanine (G), thymine (T), or cytosine (C). Many nucleotide strands become twisted to form a double helix of a DNA molecule. During duplication, linked DNA chains separate. Then new complementary chains form and link to the originals (parents). This results in two identical double helices, consisting of parent and daughter, as shown.

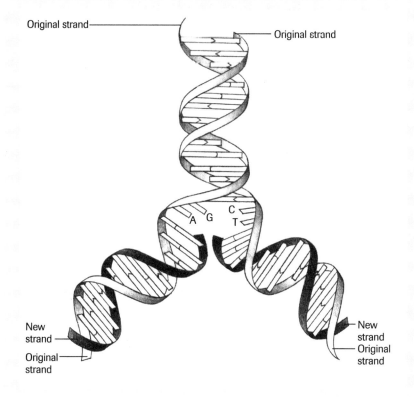

Original strand

Original strand

A G   C T

New strand

New strand

Original strand

Original strand

   – Both daughter cells are identical to each other and to the parent cell
● Cell division occurs in five phases: *interphase* (inactive phase), *prophase, metaphase, anaphase,* and *telophase* (all active phases) (see *Five phases of mitosis,* page 34)

● **Meiosis**
   ● Form of cell division that only gametes (ova and spermatozoa) undergo
   ● Genetic material mixes between homologous chromosomes (number of chromosomes in four daughter cells reduces by half)
      – Each cell has only 23 chromosomes (haploid)
      – Each cell contains genetic material from both parents due to crossover and because the chromosomes of each parent don't all move to one side of the cell during anaphase

- Cell division occurs in two major steps
  - First division has six phases
  - Second division has four phases; at the end, each parent cell has produced four daughter cells genetically different from the parent cell (see *Meiosis: Step-by-step*)

Five phases of mitosis

- Interphase: nucleus and nuclear membrane are well defined
- Prophase: nucleolus disappears and chromosomes are distinct
- Metaphase: chromosomes line up in the cell's center
- Anaphase: centromeres move apart and chromosomes move to opposite ends
- Telophase: nuclear membrane forms around each nucleus and the cell is divided in half

Five phases of mitosis

Through the process of mitosis, the nuclear content of all body cells (except gametes) reproduces and divides. The result is the formation of two new daughter cells, each containing the diploid (46) number of chromosomes.

INTERPHASE

During *interphase*, the nucleus and nuclear membrane are well defined and the nucleolus is visible. As chromosomes replicate, each forms a double strand that remains attached at the center by a centromere.

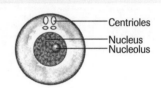

Centrioles
Nucleus
Nucleolus

PROPHASE

In *prophase*, the nucleolus disappears and the chromosomes become distinct. *Chromatids*, halves of each duplicated chromosome, remain attached by the centromere. Centrioles move to opposite sides of the cell and radiate spindle fibers.

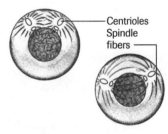

Centrioles
Spindle fibers

METAPHASE

Metaphase occurs when chromosomes line up randomly in the center of the cell between the spindles, along the metaphase plate. The centromere of each chromosome then replicates.

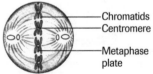

Chromatids
Centromere
Metaphase plate

ANAPHASE

Anaphase is characterized by centromeres moving apart, pulling the separate chromatids (now called *chromosomes*) to opposite ends of the cell. The number of chromosomes at each end of the cell equals the original number.

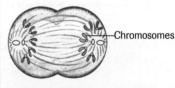

Chromosomes

TELOPHASE

During *telophase*, the final stage of mitosis, a nuclear membrane forms around each nucleus and spindle fibers disappear. The cytoplasm compresses and divides the cell in half. Each new cell contains the diploid (46) number of chromosomes.

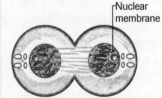

Nuclear membrane

Meiosis: Step-by-step

Meiosis has two divisions separated by a resting phase. By the end of the first division, two daughter cells exist, each containing the haploid (23) number of chromosomes. When the second division ends, each of the two daughter cells from the first division divides, resulting in four daughter cells, each containing the haploid number of chromosomes.

FIRST DIVISION

The first division has six phases. Here's what happens during each one.

Interphase

1. Chromosomes replicate, forming a double strand attached at the center by a centromere.
2. Chromosomes appear as an indistinguishable matrix within the nucleus.
3. Centrioles appear outside the nucleus.

Prophase I

1. The nucleolus and nuclear membrane disappear.
2. Chromosomes are distinct, with chromatids attached by the centromere.
3. Homologous chromosomes move close together and intertwine; exchange of genetic information (genetic recombination) may occur.
4. Centrioles separate and spindle fibers appear.

Metaphase I

1. Pairs of synaptic chromosomes line up randomly along the metaphase plate.
2. Spindle fibers attach to each chromosome pair.

Anaphase I

1. Synaptic pairs separate.
2. Spindle fibers pull homologous, double-stranded chromosomes to opposite ends of the cell.
3. Chromatids remain attached.

Telophase I

1. The nuclear membrane forms.
2. Spindle fibers and chromosomes disappear.
3. Cytoplasm compresses and divides the cell in half.
4. Each new cell contains the haploid (23) number of chromosomes.

Interkinesis

1. The nucleus and nuclear membrane are well defined.
2. The nucleolus is prominent and each chromosome has two chromatids that don't replicate.

SECOND DIVISION

The second division closely resembles mitosis and is characterized by these four phases.

Prophase II

1. The nuclear membrane disappears.
2. Spindle fibers form.
3. Double-stranded chromosomes appear as thin threads.

Metaphase II

1. Chromosomes line up along the metaphase plate.
2. Centromeres replicate.

Anaphase II

1. Chromatids separate (now a single-stranded chromosome).
2. Chromosomes move away from each other to the opposite ends of the cell.

Telophase II

1. The nuclear membrane forms.
2. Chromosomes and spindle fibers disappear.
3. Cytoplasm compresses, dividing the cell in half.
4. Four daughter cells are created, each containing the haploid (23) number of chromosomes.

Ten phases of meiosis

- Interphase: Chromosomes replicate and form a double strand
- Prophase I: Chromosomes are distinct; homologous chromosomes intertwine
- Metaphase I: Synaptic chromosomes line up
- Anaphase I: Synaptic pairs separate
- Telophase I: Nuclear membrane forms; cell divides in half
- Interkinesis: Nucleus and nuclear membrane are well defined; nucleolus is prominent
- Prophase II: Nuclear membrane disappears
- Metaphase II: Chromosomes line up
- Anaphase II: Chromosomes move to opposite ends of the cell
- Telophase II: Nuclear membrane forms; cell divides in half

TOP 5

Items to study for your next test on cell organization

1. Cellular components and their functions
2. Breakdown of ATP by mitochondria
3. Types of movement across cell membranes
4. Chromosome and DNA duplication
5. The processes of mitosis and meiosis

NCLEX CHECKS

It's never too soon to begin your NCLEX preparation. Now that you've reviewed this chapter, carefully read each of the following questions and choose the best answer. Then compare your responses with the correct answers.

1. The nurse knows that which cellular component is the control center of a cell?
- ☐ **1.** Nucleus
- ☐ **2.** Golgi apparatus
- ☐ **3.** Ribosome
- ☐ **4.** Mitochondrion

2. While explaining meiosis to a client, the nurse explains that meiosis ends during which phase?
- ☐ **1.** When two new daughter cells form, each with the haploid number of chromosomes
- ☐ **2.** When one daughter cell forms and is an exact copy of the original cell
- ☐ **3.** When four new daughter cells form, each with the haploid number of chromosomes
- ☐ **4.** When four new daughter cells form, each with the diploid number of chromosomes

3. The nurse knows that centromeres move apart and pull the separate chromosomes to opposite ends of the cell in which phase of mitosis?
- ☐ **1.** Interphase
- ☐ **2.** Prophase
- ☐ **3.** Metaphase
- ☐ **4.** Anaphase

4. The nurse knows that which type of movement requires no energy?
- ☐ **1.** Active transport
- ☐ **2.** Diffusion
- ☐ **3.** Phagocytosis
- ☐ **4.** Pinocytosis

5. While explaining cellular structures to a client, the nurse knows that which cellular structure connects all parts of the cytoplasm?
- ☐ **1.** Endoplasmic reticulum
- ☐ **2.** Lysosome
- ☐ **3.** Centriole
- ☐ **4.** Nucleolus

6. The nurse keeps in mind that which factor influences diffusion?

☐ **1.** Smaller particles diffuse more slowly than larger particles.

☐ **2.** Lipid-soluble particles diffuse more rapidly through the lipid layers of the cell membrane.

☐ **3.** Ions on one side of the membrane diffuse more slowly when ions on the other side of the membrane have the opposite electrical charge.

☐ **4.** Ions with the same electrical charge attract each other, which speeds up diffusion.

7. The nurse knows that which statement describes osmosis?

☐ **1.** Osmosis involves active transport.

☐ **2.** Water molecules move from a dilute solution to a concentrated solution.

☐ **3.** Dissolved particles move from an area of higher concentration to one of lower concentration.

☐ **4.** The size and electrical charge of the particles determine the rate of movement.

8. In the first meiotic division, the gametes undergo six phases of cell division. Place all the phases listed below in ascending chronological order. Use all the options.

1. Metaphase	
2. Anaphase	
3. Telophase	
4. Prophase	
5. Interphase	
6. Interkinesis	

9. The nurse knows that which organelle breaks down foreign or damaged material in a cell?

☐ **1.** Ribosomes

☐ **2.** Lysosomes

☐ **3.** Peroxisomes

☐ **4.** Centrosomes

10. The nurse understands that which cell structure synthesizes RNA?
☐ **1.** Plasma membrane
☐ **2.** Cytoplasm
☐ **3.** Nucleoli
☐ **4.** Nucleus

ANSWERS AND RATIONALES

1. CORRECT ANSWER: 1
Serving as the cell's control center, the nucleus plays a role in cell growth, metabolism, and reproduction. The Golgi apparatus synthesizes carbohydrate molecules, ribosomes synthesize proteins, and mitochondria are energy-producing cellular structures.

2. CORRECT ANSWER: 3
Meiosis comes to completion with the end of telophase II. The result is four daughter cells, each containing the haploid (23) number of chromosomes.

3. CORRECT ANSWER: 4
Anaphase is characterized by centromeres moving apart and pulling the separate chromatids (now called *chromosomes*) to opposite ends of the cell. The number of chromosomes at either end of the cell is the same as the original number. In interphase, the nucleus and nuclear membrane are well defined and the nucleolus is visible. The replicating chromosomes form double strands attached at the middle by a centromere. During prophase, the nucleolus disappears and the chromosomes become distinct. Chromatids are still attached by the centromere. In metaphase, the chromosomes line up in the center of the cell between the spindles, and the centromere of each chromosome replicates.

4. CORRECT ANSWER: 2
Diffusion is a form of passive transport that doesn't require cellular energy to move dissolved particles from an area of higher concentration to an area of lower concentration. Active transport uses energy from the breakdown of ATP to transport a substance across a cell membrane. Phagocytosis requires energy to engulf and ingest particles that are too large to pass through cell membranes. Pinocytosis uses energy to engulf substances in solution or very small particles in suspension.

5. CORRECT ANSWER: 1
The endoplasmic reticulum is a system of interconnecting tubular channels that connects all parts of the cytoplasm. Lysosomes are digestive bodies that break down damaged or foreign material in the cells. Centrioles are short cylinders adjacent to the nucleus that move to opposite

ends of the cell and form the mitotic spindle during cell division. Nucleoli are spherical structures in the nucleus that synthesize RNA.

6. CORRECT ANSWER: 2

Lipid-soluble particles diffuse more quickly through the lipid layers of the cell membrane. Particle size does affect diffusion, but smaller particles diffuse more quickly than larger particles. Ions move more rapidly through a membrane when the ions on either side have opposite electrical charges. Ions with the same electrical charge repel each other, slowing diffusion.

7. CORRECT ANSWER: 2

In osmosis, water molecules move across the cell membrane from a dilute solution (with a higher concentration of water molecules) to a concentrated solution (with a lower concentration of water molecules). Osmosis uses passive transport to move molecules from a solution of higher molecular concentration to a solution of lower molecular concentration. Dissolved particles move from an area of higher concentration to one of lower concentration as a result of diffusion, not osmosis. Particle size and electrical charge affect the rate of movement in diffusion, with small particles diffusing faster than large ones and ions of unlike charges attracting each other.

8. CORRECT ANSWER:

| 5. Interphase |
| 4. Prophase |
| 1. Metaphase |
| 2. Anaphase |
| 3. Telophase |
| 6. Interkinesis |

In meiosis, the first phase is interphase, during which chromosomes replicate and are attached at the center by a centromere. Next, during prophase, chromosomes align so that matching genes are side by side. The third phase is metaphase, during which the chromosomes move to the center of the cell; the two chromatids of each chromosome begin to separate but remain joined at the centromere, where spindle fibers are attached. Then, during anaphase, the homologous chromosomes (not the chromatids) of each pair separate and move to opposite poles of the cell. The fifth phase is telophase, during which nuclear membranes form around the chromosomes and the cytoplasm divides, forming two new daughter cells. Lastly, during interkinesis, the nucleus and nuclear membrane are well defined and the nucleolus is prominent. Each chromo-some has two chromatids that don't replicate.

9. CORRECT ANSWER: 2
Lysosomes are digestive bodies that break down foreign or damaged materials in cells. Ribosomes are the sites of protein synthesis. Peroxi-somes contain oxidases, enzymes capable of reducing oxygen to hydro-gen peroxide and hydrogen peroxide to water. Centrosomes contain centrioles, short cylinders adjacent to the nucleus that take part in cell division.

10. CORRECT ANSWER: 3
Nucleoli are found in the nucleus and synthesize RNA. The nucleus is the control center of the cell, directing the activities of the structures in the cytoplasm. The plasma membrane regulates the passage of certain materials in and out of the cell. Cytoplasm includes the cell's contents from the cell membrane to the nucleus.

4

Tissue organization

LEARNING OBJECTIVES

After studying this chapter, you should be able to:

● Describe the relationship between tissues and cells.

● Identify the four basic types of tissue.

● Describe the location of each tissue type.

● Understand the function of each tissue type.

● Identify special characteristics of each type of tissue.

CHAPTER OVERVIEW

The tissue level is the third level of structural organization. Tissues are groups of cells with the same general function. By knowing the location and function of each type of tissue, the nurse can gain a better understanding of the role of tissue in health, illness, and recovery. This chapter reviews epithelial, connective, muscle, and nervous tissues.

EPITHELIAL TISSUE

● **Key concepts**
  • Continuous multicellular sheet with at least two types of epithelial cells

- Covers most internal and external body surfaces, lines body cavities, and forms certain glands
- Classified by number of cell layers and shape of surface cells (see *Differentiating epithelial tissues*)

● **Cell layer types**
- Classified by number of cell layers
  - *Simple* epithelial tissue has only one layer
  - *Stratified* epithelial tissue has two or more layers
  - *Pseudostratified* epithelial tissue has only one layer but appears to have more
- Depends on location and function; for example, simple epithelium appears in areas with little wear and tear, whereas stratified epithelium appears in areas with much greater wear and tear

● **Surface cell shapes**
- Classified according to shape of surface cells
  - *Squamous* epithelial tissue has flat surface cells
  - *Columnar* epithelial tissue has tall, cylindrical, prismatic surface cells
  - *Cuboidal* epithelial tissue has cube-shaped surface cells
- Can also be *transitional;* transitional tissue has cells that change shape easily
  - Transitional tissue usually appears in stratified epithelium
  - It's located in areas that require ready distention (ability to stretch), such as the lining of the urinary bladder

● **Characteristics of epithelium**
- Some columnar epithelial cells have vertical striations (microvilli) called a *striated* (or *brush*) *border*
- Stereociliated epithelial cells have long, piriform (pear-shaped) tufts; such cells line the epididymis
- Ciliated epithelial cells possess cilia
  - *Cilia* are fine, hairlike protuberances on the free border
  - Larger than microvilli, cilia propel fluid and particles through the lumen of an organ
- *Wandering cells* are macrophages (phagocytes) that enter the epithelium from connective tissue
- Some epithelial tissues (such as the olfactory mucosa) have branches of sensory nerves piercing the underlying layer (basement lamina) of tissue
- Some types of epithelium shed (desquamate) and regenerate continuously as cells from deeper layers transform into epithelium
- Epithelial tissue on the interior of the body that has a single layer of squamous cells attached to a basement membrane is called *endothelium;* it lines the heart, lymphatic vessels, and blood vessels

Differentiating epithelial tissues

Classification of epithelial tissue (epithelium) depends on the number of cell layers and the shape of surface cells. Thus, epithelium may be simple (one-layered), stratified (multilayered), or pseudostratified (one-layered but appearing to be multilayered). It may also be squamous (containing flat surface cells), columnar (containing tall, cylindrical, prismatic surface cells), or cuboidal (containing cube-shaped surface cells). The first illustration shows how the basement membrane of simple squamous epithelium joins the epithelium to underlying connective tissues. The remaining illustrations show the five other types of epithelial tissue.

SIMPLE SQUAMOUS EPITHELIUM

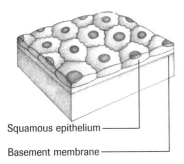

Squamous epithelium ————

Basement membrane ————

STRATIFIED COLUMNAR EPITHELIUM

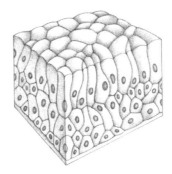

SIMPLE CUBOIDAL EPITHELIUM

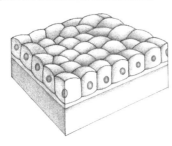

STRATIFIED SQUAMOUS EPITHELIUM

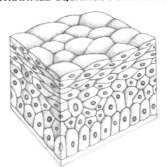

SIMPLE COLUMNAR EPITHELIUM

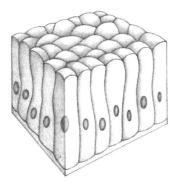

PSEUDOSTRATIFIED COLUMNAR EPITHELIUM

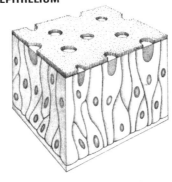

Types of epithelium

- Simple squamous
- Simple cuboidal
- Simple columnar
- Stratified columnar
- Stratified squamous
- Pseudostratified columnar

Key characteristics of glandular epithelium

- Forms glands (organs that produce secretions)
- Endocrine glands release secretions into blood or lymph
- Exocrine glands discharge secretions onto external or internal surfaces
- Mixed glands contain endocrine and exocrine cells

Key facts about connective tissue

- Connects and supports body structures
- Consists of cells, fibers, and ground substance

Types of tissue cells

- Fibroblasts: secrete substances that form matrix
- Macrophages: function as phagocytes
- Plasma cells: secrete antibodies
- Mast cells: produce histamine
- Adipocytes: store fat
- WBCs: defend against infection

● **Glandular epithelium**
- *Glands*—organs that produce secretions—are composed of a special type of epithelium called *glandular epithelium*
  - Many glands are enclosed in dense connective tissue capsules
  - Glands are divided into *lobes*, then into smaller units called *lobules*
- A gland's secretion mode determines its classification as *exocrine* or *endocrine*
  - *Secretion* is the process of elaborating a specific product—that is, creating a more complex substance out of simpler materials; it may involve separating out an element of the blood or elaborating a totally new chemical substance (such as urine secreted by kidneys)
  - *Excretion* is the process of eliminating a product from the body; for example, the urinary bladder excretes urine
  - Endocrine glands release secretions into the blood or lymph; for example, the medulla of the adrenal gland secretes epinephrine and norepinephrine into the bloodstream
  - Exocrine glands discharge secretions onto external or internal surfaces; for example, sudoriferous (sweat) glands secrete sweat onto the skin's surface
  - Mixed glands contain endocrine and exocrine cells
    - The pancreas contains alpha and beta cells (in the islets of Langerhans); these endocrine cells produce glucagon and insulin, respectively
    - The pancreas also contains acinar cells; these exocrine cells secrete digestive juices

CONNECTIVE TISSUE

● **Key concepts**
- Binds together and supports body structures
- Composed of cells, fibers, and ground substance

● **Tissue cells**
- Include fibroblasts, macrophages, plasma cells, mast cells, adipocytes, and white blood cells (WBCs)
- Each type of cell performs a distinct function
  - *Fibroblasts* secrete substances that form the matrix
  - *Macrophages* function as phagocytes
  - *Plasma cells* secrete antibodies
  - *Mast cells* produce histamine and contain heparin
  - *Adipocytes* store fat
  - *WBCs* act as a defense mechanism against infection

- May be fixed or wandering
  - *Fixed cells* are typical cells that remain in place
  - *Wandering cells* may move from one site to another

● **Tissue matrix**
- Separates cells from each other, preventing them from touching the way epithelial cells touch
- Has two components: fibers and ground substance
  - *Fibers*, which provide strength and support, come in three types: *collagenous*, *reticular*, and *elastic*
  - *Ground substance* includes extracellular fluid chemicals and large molecules (such as hyaluronic acid and proteins)

● **Classification**
- Connective tissue may be classified as loose, dense, cartilage, bone (osseous), or blood
- *Loose connective tissue* develops from the mesenchyme after other embryonic tissues have formed
  - Large spaces separate its fibers and cells; it contains much intercellular fluid
  - Types of loose connective tissue include *areolar*, *adipose*, and *reticular*
- *Dense connective tissue* has a greater concentration of fibers than loose connective tissue
  - This tissue type provides structural support
  - It occurs as dense regular, dense irregular, and elastic connective tissue
    · *Dense regular connective tissue* consists of tightly packed fibers arranged in a consistent pattern; it includes tendons, ligaments, and aponeuroses
    · *Dense irregular connective tissue* consists of tightly packed fibers arranged in an inconsistent pattern; it's found in the dermis, GI tract submucosa, fibrous capsules, and fascia
    · *Elastic connective tissue* consists of freely branching elastic fibers; it's found in lung tissues, arterial walls, bronchial tubes, and other structures that must stretch
- *Cartilage* and *bone tissues* are connective tissue of the skeletal system
- *Blood (vascular) tissue* is an opaque, viscous fluid that circulates through the heart, arteries, capillaries, and veins
  - Blood uses plasma as the liquid matrix
  - Formed elements (blood cells) are suspended in the plasma (see chapter 13, Hematologic system)
- Some types of connective tissue have special properties

Key facts about tissue matrix

- Separates cells from each other
- Prevents cells from touching
- Two components: fibers and ground substance

Key characteristics of loose connective tissue

- Has large spaces between fibers and cells
- Contains much intercellular fluid
- Types include areolar, adipose, and reticular

Key characteristics of dense connective tissue

- Contains greater concentration of fibers
- Provides structural support
- Dense regular: has tightly packed fibers in a consistent pattern; found in tendons, ligaments, and aponeuroses
- Dense irregular: has tightly packed fibers in an inconsistent pattern; found in dermis, GI tract submucosa, fibrous capsules, and fascia
- Elastic: contains freely branching elastic fibers; found in lungs, arterial walls, and bronchial tubes

Key characteristics of blood tissue

- Opaque, viscous fluid
- Uses plasma as the liquid matrix
- Formed elements are suspended in the plasma

– *Mucous connective tissue* (Wharton's jelly) of the umbilical cord is a temporary tissue that derives from the mesenchyme; it supports the umbilical cord
– *Elastic connective tissue* of the vocal cords permits speech
– *Pigmented connective tissue* of the sclera gives the eyeball its white color

● **Membranes**
  • *Epithelial membrane* is the plane of contact between an epithelial layer and the connective tissue layer beneath it; three main types are *mucous*, *serous*, and *cutaneous*
  • *Synovial membrane* contains connective tissue only; it lines joint cavities, bursae, and tendons

MUSCLE TISSUE

● **Key concepts**
  • Consists of well-vascularized muscle cells
    – Cylindrical cells may measure several centimeters long; elongated shape enhances their ability to contract (contractility)
    – *Myofibrils* (muscle fibers) of muscle tissue contain the contractile proteins *actin* and *myosin*
  • Three basic types of muscle tissue are skeletal, cardiac, and smooth

● **Skeletal muscle**
  • Has characteristic striped (striated) appearance
    – Striated muscle fibers are multinucleated masses of protoplasm innervated by cerebrospinal nerves
    – Contains specialized myofibrils—bundles of fine fibers made up of even finer fibers called *thin* and *thick filaments*
      · Thin filaments contain the contractile protein actin
      · Thick filaments contain the contractile protein myosin
  • Includes all striated muscle tissue capable of voluntary contraction

● **Cardiac muscle**
  • Striated muscle of the heart
    – Cardiac muscle fibers are separate cellular units; they aren't multinucleated like other striated muscle fibers
    – Sometimes cardiac muscle is classified as striated muscle rather than as a separate category; however, unlike other striated muscle, it contracts involuntarily
  • Connected by interwoven, intercalated disks that mediate synchronized cardiac muscle contraction

Types of membranes

• Epithelial: contact between an epithelial layer and connective tissue; three types are mucous, serous, and cutaneous
• Synovial: connective tissue only; lines joint cavities, bursae, and tendons

Key facts about muscle tissue

• Consists of well-vascularized muscle cells
• Types include skeletal, cardiac, and smooth

Key characteristics of skeletal muscle

• Has characteristic striated appearance
• Capable of voluntary contraction

Key characteristics of cardiac muscle

• Striated muscle of the heart
• Consists of separate cellular units (not multinucleated like other striated muscle fibers)
• Contracts involuntarily

Smooth muscle

- Composed of long spindle-shaped cells; it lacks the characteristic striped pattern of striated muscle
- Activity not under voluntary control because of autonomic nervous system innervation
- Serves several functions, including lining the walls of many internal organs
  - Smooth muscle lines the digestive tract from the middle of the esophagus to the internal anal sphincter, forming the contractile portion of the GI tract
  - It lines the walls of respiratory passages from the trachea to the alveolar ducts
  - It also lines urinary and genital ducts, walls of arteries and veins, and larger lymphatic trunks
  - In the skin, smooth-muscle fibers form *arrectores pilorum*, tiny muscles whose contraction causes hair to stand erect
  - In the mammary glands, smooth muscle causes the nipples to become erect; in the scrotum, it wrinkles the skin to help elevate the testes
  - In the ciliary body of the eye, smooth muscle plays a role in accommodation; contraction in the iris results in pupil dilation

Key characteristics of smooth muscle

- Lacks the characteristic striated appearance
- Not under voluntary control
- Lines the walls of many internal organs

NERVOUS TISSUE

Key concepts

- Main function is communication (see chapter 9, Nervous system)
- Has two basic attributes: irritability and conductivity
  - *Irritability* is the capacity to react to various physical and chemical agents
  - *Conductivity* is the ability to transmit the resulting reaction from one point to another

Cell types

- Nervous tissue includes two types of cells: neurons and neuroglia
- Highly specialized *neurons* receive and transmit nerve impulses
  - A typical neuron consists of a cell body with cytoplasmic extensions—several dendrites on one pole and a single insulated axon on the opposite pole
  - Cytoplasmic extensions allow the neuron to conduct impulses over long distances
- *Neuroglia* form the support structure of nervous tissue
  - These cells insulate and protect neurons
  - They occur only in the central nervous system

Key facts about nervous tissue

- Main function is communication
- Reacts to physical and chemical agents (irritability)
- Transmits reactions from one point to another (conductivity)
- Neurons receive and transmit impulses
- Neuroglia form the support structure

NCLEX CHECKS

It's never too soon to begin your NCLEX preparation. Now that you've reviewed this chapter, carefully read each of the following questions and choose the best answer. Then compare your responses with the correct answers.

1. The nurse knows that which are the four basic types of tissue in the human body?
- ☐ **1.** Muscle, tendons, glands, and connective tissue
- ☐ **2.** Neurons, cartilage, glands, and adipose tissue
- ☐ **3.** Neuroglia, skeletal muscle tissue, dense connective tissue, and stereociliated epithelial cells
- ☐ **4.** Epithelial, connective, muscle, and nervous tissue

2. The nurse knows that squamous epithelial tissue has surface cells that are which shape?
- ☐ **1.** Flat
- ☐ **2.** Cylindrical
- ☐ **3.** Cuboidal
- ☐ **4.** Tall

3. The nurse is caring for a client who can't sweat. The nurse explains to the client that he has a disorder in which type of gland?
- ☐ **1.** Endocrine
- ☐ **2.** Exocrine
- ☐ **3.** Mixed
- ☐ **4.** Islets of Langerhans

4. The nurse is obtaining a client's blood sample for laboratory tests to determine his ability to fight infection. For which connective tissue is the laboratory most likely evaluating?
- ☐ **1.** Fibroblasts
- ☐ **2.** Mast cells
- ☐ **3.** Adipocytes
- ☐ **4.** WBCs

5. When the nurse helps a client perform range-of-motion exercises, which type of muscle tissue is the client exercising?
- ☐ **1.** Skeletal
- ☐ **2.** Cardiac
- ☐ **3.** Smooth
- ☐ **4.** Myosin

6. The nurse is assessing a client's neurologic function. The nurse knows that a neuron has which structures?
- ☐ **1.** One axon and one dendrite
- ☐ **2.** One axon and many dendrites
- ☐ **3.** Many axons and one dendrite
- ☐ **4.** Many axons and many dendrites

7. The nurse is explaining to a client that damage to the single layer of squamous cells lining the blood vessels can lead to atherosclerotic heart disease. The nurse is referring to which cells?
☐ **1.** Cilia
☐ **2.** Wandering cells
☐ **3.** Endothelium
☐ **4.** Microvilli

8. A client is undergoing synovial membrane biopsy to diagnose the cause of a knee joint infection. In answer to the client's questions, the nurse explains that the synovial membrane is which type of tissue?
☐ **1.** Epithelial
☐ **2.** Muscle
☐ **3.** Nervous
☐ **4.** Connective

9. The nurse knows that epithelium has which characteristic structures? Select all that apply.
☐ **1.** Microvilli
☐ **2.** Matrix
☐ **3.** Piriform tufts
☐ **4.** Actin
☐ **5.** Cilia
☐ **6.** Neuroglia

10. When teaching a client how to perform deep-breathing exercises, the nurse understands that lung tissue contains which type of connective tissue?
☐ **1.** Loose connective tissue
☐ **2.** Dense regular connective tissue
☐ **3.** Dense irregular connective tissue
☐ **4.** Elastic connective tissue

ANSWERS AND RATIONALES

1. CORRECT ANSWER: 4
The human body contains four basic types of tissue: epithelial, connective, muscle, and nervous. Tendons, cartilage, adipose, and dense connective tissue are types of connective tissue. Glands and stereociliated epithelial cells are types of epithelial tissue. Neurons and neuroglia are types of nerve tissues. Skeletal muscle is a type of muscle tissue.

2. CORRECT ANSWER: 1
Squamous epithelial tissue has flat surface cells. Columnar epithelial tissue has tall, cylindrical, prismatic surface cells. Cuboidal epithelial tissue has cube-shaped surface cells.

3. CORRECT ANSWER: 2

Sudoriferous (sweat) glands are exocrine glands that secrete sweat onto the surface of the skin. Endocrine glands release secretions into the blood or lymph. Mixed glands consist of both endocrine and exocrine cells. The islets of Langerhans contain endocrine cells.

4. CORRECT ANSWER: 4

Connective tissue cells include fibroblasts, macrophages, plasma cells, mast cells, adipocytes, and WBCs. WBCs act as a defense mechanism against infection. Fibroblasts secrete substances that form matrix. Mast cells produce histamine and contain heparin. Adipocytes store fat.

5. CORRECT ANSWER: 1

The three basic types of muscle tissue are skeletal, cardiac, and smooth. Skeletal muscle, the type of muscle the client is exercising, includes all striated muscle capable of voluntary contraction. Cardiac muscle is the striated muscle of the heart. Smooth-muscle tissue lines the walls of many internal organs. Myosin, along with actin, is the contractile protein in muscle tissue.

6. CORRECT ANSWER: 2

Neurons are highly specialized cells that generate and conduct nerve impulses. A typical neuron has a cell body with one axon and many dendrites.

7. CORRECT ANSWER: 3

The endothelium consists of epithelial tissue with a single layer of squamous cells attached to a basement membrane. It lines the heart, lymphatic vessels, and blood vessels. Cilia are fine, hairlike projections on epithelial cells. Wandering cells are macrophages that enter the epithelium from connective tissue. Microvilli are vertical striations found on some columnar epithelial cells.

8. CORRECT ANSWER: 4

Connective tissue binds together and supports body structures. It includes the synovial membrane, which lines joint cavities, bursae, and tendons. Epithelial tissue, a continuous multicellular sheet with at least two types of epithelial cells, covers the surface of the body, lines body cavities, and forms certain glands. Muscle tissue consists of well-vascularized striated, cardiac, and smooth-muscle cells. Nervous tissue includes neurons and neuroglia.

9. CORRECT ANSWER: 1, 3, 5

Epithelium has columnar epithelial cells with vertical striations (microvilli); stereociliated epithelial cells with long, pear-shaped tufts (piriform); and fine, hairlike projections on the free border (cilia). Matrix is a connective tissue that separates cells from each other. Actin is a contractile protein in muscle tissue. Neuroglia form the structural support of nervous tissue.

10. CORRECT ANSWER: 4

The lungs contain elastic connective tissue that allows them to expand and recoil with deep-breathing exercises. Loose connective tissue has large spaces that separate the fibers and cells, contains much intercellular fluid, and is found in areolar and adipose tissue. Dense regular connective tissue consists of tightly packed fibers arranged in a consistent pattern and includes ligaments, tendons, and aponeuroses (flat fibrous sheets that attach muscles to bones or other tissues). Dense irregular connective tissue has tightly packed fibers arranged in an inconsistent pattern and is found in the dermis, GI tract submucosa, fibrous capsules, and fasciae.

5

Genetics

LEARNING OBJECTIVES

After studying this chapter, you should be able to:

● Describe the role of chromosomes and genes in heredity.
● Explain the difference between autosomes and sex chromosomes.
● Understand factors that determine trait dominance.
● Discuss the structure and function of deoxyribonucleic acid (DNA) in genetics.
● Discuss the types and functions of ribonucleic acid (RNA).

CHAPTER OVERVIEW

Genetics is the study of heredity—the passing of traits from biological parents to their children. A knowledge of genetics can help the nurse better understand how people inherit not only physical traits, such as eye color, but also biochemical and physiologic traits, including the tendency to develop certain diseases. This chapter reviews cellular genetic material, including chromosomes and genes. It also examines DNA and RNA and their roles in the genetic expression of inherited traits.

CELLULAR GENETIC MATERIAL

● **Chromosomes**
- *Chromosomes* contain the genetic material of the cell
- Composed of DNA and protein, chromosomes control cell activities in the nucleus; they also direct protein synthesis using ribosomes in cytoplasm
- In the nondividing cell, chromosomes appear as a network of granules (*chromatin*)
- They exist in pairs except in gametes (male and female reproductive cells)—one chromosome from each pair comes from the male parent; the other, from the female parent
- Normal cells contain 23 pairs of chromosomes
  - Twenty-two pairs are sets of homologous chromosomes (*autosomes*) that contain genetic information, which controls the same characteristics or functions
  - One pair is composed of sex (X and Y) chromosomes; the composition of these chromosomes determines sex
    - XY is genetically male
    - XX is genetically female
      - In females, genetic activity of both X chromosomes is essential only during the first few weeks of embryonic development; later development requires only one functional X chromosome
      - The other X chromosome is inactivated and appears as a dense chromatin mass called a *Barr body* (or *sex chromatin body*), which is attached to the nuclear membrane in the cells of a normal female
      - The Barr body is absent in the cells of a normal male who has only one functional X chromosome
- Complete set of chromosomes containing all genetic information for one person is called a *genome* (see *The genome at a glance*)
- Disorders may result from chromosomal aberrations, deviations in either the structure or number of chromosomes

The genome at a glance

The human genome is composed of a set of long deoxyribonucleic acid (DNA) molecules, one for each chromosome. DNA has four different chemical building blocks, called *bases*. Each human genome contains about 3 billion of these bases, arranged in an order that's unique for each person. DNA molecules have more than 30,000 genes along them.

Key facts about chromosomes

- Contain the genetic material of the cell
- Composed of DNA and protein
- Exist in pairs except in gametes
- Normal cells contain 23 pairs of chromosomes
- Complete set of chromosomes is called a *genome*

Key facts about the human genome

- Composed of one set of DNA molecules for each chromosome
- DNA has four chemical building blocks (bases) and more than 30,000 genes
- Contains 3 billion bases with a unique order for each person

Key facts about genes

- The segments of DNA responsible for inherited traits
- Occur in pairs on homologous chromosomes
- Gene locus: the location of a specific gene on a chromosome
- Alleles: alternate forms of a gene that occupy a particular locus
- Gene expression: the effect that the gene has on cell structure or function

Types of gene expression

- Dominant: can be expressed and transmitted to offspring even if only one parent has it
- Recessive: expressed only when both parents transmit it to their offspring
- Codominant: allows expression of both alleles
- Sex-linked: carried on sex chromosomes; recessive

● Genes

- *Genes* are segments of chromosomal DNA chains that are responsible for inherited traits; they're arranged in a line on chromosomes like beads on a string
- The location of a specific gene on a chromosome is called the *gene locus*
  - Genetic information stored at a gene locus determines the genetic constitution, or *genotype* of a person
  - Detectable, outward manifestation of a genotype is called the *phenotype*
- *Alleles* are alternate forms of a gene that can occupy a particular locus on a chromosome (only one allele can occupy a specific gene locus)
- Genes occur in pairs on homologous chromosomes (because chromosomes are paired), with one allele at the locus on both homologous chromosomes
  - If both chromosomes have the same alleles for a particular gene, a person is *homozygous* for that gene
  - If the chromosomes have different alleles, a person is *heterozygous* for the gene
- The effect that the gene has on cell structure or function is called *gene expression,* which varies with the gene (see *How genes express themselves*)
  - *Dominant* genes are expressed in the heterozygous state
    · A dominant gene is expressed even if only one parent transmits it to the offspring (see *Understanding autosomal dominant inheritance*)

How genes express themselves

Genes account for inherited traits. *Gene expression* refers to a gene's effect on cell structure or function; however, the effects vary with the gene.

DOMINANT GENE
A dominant gene (such as the one for dark hair) can be expressed and transmitted to the offspring even if only one parent possesses the gene.

RECESSIVE GENE
Unlike a dominant gene, a recessive gene (such as the gene for blond hair) is expressed only when both parents transmit the gene to the offspring.

CODOMINANT GENE
A codominant gene (such as the gene that directs specific types of hemoglobin synthesis in red blood cells) allows expression of both alleles.

SEX-LINKED GENE
A sex-linked gene is carried on the sex chromosomes. Almost all sex-linked genes appear on the X chromosome and are recessive. In the male, sex-linked genes behave like dominant genes because no second X chromosome exists.

• Dark hair and eyes result from dominant genes
– *Recessive* genes are expressed in the homozygous state
• A recessive gene is expressed only when both parents transmit it to the offspring (see *Understanding autosomal recessive inheritance*)

Understanding autosomal dominant inheritance

This diagram shows the possible offspring of a parent with recessive normal genes (aa) and a parent with an altered dominant gene (Aa). *Note:* With each pregnancy, the offspring has a 50% chance of being affected.

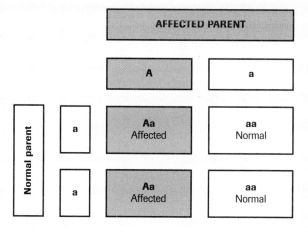

Understanding autosomal recessive inheritance

This diagram shows the possible offspring of two unaffected parents, each with an altered recessive gene (a) on an autosome. Each offspring will have a one-in-four chance of being affected and a two-in-four chance of being a carrier.

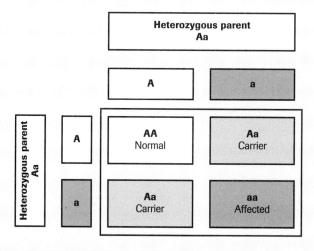

· Blond hair and blue eyes result from recessive genes
– *Codominant* genes allow expression of both alleles (such as the genes that direct specific types of hemoglobin synthesis in red blood cells)
– *Sex-linked* genes are carried on sex chromosomes
   · Almost all appear on the X chromosome and are recessive (see *Understanding X-linked recessive inheritance*)
   · In the male, sex-linked genes behave like dominant genes because males have no second X chromosome (see *Understanding X-linked dominant inheritance*)

DNA

Key concepts
• DNA, a large nucleic acid molecule found in chromosomes in the nucleus, carries genetic information in living cells
• Basic structural unit is the *nucleotide,* which consists of a phosphate group linked to *deoxyribose* (a five-carbon sugar similar to ribose except that it has hydrogen instead of hydroxyl connected to a carbon atom) joined to a nitrogen-containing compound called a *base*
• Four different DNA nucleotides exist, differing only in the base joined to deoxyribose
   – *Adenine* and *guanine* are double-ring compounds classified as purines
   – *Thymine* and *cytosine* are single-ring compounds classified as pyrimidines
   – Adenine bonds only with thymine; guanine bonds only with cytosine (bases that can link with each other are called *complementary*)

DNA chains
• Nucleotides are joined into long chains by chemical bonds between the phosphate group of the nucleotide and a carbon atom in the deoxyribose molecule of the adjacent nucleotide
• Nitrogen bases project from the deoxyribose molecule at right angles to the long axis of the chain
• DNA chains exist in pairs; weak chemical attractions (hydrogen bonds) between the nitrogen bases on adjacent chains hold them together
• Linked chains form a spiral structure (double helix), which resembles a spiral staircase
   – Deoxyribose and phosphate groups form the railings
   – Nitrogen base pairs form the steps

Key facts about DNA
• Carries genetic information
• Basic structural unit is the nucleotide
• Nucleotides are joined into long chains by chemical bonds
• DNA chains exist in pairs and form a spiral structure (double helix)
• Sequencing of nucleotide bases forms the genetic code

Types of DNA nucleotides
• Adenine and guanine (purines): double-ring compounds
• Thymine and cytosine (pyrimidines): single-ring compounds

Understanding X-linked recessive inheritance

This diagram shows the possible offspring of a normal parent and a parent with a recessive gene on the X chromosome (shown by an open dot). All of the female offspring of an affected male will be carriers. The son of a female carrier may inherit a recessive gene on the X chromosome and be affected by the disease.

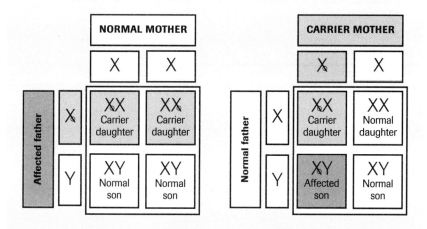

Understanding X-linked dominant inheritance

This diagram shows the possible offspring of a normal parent and a parent with an X-linked dominant gene on the X chromosome (shown by a dot). When the father is affected, only his daughters have the abnormal gene. When the mother is affected, both male and female offspring may be affected.

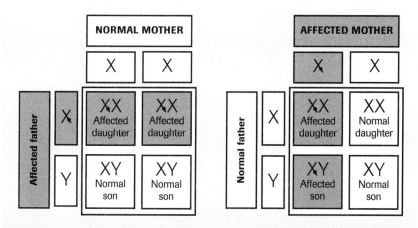

- Sequencing of nucleotide bases forms the genetic code (series of coded messages)
- Each group of three bases (called a *codon*) specifies the synthesis of a specific amino acid, which is carried to the ribosomes to synthesize protein

RNA

● Key concepts

- RNA transfers genetic information from nuclear DNA to ribosomes in cytoplasm (where protein synthesis occurs); several types of RNA take part in this process
- RNA consists of nucleotide chains, which contain the five-carbon sugar *ribose* (rather than deoxyribose)
  - Adenine bonds with uracil (not thymine, as in DNA)
  - Guanine bonds with cytosine

● Types of RNA

- Nucleus produces three types of RNA, which pass into cytoplasm: *ribosomal RNA* (rRNA), *messenger RNA* (mRNA), and *transfer RNA* (tRNA) (see *Types of RNA*)
  - rRNA makes ribosomes in the endoplasmic reticulum of cytoplasm (where the cell produces proteins)
  - mRNA specifies the arrangement of amino acids to make proteins at ribosomes
  - tRNA carries specific amino acids during protein synthesis

● Protein synthesis in cytoplasm

- One or more ribosomes attach themselves to the mRNA strand that contains instructions for protein synthesis

---

Types of RNA

Three types of ribonucleic acid (RNA) exist: ribosomal (rRNA), messenger (mRNA), and transfer (tRNA). Each has its own specific function.

RIBOSOMAL RNA
rRNA makes ribosomes in the endoplasmic reticulum of the cytoplasm, where the cell produces proteins.

MESSENGER RNA
mRNA directs the arrangement of amino acids to make proteins at the ribosomes. Its single strand of nucleotides is complementary to a segment of the deoxyribonucleic acid chain that contains instructions for

protein synthesis. Its chains pass from the nucleus into the cytoplasm, attaching to ribosomes there.

TRANSFER RNA
tRNA consists of short nucleotide chains, each of which is specific for an individual amino acid. tRNA transfers the genetic code from mRNA for the production of a specific amino acid.

Key facts about RNA

- Consists of nucleotide chains containing ribose (rather than deoxyribose)
- Transfers genetic information from nuclear DNA to ribosomes
- Three types involved in protein synthesis

Types of RNA

- Ribosomal: makes ribosomes
- Messenger: makes proteins at ribosomes
- Transfer: carries amino acids during protein synthesis

Key facts about protein synthesis

- Ribosomes attach to mRNA strand
- tRNA attaches to amino acids
- Ribosomes join amino acids into a chain
- Protein is released and mRNA detaches from ribosomes

- tRNA chains attach themselves to amino acids in cytoplasm and transfer them to ribosomes
- Ribosomes join amino acids into a chain according to sequence of bases on the mRNA strand to form a protein
- When the chain is complete, new protein is released and the mRNA strand detaches from ribosomes

NCLEX CHECKS

It's never too soon to begin your NCLEX preparation. Now that you've reviewed this chapter, carefully read each of the following questions and choose the best answer. Then compare your responses with the correct answers.

1. The nurse is counseling a pregnant client and her spouse about genetic disorders. The nurse correctly explains that the fertilized cell has which total number of chromosomes?

☐ **1.** 12
☐ **2.** 23
☐ **3.** 46
☐ **4.** 52

2. The nurse is reviewing the genetic transmission of traits to expectant parents. The parents want to know if it's possible for their child to have blond hair. Which response by the nurse correctly answers their question?

☐ **1.** "Both parents must transmit the gene for blond hair."
☐ **2.** "One parent transmits the gene for blond hair."
☐ **3.** "One grandparent must have blond hair."
☐ **4.** "Neither parent must have the gene for blond hair."

3. A child has brown eyes and brown hair. The nurse explains to the parents that this description reveals the child's:

☐ **1.** phenotype.
☐ **2.** genotype.
☐ **3.** genome.
☐ **4.** autosome.

4. While counseling expectant parents, the nurse learns that the father has an X-linked dominant disorder and the mother is normal. The nurse knows that which percentage represents the chance that the parents will have a daughter with the disorder?

☐ **1.** 25%
☐ **2.** 50%
☐ **3.** 75%
☐ **4.** 100%

TOP 7

Items to study for your next test on genetics

1. Role of chromosomes
2. Chromosome pairing
3. Comparison of autosomes and sex chromosomes
4. Genetic expression
5. Structure of DNA and RNA
6. Types of RNA
7. Process of protein synthesis in the cytoplasm

5. In order to have an offspring with blond hair, the nurse tells the pregnant client that the child must have the same gene on both chromosomes. The nurse knows that which is the term for this?

☐ **1.** Complementary
☐ **2.** Codominant
☐ **3.** Heterozygous
☐ **4.** Homozygous

6. The nurse knows that which of the following directs the arrangement of amino acids to make proteins at the ribosomes?

☐ **1.** rRNA
☐ **2.** mRNA
☐ **3.** tRNA
☐ **4.** DNA

7. The nurse is explaining normal cells to the client. The nurse knows that which statement is true of normal cells?

☐ **1.** They contain 23 pairs of autosomes.
☐ **2.** They contain 23 pairs of sex chromosomes.
☐ **3.** They contain 22 pairs of autosomes.
☐ **4.** They contain 22 pairs of sex chromosomes.

8. The nurse knows that which of the following are characteristics of female sex chromosomes? Select all that apply.

☐ **1.** XX is genetically female.
☐ **2.** One X chromosome is inactivated.
☐ **3.** Female chromosomes consist of 22 pairs.
☐ **4.** Only one X chromosome is required after the first few weeks of embryonic life.
☐ **5.** XY is genetically female.

9. Parents ask the nurse why their offspring has brown hair when only one parent has this trait. The nurse responds that a gene that's expressed when only one parent transmits it to the offspring is called:

☐ **1.** a sex-linked gene.
☐ **2.** a codominant gene.
☐ **3.** a recessive gene.
☐ **4.** a dominant gene.

10. The nurse knows that which is the structural unit of DNA?

☐ **1.** Nucleotide
☐ **2.** Genetic code
☐ **3.** Codon
☐ **4.** Base

ANSWERS AND RATIONALES

1. CORRECT ANSWER: 3
There are 46 chromosomes (23 pairs) in the nucleus of a fertilized cell. Gametes (ova and spermatozoa) have 23 chromosomes.

2. CORRECT ANSWER: 1
Because the trait for blond hair is recessive, it's expressed only when both parents transmit it to their offspring. One grandparent having blond hair doesn't guarantee that both parents will have the gene for blond hair to transmit to the child.

3. CORRECT ANSWER: 1
Phenotype refers to the outward, detectable manifestation of a person's genetic makeup, or genotype. The genome is the complete set of chromosomes containing all the genetic information for one person. An autosome is any chromosome other than the sex chromosomes. Twenty-two of the human chromosome pairs are autosomes.

4. CORRECT ANSWER: 4
When the father has an X-linked dominant gene and the mother is normal, 100% of the daughters will be affected and the sons will be unaffected.

5. CORRECT ANSWER: 4
If both chromosomes have the same alleles for a particular gene, the person is homozygous for that gene. If the chromosomes have different alleles, the person is heterozygous for the gene. The base pairs that link with each other to form DNA chains are called *complementary pairs*. Codominant genes allow expression of both alleles.

6. CORRECT ANSWER: 2
mRNA directs amino acid arrangement to make proteins at the ribosomes. rRNA makes ribosomes in the endoplasmic reticulum of the cytoplasm, where the cell produces proteins. tRNA transfers the genetic code from mRNA for the production of a specific amino acid. DNA carries genetic information and provides the blueprint for protein synthesis.

7. CORRECT ANSWER: 3
Normal cells contain 23 pairs of chromosomes; 22 pairs are autosomes and one pair is composed of sex chromosomes.

8. CORRECT ANSWER: 1, 2, 4
XX is genetically female; XY is genetically male. In females, one X chromosome is inactivated and appears as a dense chromatic mass called a *Barr body*. Normal cells contain 23 pairs of chromosomes: 22 pairs are autosomes and one pair contains the sex chromosomes. The genetic ac-

tivity of both X chromosomes is essential only during the first few weeks of embryonic development.

9. CORRECT ANSWER: 4

A dominant gene is expressed even if only one parent transmits it to the offspring. A sex-linked gene is carried on the sex chromosomes; almost all appear on the X chromosome and are recessive. With a codominant gene, expression of both alleles occurs. A recessive gene is expressed only when both parents transmit it to the offspring.

10. CORRECT ANSWER: 1

The basic structural unit of DNA is the nucleotide. The sequence of nucleotide bases in DNA chains forms the genetic code. A codon, composed of three bases, specifies the synthesis of a specific amino acid. A nucleotide consists of a phosphate group linked to deoxyribose, joined to a nitrogen-containing compound called a base.

6

Integumentary system

LEARNING OBJECTIVES

After studying this chapter, you should be able to:

- Explain the basic functions of the skin.
- Describe changes in the skin across the life span.
- Describe the cells and layers of the epidermis.
- Identify the cells and regions of the dermis.
- Discuss the components and functions of the skin derivatives.
- Explain the role of the skin in thermoregulation.

CHAPTER OVERVIEW

The integumentary system consists of the skin, hair, nails, and certain glands. One of the largest and most visible organs of the body, the integumentary system is commonly affected by changes in other systems. Understanding the anatomy and physiology of the integumentary system can help the nurse quickly detect signs of disease and recovery. This chapter reviews the skin and its derivatives and the process of thermoregulation.

Key facts about the skin

- Integumentary system consists of skin, hair, nails, and glands
- Epidermis and dermis are separated by the basement membrane
- Skin cells die and are replaced continuously

Key functions of the skin

- Protects the body chemically, physically, and biologically
- Excretes waste products
- Helps regulate body temperature
- Provides cutaneous sensation
- Participates in vitamin D synthesis
- Acts as a reservoir for blood

SKIN

● **Key concepts**
- The integumentary system consists of skin and its derivatives—hair, nails, and the sudoriferous, sebaceous, and ceruminous glands
- Also called *integument,* skin weighs about 9 lb (4.1 kg) and covers a surface area of roughly 15 to 20 ft^2 (1.5 to 2 m^2)
- Every square inch (6.5 cm^2) contains approximately 15' (4.6 m) of blood vessels, 12' (3.7 m) of nerves, 650 sweat glands, 100 oil glands, 1,500 sensory receptors, and 3 million cells
- Thickness varies from $1/3$" to $1/8$" (3 to 8.5 mm); skin is quite thin on the eyelids and quite thick on the palms and soles
- Two fused layers—epidermis and dermis—are separated by the *basement membrane*
- Skin cells die and are replaced continuously

● **Functions of the integumentary system**
- Skin and its derivatives protect the body chemically, physically, and biologically
  - Chemically, acidic skin secretions inhibit bacteria from multiplying on body's surface
    · Bactericidal substances in the *sebum* (sebaceous gland secretion) kill some bacteria
    · *Melanin* (chemical pigment) shields skin from the sun's ultraviolet rays
  - Physically, *keratinized cells* of the epidermis, hair, and nails provide a barrier to invading organisms
  - Biologically, the epidermis contains macrophage-like *Langerhans cells* that play a role in immunity; dermal macrophages serve as second line of defense against bacteria and viruses; melanocytes produce melanin, which filters ultraviolet (UV) light
- Skin excretes waste products
  - Small amount of waste is excreted in sweat (most nitrogenous wastes are eliminated in urine)
  - Large amounts of sodium chloride are excreted through profuse sweating
- Skin helps regulate body temperature (thermoregulation)
- Skin provides *cutaneous* sensation
  - It contains sensory receptors—Meissner's corpuscles, pacinian corpuscles, and free nerve endings
  - Sensory nerve fibers originate in the nerve roots along the spine and supply sensation to specific areas of the skin called *dermatomes*
  - These receptors receive stimuli that the brain interprets as temperature, pressure, or presence of tissue-damaging elements

- Skin participates in vitamin D synthesis
  - When exposed to UV rays, skin converts cholesterol molecules to vitamin D
  - Vitamin D, in turn, participates in calcium metabolism
- Skin also acts as a reservoir for blood; when needed, blood can be shunted to the general circulation (such as to supply vigorously working muscles)

Developmental considerations
- In the embryo, the epidermis and dermis develop from *ectodermal* and *mesodermal* germ layers (respectively)
- A neonate's skin is covered with *vernix caseosa* (white, cheesy substance that protects skin from amniotic fluid in utero)
- During adolescence, sebaceous glands become more active from excessive hormonal secretions
- With advanced age, skin and its derivatives change
  - Skin loses elasticity, develops wrinkles, undergoes pigmentation changes, and heals more slowly; because of this, elderly people are more likely to develop skin cancer, pressure ulcers, and shingles than younger people
  - Hair loses pigmentation and grows more slowly; nails also grow more slowly
  - Sweat and oil production diminishes

Epidermis
- Surface layer of skin and the outermost protective covering of the body, the *epidermis* is composed of keratinized, stratified squamous epithelium
- Cells include keratinocytes, melanocytes, Merkel cells, and Langerhans cells
  - *Keratinocytes* are the most abundant type of epidermal cell; their chief role is to produce keratin, a water-insoluble protein that hardens structures (such as hair follicles)
  - *Melanocytes* are clear cells that synthesize tyrosinase and melanin
  - *Merkel cells* are cup-shaped tactile nerve endings that serve as touch receptors
  - *Langerhans cells* are branched, star-shaped cells that resemble melanocytes but don't synthesize tyrosinase; arising in bone marrow, they migrate to the epidermis in a macrophage-like fashion
- Epidermis consists of five layers, or *strata* (see *Skin layers,* page 66)
  - *Stratum basale* (basal layer) is the deepest layer of the epidermis
    - Most cells are keratinocytes (arranged perpendicularly)
    - Merkel cells occasionally appear among keratinocytes
    - Melanocytes make up about 25% of its cells

Key developmental changes of the skin
- Develops from ectodermal and mesodermal germ layers in the embryo
- Covered with vernix caseosa at birth
- Sebaceous glands become more active in adolescence
- Loses elasticity and heals slower with advanced age

Key characteristics of the epidermis
- Outermost protective covering
- Composed of keratinized, stratified squamous epithelium

Types of cells in the epidermis
- Keratinocytes: most abundant; produce keratin
- Melanocytes: synthesize tyrosinase and melanin
- Merkel cells: serve as touch receptors
- Langerhans cells: arise in bone marrow and migrate to the epidermis

Layers of the epidermis

- Stratum basale: deepest layer
- Stratum spinosum: thicker than stratum basale and lies just above it
- Stratum granulosum: thin layer above stratum spinosum
- Stratum lucidum: translucent band just above stratum granulosum
- Stratum corneum: outermost layer

Skin layers

The epidermis has five layers, or strata: the stratum basale, stratum spinosum, stratum granulosum, stratum lucidum, and stratum corneum. The dermis has a papillary region and a reticular region. Subcutaneous tissue, found beneath the dermis, is a layer of loose connective tissue that attaches the skin to underlying structures. Within these layers are hair follicles, glands, and other skin structures.

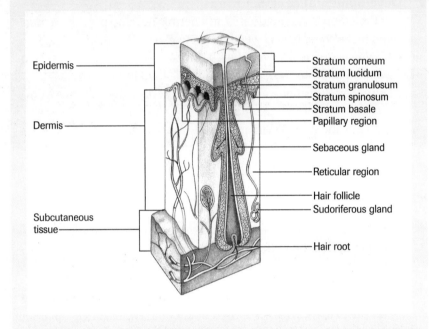

- *Stratum spinosum* (spiny layer) is thicker than the stratum basale and lies just above it
    - This layer contains Langerhans cells in addition to keratinocytes
    - Collectively, stratum basale and stratum spinosum are called *stratum germinativum* (growth layer) because epidermal growth occurs in these layers
- *Stratum granulosum* (granular layer) is a thin layer above stratum spinosum
    - It's composed of flattened cells and some Langerhans cells
    - Its name derives from the granular substance (keratohyalin) found within flattened cells
    - *Keratinization* (production of keratin) begins here
- *Stratum lucidum* (clear layer) is a translucent band just above stratum granulosum consisting of several rows of flattened keratinocytes with indistinct or absent nuclei
- *Stratum corneum* (horny layer) is the outermost epidermal layer

TIME-OUT FOR TEACHING

Teaching a patient with skin cancer

When teaching a patient with skin cancer, make sure you:
- explain the disorder
- prepare the patient for diagnostic testing (including skin biopsy)
- describe the procedures he may undergo during and after treatment, such as chemotherapy, chemo-surgery, curettage and electrodessication, immunotherapy, and radiation therapy

- emphasize the importance of using sunblock and wearing layered clothing when outdoors
- demonstrate how to self-monitor for lesions and moles that don't heal or that change characteristics
- stress the need for regular skin checkups by a health care professional.

- It contains 20 to 30 layers of flattened, cornified, nonnucleated cells
- It accounts for 75% of epidermal thickness (see *Teaching a patient with skin cancer*)

● **Dermis**
- The layer of skin just below the epidermis, the *dermis* (also called *corium*) forms the bulk of skin
- It's composed of strong, flexible connective tissue that has a matrix heavily embedded with *collagen* (protein that gives strength to dermis), *elastin* (makes skin pliable), and *reticular fibers* (bind collagen and elastin fibers together)
- Dermis contains many blood vessels, nerve fibers, and lymphatic vessels as well as most of the body's hair follicles, sweat glands, and oil glands
- Sometimes called the *true skin,* the dermis nourishes the epidermis (which lacks blood vessels, lymphatic vessels, and connective tissue)
- Cells include fibroblasts, macrophages and, occasionally, mast cells and white blood cells (WBCs)
  - *Fibroblasts* are differentiated cells of adult connective tissue
  - *Macrophages* are large, highly phagocytic cells
  - *Mast cells* are connective tissue cells that can elaborate basophilic cytoplasmic granules containing histamine and heparin
  - *WBCs* (leukocytes) are formed elements of blood involved in inflammatory and immune responses
- Dermis may tear with excessive skin stretching; such damage results in silvery white scars called *striae* (commonly called *stretch marks*), which occur especially during pregnancy

Two regions of the dermis

- Papillary: contains dermal papillae, which make blood vessels and nerves available to the skin surface
- Reticular: contains dense, irregular connective tissue, which provides flexibility and strength

Key facts about skin derivatives

- Consist of hair, nails, and sudoriferous, sebaceous, and ceruminous glands
- Originate from epidermis
- Help maintain homeostasis

Key facts about hair

- Protects the body from heat loss and UV rays
- Shields the eyes and helps keep dust out of the upper respiratory tract
- Follicles extend into the dermis
- Nutrition and hormones affect growth and distribution

- *Subcutaneous tissue* (also called *hypodermis* or *superficial fascia*) lies beneath the dermis
  - It consists of loose connective tissue that attaches skin to underlying structures
  - Fat in subcutaneous tissue insulates the body
- Dermis has two regions: papillary and reticular
  - *Papillary region* (upper region) accounts for about 20% of dermal thickness; its surface contains small, fingerlike projections called *dermal papillae*
    - Many dermal papillae contain capillary loops; others contain free nerve endings (pain or touch receptors)
    - Dermal papillae make blood vessels and nerves more readily available to skin surface
  - *Reticular region* (lower region) is composed of dense, irregular collagenous connective tissue; its irregular arrangement makes dermis flexible and strong

SKIN DERIVATIVES

● **Key concepts**
- Skin derivatives—hair, nails, and sudoriferous, sebaceous, and ceruminous glands—originate from the epidermis
- They help maintain *homeostasis* (equilibrium of the body's internal environment)

● **Hair**
- Hair covers most body parts; only the lips, nipples, palms, soles, and parts of the external genitalia totally lack hair
  - Hair protects the body from heat loss and UV rays
  - It also shields the eyes and helps keep dust out of the upper respiratory tract
- Follicles extend into the dermis
  - Nerve ending surrounds the bulb of each hair follicle
  - Sebaceous glands secrete oily sebum directly onto the hair follicle, lubricating the hair shaft
  - Smooth-muscle fibers (called *arrectores pilorum)* cause *cutis anserina* (gooseflesh); each tiny arrector pili muscle moves the individual hair when it contracts
- Nutrition and hormones affect hair growth and distribution
  - Poor nutrition leads to less nourishing blood supply to hair
  - The male hormone testosterone encourages hair growth
  - Abnormal hair growth may indicate the presence of a hormone-producing tumor

Cross section of a fingernail

This illustration shows the anatomic components of a fingernail.

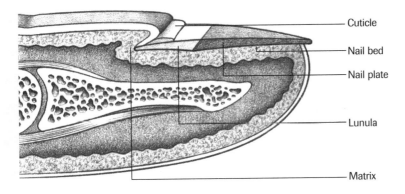

- Cuticle
- Nail bed
- Nail plate
- Lunula
- Matrix

- **Nails**
  - Nails are modified, heavily keratinized epidermal protective coverings on the dorsal surface at the end of each finger and toe (see *Cross section of a fingernail*)
  - *Cuticle* is the skin fold over the proximal portion of the nail
  - *Lunula* is the white, crescent-shaped region at the base of the nail plate

- **Sudoriferous glands**
  - Also known as sweat glands, *sudoriferous glands* are long, coiled tubes located in the dermis or subcutaneous tissue that secrete sweat through a duct on the body's surface
  - These glands play a crucial role in maintaining normal body temperature; sympathetic division of autonomic nervous system regulates their function
  - About 2.5 million are in the body; only the lips, nipples, and parts of the external genitalia lack these glands
  - Sudoriferous glands are classified as eccrine or apocrine
    - *Eccrine glands* are distributed over nearly the entire body surface
      - They're most abundant on the palms, soles, and forehead (more numerous than apocrine glands)
      - Gland's secretory coil originates in the dermis, with a duct extending up to a funnel-shaped pore on the skin's surface

Key characteristics of apocrine glands

- Appear mainly in axillary, anal, and genital areas
- Ducts terminate in upper portion of hair follicles
- Mammary glands (modified apocrine glands) secrete milk

Key characteristics of sebaceous glands

- Secrete sebum, which lubricates hair and skin via ducts to hair follicles
- Appear everywhere on the body except for palms of hands and soles of feet

Key facts about thermoregulation

- Skin keeps body temperature around 98.6° F (37° C)
- Occurs by negative feedback mechanisms
- Skin senses temperature stimulus, sends impulse to the brain; the brain transmits impulses to sweat glands and blood vessels

- Eccrine glands promote cooling through evaporation of secretions; in the palms and soles, they secrete fluid mainly in response to stress
  – *Apocrine glands* appear mainly in axillary, anal, and genital areas
  - Large, branched, and specialized, apocrine glands empty into ducts, which terminate in the upper portion of hair follicles rather than on the skin's surface
  - Mammary glands (modified apocrine glands) secrete milk

● **Sebaceous glands**
- Also called oil glands, sebaceous glands are simple alveolar glands that secrete *sebum* (oil)
- Sebum softens and lubricates hair and skin, preventing hair from becoming brittle and impeding water loss from skin; it also acts as a bactericide
- Sebum usually travels via a duct to a hair follicle
  – Duct blocked by sebum forms a whitehead
  – As duct contents oxidize and dry, they form a blackhead
- Only palms and soles lack sebaceous glands
- Hormones influence secretion; sex hormones cause sebaceous glands to hypertrophy during puberty and atrophy in old age

● **Ceruminous glands**
- Modified apocrine glands, ceruminous glands line the external ear canal
- Combination of ceruminous and sebaceous gland secretions is called *cerumen* (earwax)

THERMOREGULATION

● **Key concepts**
- Skin normally keeps body temperature around 98.6° F (37° C); this homeostatic process is called *thermoregulation*
- Thermoregulation occurs by negative feedback mechanisms

● **Feedback mechanisms**
- When skin receptors sense temperature stimulus (environmental heat or cold), they send impulses (input) to the control center in the brain (see *The skin's role in thermoregulation*)
- Brain transmits impulses (output) to effector organs (sweat glands and blood vessels)
- Effector organs respond to the brain's message
  – When the body is hot, sweat glands produce perspiration and blood vessels dilate
    - Evaporation of sweat from the surface dissipates heat
    - Vasodilation brings more warm blood to skin, where it's cooled

GO WITH THE FLOW

The skin's role in thermoregulation

Abundant nerves, blood vessels, and eccrine glands within the skin's deeper layer aid thermoregulation (control of body temperature). The first part of this flow chart shows how the body conserves heat. The second part shows how the body cools off.

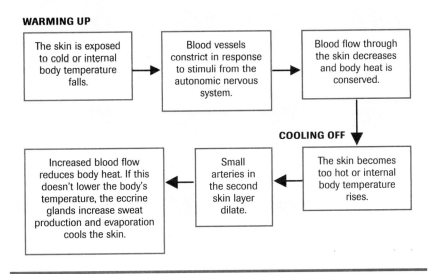

WARMING UP

| The skin is exposed to cold or internal body temperature falls. | → | Blood vessels constrict in response to stimuli from the autonomic nervous system. | → | Blood flow through the skin decreases and body heat is conserved. |

COOLING OFF ▼

| Increased blood flow reduces body heat. If this doesn't lower the body's temperature, the eccrine glands increase sweat production and evaporation cools the skin. | ◄ | Small arteries in the second skin layer dilate. | ◄ | The skin becomes too hot or internal body temperature rises. |

TOP 5

Items to study for your next test on the integumentary system

1. Major functions of the skin
2. Cells of the epidermis
3. Epidermal layers
4. Structure and function of the dermis
5. Structure and function of hair

– When the body is cold, blood vessels constrict to prevent heat loss

NCLEX CHECKS

It's never too soon to begin your NCLEX preparation. Now that you've reviewed this chapter, carefully read each of the following questions and choose the best answer. Then compare your responses with the correct answers.

1. When teaching a client about skin care, the nurse tells the client that the main functions of the skin include which of the following? Select all that apply.

- ☐ **1.** Support
- ☐ **2.** Protection
- ☐ **3.** Motor response
- ☐ **4.** Sensory perception
- ☐ **5.** Nourishment
- ☐ **6.** Temperature regulation

2. The nurse is teaching a class on preventing skin cancer and correctly explains that which is the outermost layer of the skin?
- [ ] **1.** Epidermis
- [ ] **2.** Dermis
- [ ] **3.** Hypodermis
- [ ] **4.** Papillary dermis

3. While performing a skin assessment, the nurse should consider which integumentary structure an epidermal appendage?
- [ ] **1.** Blood vessel
- [ ] **2.** Nerve
- [ ] **3.** Stratum basale
- [ ] **4.** Hair

4. The nurse is teaching an adolescent about acne. Which statement would the nurse make to this client?
- [ ] **1.** "Sebum causes the hair to become brittle."
- [ ] **2.** "Sebaceous glands are found on the soles and palms."
- [ ] **3.** "Whiteheads occur when sebum blocks a duct."
- [ ] **4.** "Sebaceous glands atrophy during puberty."

5. A client tells the nurse that his palms sweat profusely when he's feeling stressed. The nurse explains that which sweat glands are responsible for this reaction?
- [ ] **1.** Apocrine
- [ ] **2.** Eccrine
- [ ] **3.** Mammary
- [ ] **4.** Sebaceous

6. Which mechanism aids thermoregulation?
- [ ] **1.** Sweat evaporation
- [ ] **2.** Blood vessel constriction
- [ ] **3.** Blood vessel dilation
- [ ] **4.** Parasympathetic nervous stimulation

7. A client has just delivered a baby and asks the nurse about the white substance covering the baby's skin. The nurse responds that this substance is called:
- [ ] **1.** keratin.
- [ ] **2.** melanin.
- [ ] **3.** sebum.
- [ ] **4.** vernix caseosa.

8. Which age-related change in the integumentary system can a nurse expect when assessing an elderly client?
- [ ] **1.** More-active sebaceous glands
- [ ] **2.** More-elastic skin
- [ ] **3.** Altered pigmentation
- [ ] **4.** Quicker nail growth

9. The nurse is teaching an adolescent about hair care. Which statement by the nurse would be appropriate?

- ☐ **1.** "Good nutrition has no effect on blood supply to the hair."
- ☐ **2.** "Testosterone reduces hair growth."
- ☐ **3.** "Sebum dries out the hair."
- ☐ **4.** "Hair doesn't cover the lips, nipples, palms, soles, and parts of the genitalia."

10. The nurse is removing excess cerumen from a client's ear. The nurse explains to the client that cerumen:

- ☐ **1.** lines the internal auditory canal.
- ☐ **2.** contains fibroblasts and macrophages.
- ☐ **3.** is a combination of ceruminous and sudoriferous gland secretions.
- ☐ **4.** is also called *earwax*.

ANSWERS AND RATIONALES

1. CORRECT ANSWER: 2, 4, 6
The skin's main functions include protection from injury, noxious chemicals, and bacterial invasion; sensory perception of touch, temperature, and pain; and regulation of body heat. Other major functions of the skin are excreting wastes, synthesizing vitamin D, and serving as a reservoir for blood.

2. CORRECT ANSWER: 1
The epidermis is the skin's surface layer and the body's outermost protective covering. The dermis lies just below the epidermis. The loose, connective tissue of the hypodermis (subcutaneous tissue) attaches the skin to underlying structures. The papillary region is the uppermost region of the dermis.

3. CORRECT ANSWER: 4
The appendages of the epidermis are the nails, hair, sebaceous glands, eccrine glands, and apocrine glands. The dermis contains blood vessels and nerve fibers as well as lymphatic vessels, hair follicles, and sudoriferous and sebaceous glands. The stratum basale is the deepest layer of the epidermis.

4. CORRECT ANSWER: 3
A whitehead forms when sebum blocks a duct. Sebum softens and lubricates the hair, preventing it from becoming brittle. The only body areas lacking sebaceous glands are the palms and soles. During puberty, sebaceous glands hypertrophy and become overactive.

5. CORRECT ANSWER: 2

Eccrine glands are widely distributed throughout the body and produce an odorless, watery fluid. Eccrine glands in the palms and soles secrete this fluid mainly in response to emotional stress. Apocrine glands occur mainly in the axillary, anal, and genital areas. Mammary glands, a type of apocrine gland, secrete milk. Sebaceous glands secrete oil and occur all over the body except for the palms and soles.

6. CORRECT ANSWER: 2

When hypothermia occurs, blood vessels constrict to prevent heat loss. When the body becomes too hot, sweat glands produce perspiration, which cools the body as it evaporates, and blood vessels dilate to bring warm blood to the skin, where the blood cools. Excessive cold stimulates the autonomic nervous system (not the parasympathetic nervous system), causing blood vessels to constrict.

7. CORRECT ANSWER: 4

A neonate's skin is covered with vernix caseosa, a white, cheesy substance that protects the skin from amniotic fluid in the uterus. Keratin is a water-insoluble protein that hardens structures such as hair follicles. Melanin is a chemical pigment that shields the skin from the sun's UV rays. Sebum is a type of oil secreted from the sebaceous glands.

8. CORRECT ANSWER: 3

In elderly clients, pigmentation changes are common. Sebaceous gland activity increases during adolescence and decreases in advanced age. The skin becomes less elastic, and nails grow more slowly.

9. CORRECT ANSWER: 4

Hair covers most parts of the body; only the lips, nipples, palms, soles, and parts of the external genitalia totally lack hair. Poor nutrition leads to a less nourishing blood supply to the hair. The male hormone testosterone promotes hair growth. Sebum, secreted by the sebaceous glands, lubricates the hair shaft.

10. CORRECT ANSWER: 4

Cerumen, a combination of ceruminous and sebaceous gland secretions, is also called *earwax*. Cerumen lines the external auditory canal. Fibroblasts and macrophages are cells in the dermis.

7

Skeletal system

LEARNING OBJECTIVES

After studying this chapter, you should be able to:

● Describe the classification of bones and their functions.

● Understand bone formation, remodeling, and resorption.

● Discuss changes in the skeletal system across the life span.

● Explain the types of cartilage and their functions.

● Identify the bones of the axial and appendicular skeletons.

● Identify the types of joints and their functions.

CHAPTER OVERVIEW

The skeletal system forms the framework that supports and protects the body. It's made up of four types of bones and three types of cartilage. Together with the muscular and nervous systems, the skeletal system controls body movement. The nurse needs a full understanding of skeletal anatomy and physiology to provide comprehensive care for patients with musculoskeletal disorders or injuries and related health problems. This chapter reviews bone, cartilage, the axial and appendicular skeleton, and joints.

BONE

● Key concepts
- The skeleton consists of 206 bones
- Bone, a hard form of connective tissue, is composed of one of two types of osseous (bony) tissue
  - *Compact* bone tissue is dense and smooth
  - *Cancellous* (spongy) bone tissue has a spongy or latticelike structure

Key facts about bones
- Hard form of connective tissue
- Each bone consists of two types of tissue: compact and cancellous

Viewing a long bone

The main parts of a long bone, shown here, are the *diaphysis* (main shaft) and the *epiphyses* (ends). The *metaphysis* lies between the epiphysis and diaphysis in the developing long bone. Periosteum, a tough fibrous membrane sheath, surrounds the diaphysis; endosteum lines the medullary cavity. At the epiphyseal line, cartilage separates the epiphyses from the diaphysis.

TWO TYPES OF BONE TISSUE
Each bone consists of an outer layer of dense, smooth, compact bone that contains central (haversian) canals, and an inner layer of spongy cancellous bone that lacks these canals.

Cancellous bone
Cancellous bone consists of *trabeculae* (tiny spicules that form a meshwork) that interlace to form a latticework. Red marrow fills the spaces between the trabeculae of some bones.

Key characteristics of cancellous bone
- Spongy inner layer
- Consists of trabeculae
- Red marrow fills spaces

Key characteristics of compact bone
- Hard and smooth outer layer
- Consists of calcified matrix layers

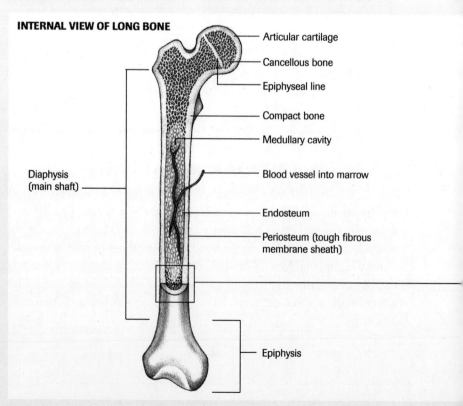

INTERNAL VIEW OF LONG BONE

- Articular cartilage
- Cancellous bone
- Epiphyseal line
- Compact bone
- Medullary cavity
- Blood vessel into marrow
- Endosteum
- Periosteum (tough fibrous membrane sheath)

Diaphysis (main shaft)

Epiphysis

- Bones support and protect the body, allow movement and *hematopoiesis* (blood cell formation), and act as a mineral reservoir; they constantly undergo formation and breakdown
- Bones are classified by shape as long, short, flat, or irregular

● **Classification by shape**
- *Long bones* are longer than they are wide (see *Viewing a long bone*)
  – Long bones of the upper body include the clavicle, humerus, radius, and ulna; long bones of the lower body include the femur, tibia, and fibula as well as the metatarsals, metacarpals, and phalanges

Cancellous bone fills the central regions of the epiphyses and the inner portions of short, flat, and irregular bones.

Compact bone
Compact bone is found in the diaphyses of long bones and the outer layers of short, flat, and irregular bones. Compact bone consists of layers of calcified matrix containing spaces occupied by osteocytes (bone cells). *Lamellae* (bone layers) are arranged around haversian canals. Small cavities called *lacunae*, which lie between the lamellae, contain osteocytes. *Canaliculi* (tiny canals) connect the lacunae, forming the structural units of the bone. Canaliculi also provide nutrients to bone tissue. *Volkmann's canals* allow for the passage of blood vessels through the bone.

Key characteristics of long bones

- Longer than they are wide
- Consist of a shaft and two extremities
- Diaphysis contains a medullary cavity filled with yellow marrow
- Epiphyses are separated from the diaphysis by cartilage at the epiphyseal line

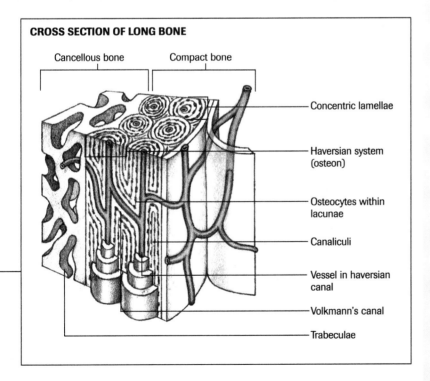

CROSS SECTION OF LONG BONE

Cancellous bone   Compact bone

Concentric lamellae

Haversian system (osteon)

Osteocytes within lacunae

Canaliculi

Vessel in haversian canal

Volkmann's canal

Trabeculae

Key characteristics of short bones

- Lack a long axis and are typically cuboidal
- Composed of spongy bone and marrow enclosed by a thin layer of compact bone
- Sesamoid bones: type of short bone embedded in tendons

Key characteristics of flat bones

- Thin and usually curved
- Consist of two layers of compact bone separated by spongy bone and marrow
- Examples: sternum, ribs, skull bones

Key characteristics of irregular bones

- Consist of spongy bone enclosed by thin layers of compact bone
- Examples: vertebrae, hip bones, some skull bones

Key bone functions

- Support and stabilize the body
- Protect internal organs
- Allow movement
- Act as mineral reservoir
- Promote blood cell formation

– Each long bone consists of a shaft *(diaphysis)* and two extremities *(epiphyses)*, which are usually articulated, or jointed; between the shaft and each extremity is a portion of developing long bone called the *metaphysis*

– The *diaphysis*, a tube of compact bone, contains a *medullary cavity* filled with yellow marrow (may also contain varying amounts of red marrow, depending on the growth stage)

· A thin layer of cells *(endosteum)* lines the inner surface of compact bone, defining the medullary cavity

· A tough, fibrous membrane sheath *(periosteum)* surrounds the diaphysis

– Epiphyses are separated from the diaphysis by cartilage at the *epiphyseal line*

- *Short bones* lack a long axis and are typically cuboidal (such as ankle and wrist bones)

– They're composed of spongy bone and marrow enclosed by a thin layer of compact bone; periosteum surrounds the compact bone (except on articular surfaces)

– *Sesamoid bones* are a special type of short bone embedded in tendons; the kneecap (patella) is an example

- *Flat bones* are thin and usually curved (not flat)

– They consist of two layers of compact bone separated by spongy bone and marrow

– Examples include the sternum, ribs, and most skull bones

- *Irregular bones* don't fit any other classification

– They consist of spongy bone enclosed by thin layers of compact bone

– Examples include the vertebrae, hip bones, and some skull bones

● Bone functions

- Support and stabilize the body, contributing to its shape
- Protect internal organs from injury
- Act as levers for skeletal muscles to move the body and its parts; permit locomotion, grasping of objects, and breathing
- Serve as a reservoir for such minerals as calcium, copper, magnesium, phosphorus, potassium, sodium, and sulfur; bone cavities act as storage sites for fat
- Play a role in *hematopoiesis* (blood cell formation), which occurs chiefly in the red marrow of certain bones

● Bone formation

- Bone formation occurs through either *endochondral or intramembranous ossification;* areas of bone formation are called *centers of ossification*

– *Osteoblasts* are the active bone-forming cells in both types of formation (see *Bone growth and remodeling*)

Bone growth and remodeling

The ossification of cartilage into bone, or *osteogenesis*, begins at about the ninth week of fetal development. The diaphyses of long bones form by birth, and the epiphyses begin to ossify at about that time. These illustrations show the stages of bone growth and remodeling of the epiphyses of a long bone.

CREATION OF AN OSSIFICATION CENTER

At about the ninth week of fetal development, an ossification center develops in the epiphysis. Some cartilage cells enlarge and stimulate ossification of surrounding cells. The enlarged cells then die, leaving small cavities. New cartilage continues to develop.

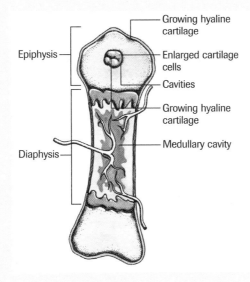

Epiphysis

Diaphysis

Growing hyaline cartilage

Enlarged cartilage cells

Cavities

Growing hyaline cartilage

Medullary cavity

OSTEOBLASTS FORM BONE

Osteoblasts begin to form bone on the remaining cartilage, creating the trabeculae network of cancellous bone. Cartilage continues to form on the outer surfaces of the epiphysis and along the upper surface of the epiphyseal plate.

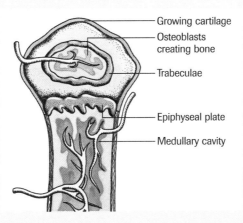

Growing cartilage

Osteoblasts creating bone

Trabeculae

Epiphyseal plate

Medullary cavity

– Osteoblasts produce an organic matrix for bones and secrete the enzyme *alkaline phosphatase*, which liberates phosphate ions from compounds at the site of bone formation
– Phosphate ions combine with calcium ions to form calcium phosphate, which is deposited in bone matrix, causing the bone to become rigid
– Osteoblasts become incorporated into the bone as it forms; then they are transformed into osteocytes
• In endochondral bone formation, a cartilage model forms first; then osteoblasts invade the cartilage and convert it into bone

Key facts about intramembranous ossification

- Osteoblasts differentiate from precursor cells in connective tissue
- Bone formation occurs directly within connective tissue, without a preliminary cartilage mass
- Bone grows by adding newly formed bone from the periosteum, with simultaneous resorption near the marrow cavity

Key facts about bone remodeling

- Involves the replacement of old bone tissue with new
- Requires hormones, minerals, and vitamins
- Stress on a bone affects its strength and thickness

– In a long bone, ossification begins first in the shaft (diaphysis); then centers of ossification form in the ends of the bone (epiphyses)

– The actively growing zone of cartilage between the diaphysis and epiphyses is called the *epiphyseal plate*

- Intramembranous bone formation occurs in many of the flat bones of the skull and in the clavicle; osteoblasts form these bones directly, without a preliminary cartilage mass

– Bone-forming cells differentiate from precursor cells in connective tissue and begin to produce bone directly within the connective tissue

– The initial centers of ossification extend peripherally and eventually convert all the connective tissue to bone

- Bone increases in length and thickness as an individual grows

– In endochondral formation, bone grows in length by continuous production of cartilage at the distal end of the epiphyseal plate and conversion of cartilage into bone in the proximal part of the epiphyseal plate; this is followed by remodeling of the bone to maintain its configuration

  · Toward the end of adolescence, the epiphyseal lines are converted into bone, a process called *closure of the epiphyses*

  · After closure occurs, no further increase in bone length can occur

– Bone also increases in thickness in endochondral formation and is remodeled as it grows

  · Addition of newly formed bone from the periosteum increases long bone diameter

  · Simultaneous *resorption* of bone near the marrow cavity also increases long bone diameter

– In intramembranous formation, bone grows by the addition of newly formed bone from the periosteum and simultaneous resorption of bone near the marrow cavity (process is similar to long bone growth, except that epiphyseal plates don't form)

● **Bone remodeling**

- Through *bone remodeling,* new bone tissue replaces old bone tissue
- In this process, *osteoclasts* constantly break down old bone tissue, while osteoblasts build new bone
- Bone remodeling requires hormones (such as growth and sex hormones), minerals (such as calcium and phosphorus), and vitamins (such as vitamin D)
- Stresses on the bone affect bone strength and thickness; heavy physical activity and weight bearing promote heavier, stronger bones by stimulating osteoblast formation and bone matrix production and by inhibiting osteoclast activity

Bone resorption

- Osteoclasts carry out bone resorption; they promote bone remodeling by removing unwanted bone while new bone forms in other areas
  - Osteoclasts secrete protein-digesting lysosomal enzymes, which digest the organic bone matrix; they also secrete lactic and citric acids, which dissolve calcium phosphate and other bone minerals
  - Osteoclasts also use phagocytosis to digest small bone fragments
  - Calcium and phosphate ions are then released into the bloodstream, where they become part of the body's ion pool
- Adrenal cortical hormones promote bone resorption

Developmental considerations

- Bone formation exceeds resorption during childhood and adolescence, allowing the bones to grow
- In young and middle adulthood, bone formation and resorption are balanced closely; bone size and density don't change
- In old age, bone breakdown exceeds formation, causing a gradual decrease in bone density
  - When bone breakdown greatly outstrips bone formation, osteoporosis can occur
  - Osteoporosis is marked by decreased bone mass and an increased tendency to develop fractures, especially pathologic ones (for teaching tips, see *Teaching a patient with osteoporosis*)

TIME-OUT FOR TEACHING

Teaching a patient with osteoporosis

Make sure you teach a patient with osteoporosis:

- how imbalance between bone formation and resorption leads to osteoporosis
- the risk factors for osteoporosis and how lifestyle modifications can reduce the risk
- what diagnostic tests to expect, such as bone mineral density testing and X-rays
- what treatments to expect, including drug and hormone replacement therapy, weight-bearing exercise, and a diet high in calcium and vitamin D
- ways to prevent injury, such as wearing a back brace, sleeping on a firm mattress, and using proper body mechanics
- what signs and symptoms to report, such as new pain (especially after trauma) and vaginal bleeding (for female patients receiving hormone therapy)
- how to perform monthly breast self-examination (for female patients receiving hormone therapy)
- where to find sources of information and support.

CARTILAGE

● **Key concepts**
- Cartilage—a tough, resilient type of connective tissue—consists of a dense network of collagenous and elastic fibers embedded in a gellike substance
- New cartilage forms from cells called *chondroblasts;* mature cartilage cells are called *chondrocytes*
- Cartilage supports and shapes various body structures; it also cushions bone
- Cartilage is avascular (bloodless) and isn't innervated

● **Types of cartilage**
- Three types of cartilage are hyaline cartilage, fibrocartilage, and elastic cartilage
- *Hyaline cartilage* has a characteristic translucent appearance
  - The most abundant type, hyaline cartilage provides flexibility and support
  - It forms the nose, larynx, trachea, bronchi, and bronchial tubes; it also forms the epiphyseal discs and most articular cartilages
  - This type of cartilage appears at joints over the ends of long bones and at the ventral ends of the ribs
- *Fibrocartilage* consists of bundles of collagenous fibers
  - It provides strength and rigidity
  - Fibrocartilage occurs in such joints as the temporomandibular joint; it's also a component of intervertebral disks, which act as cushions between vertebrae
- *Elastic cartilage* is more opaque, flexible, and elastic than hyaline cartilage; it lends strength and helps maintain the shape of certain organs, such as the auricle (external ear), auditory tube, and larynx

AXIAL SKELETON

● **Key concepts**
- The *axial skeleton* consists of the bones that form the longitudinal axis of the body—those of the head, neck, and trunk
- Its 80 bones are located in three major regions—the skull, vertebral column, and bony thorax (see *Bones of the human skeleton*)

● **Skull**
- Also called the *cranium,* the skull has several functions
  - It protects the brain
  - It provides cavities for sensory organs, such as the eyes, ears, and nose
  - It has openings that allow the passage of air and food

Key facts about cartilage
- Supports and shapes body structures
- Is avascular and isn't innervated
- Three types: hyaline, fibrocartilage, and elastic

Key characteristics of hyaline cartilage
- Most abundant
- Provides flexibility and support
- Forms the nose, larynx, trachea, and bronchi

Key characteristics of fibrocartilage
- Provides strength and rigidity
- Occurs in some joints and in intervertebral disks

Key characteristics of elastic cartilage
- More opaque, flexible, and elastic than hyaline
- Found in auricle, auditory tube, and larynx

Key facts about the axial skeleton
- Forms the longitudinal axis of the body
- Includes the skull, vertebrae, and bony thorax

Bones of the human skeleton

The skeleton accounts for roughly 20% of body mass. Composed of 206 bones, it's divided into the axial and appendicular groups. The axial skeleton includes the skull, vertebrae, and bony thorax. The appendicular skeleton includes the bones of the shoulder and pelvic girdles and the upper and lower limbs. This illustration shows the major bones of both groups.

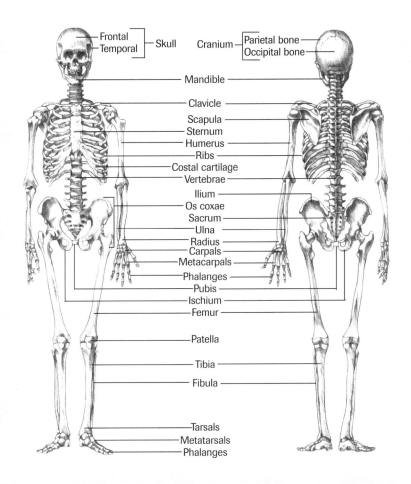

Frontal
Temporal — Skull
Cranium — Parietal bone
Occipital bone
Mandible
Clavicle
Scapula
Sternum
Humerus
Ribs
Costal cartilage
Vertebrae
Ilium
Os coxae
Sacrum
Ulna
Radius
Carpals
Metacarpals
Phalanges
Pubis
Ischium
Femur
Patella
Tibia
Fibula
Tarsals
Metatarsals
Phalanges

Key facts about the human skeleton

- Makes up 20% of body mass
- Composed of 206 bones
- Divided into axial and appendicular groups

Key facts about the skull

- Protects the brain
- Consists of cranial and facial bones

Key characteristics of cranial bones

- Eight bones consisting of paired and unpaired bones
- Paired: parietal and temporal bones
- Unpaired: frontal, sphenoid, ethmoid, and occipital bones

  – It contains teeth and jaws for mastication
- The skull consists of *cranial bones* (cranial vault, or calvaria) and *facial bones*
- The eight cranial bones include the paired parietal and temporal bones and the unpaired frontal, sphenoid, ethmoid, and occipital bones
  – These irregular bones consist of a spongy layer between internal and external tables (flat layers) of compact bone

Views of the skull

The cranium is composed of eight bones—the frontal, sphenoid, ethmoid, and occipital bones as well as two parietal and two temporal bones.

ANTERIOR VIEW

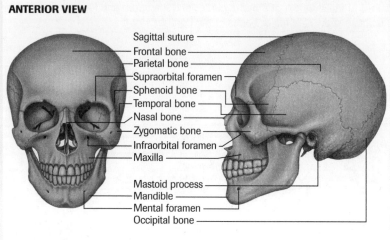

- Sagittal suture
- Frontal bone
- Parietal bone
- Supraorbital foramen
- Sphenoid bone
- Temporal bone
- Nasal bone
- Zygomatic bone
- Infraorbital foramen
- Maxilla
- Mastoid process
- Mandible
- Mental foramen
- Occipital bone

INFERIOR VIEW

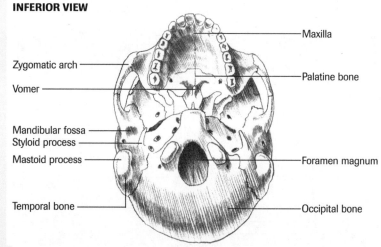

- Maxilla
- Zygomatic arch
- Vomer
- Palatine bone
- Mandibular fossa
- Styloid process
- Mastoid process
- Foramen magnum
- Temporal bone
- Occipital bone

Key characteristics of facial bones

- Forehead formed by frontal bone
- Orbits house the eyes
- Zygomatic bones form the cheeks
- Maxillae and mandible form upper and lower jaws
- Nasal bones and maxillae form piriform aperture
- Four pairs of sinuses: frontal, ethmoid, sphenoid, maxillary
- Hyoid bone lies between mandible and larynx

– Internally, bony ridges divide the cranial bones at the base of the skull into three *fossae*, or depressed regions
- Viewing the skull from different positions allows study of the facial bones (see *Views of the skull*)
  – In an anterior view, prominent skull features include the forehead, nasion, superciliary arch, orbits, zygomatic bones, piriform aperture, upper and lower jaws, and paranasal sinuses
    · The forehead is formed by the frontal bone

- The *nasion* (depression at the root of the nose) is formed by the intersection of the frontal bone and the two nasal bones
- The *superciliary arch* is the elevation that extends laterally from the *glabella* (region above the nasion and between the eyebrows)
- *Orbits* are the bony cavities that house the eyes
- The *zygomatic (malar) bones* form the prominences of the cheeks
- The nasal bones and maxillae (upper jaw bones) form the *piriform aperture*
- The *maxillae* and *mandible* form, respectively, the upper and lower jaws
- The four pairs of paranasal sinuses are named for the bones they're found in: *frontal, ethmoid, sphenoid,* and *maxillary*

– In a lateral view, the frontal, parietal, occipital, ethmoid, sphenoid, and temporal bones can be seen
- Laterally, the most prominent feature is the *zygomatic process*, which articulates with the temporal process of the zygomatic bone, the coronoid process, and the mandibular condyle
- The *mastoid* and *styloid processes* of the temporal bone are also visible
- The *mental foramen* (an opening for passage of the mental nerve and vessels) appears in the mandible

– In a posterior view, the paired parietal bones join the occipital and mastoid parts of the temporal bones
- When viewed inferiorly, the mastoid processes are prominent bilaterally
- When viewed superiorly, the sagittal suture joins the lambdoid suture

- Skull *sutures* (joints between skull bones) have closely united opposing surfaces, similar to sutures found elsewhere in the body
  – Skull sutures include the *coronal, sagittal, lambdoid,* and *squamous* sutures
  – In adults, skull joints can't move, except for the mandible; connected to the skull by paired synovial joints, the mandible moves freely
- The *hyoid bone*, which lacks direct articulation with any other bone, is in the front of the neck between the mandible and larynx
  – Although not part of the skull, the hyoid is commonly described in conjunction with it because of its relationship to the mandible and temporal bones

Key skull sutures

- Coronal
- Sagittal
- Lambdoid
- Squamous

– The hyoid serves as a movable base for the tongue and an attachment for the neck muscles that help elevate the larynx during swallowing and speech

● **Vertebral column**
  • The *vertebral column* (spine) extends from the skull to the pelvis
    – It provides the primary axial support for the body
    – It consists of 26 irregular bones called *vertebrae;* 24 of these are movable
    – The vertebral column has sagittal curves in the cervical, thoracic, lumbar, and sacral regions
      · The cervical and lumbar curves are convex anteriorly; the thoracic and sacral curves are convex posteriorly
      · These curves increase the strength, resilience, balance, and flexibility of the spine
  • A typical vertebra consists of an ovoid body (centrum), a vertebral arch (the lamina make up the posterior portion of this arch), two transverse processes, two superior articular processes, two inferior articular processes, and one spinous process (see *Structures of the vertebra*)
    – Muscle attaches at the spinous process and the two transverse processes
    – The superior and inferior articular processes articulate with the vertebrae immediately above and below them
  • The vertebral column has seven cervical vertebrae, 12 thoracic vertebrae, five lumbar vertebrae, the sacrum (formed by the fusion of five vertebrae), and the coccyx (formed by the fusion of four vertebrae)
    – The *cervical vertebrae* (designated C1 to C7) constitute the skeleton of the neck; they're smaller than the other vertebrae
      · C1, called the *atlas,* is highly modified (different from other cervical vertebrae); a ring of bone, it lacks a body or spinous process
      · C2, called the *axis,* has a toothlike process called the *dens* that projects superiorly from the body; the dens forms a specialized type of articulation with the atlas above it
      · C3 through C7 consist of a body (the discoid, weightbearing portion) anteriorly and a vertebral arch posteriorly
        - The body and arch form the *vertebral foramen;* collectively, these openings form the vertebral canal, which houses the spinal cord
        - Each of these vertebrae contains two *transverse processes,* lateral projections from the vertebral arch; and one *spinous process,* a posterior projection in the midline

Structures of the vertebra

Most vertebrae share several important features. The body (centrum) is the disk-shaped, weight-bearing, ventral portion. Laminae are flat, broad structures that fuse to form the posterior portion of the vertebral arch. Pedicles project posteriorly from the vertebral body, forming the sides of the vertebral foramen, a large opening in the center of the vertebra formed by its body and arch; collectively, the vertebral foramens compose the spinal canal (which houses the spinal cord). Processes project laterally at the points where a lamina and pedicle join; a spinous process projects posteriorly and inferiorly from the junction of the laminae. Two superior articular processes project upward from the laminae and articulate with the immediately superior vertebra; two inferior articular processes project downward from the laminae and articulate with the immediately inferior vertebra.

Key vertebral structures

- Body: weight-bearing, ventral portion
- Laminae: flat structures that form the posterior vertebral arch
- Pedicles: form the sides of vertebral foramen
- Vertebral foramens: large openings at the center of vertebrae; collectively form the spinal canal
- Spinous processes: project from the junction of the laminae
- Superior articulated processes: project upward from the laminae; articulate with superior vertebra
- Inferior articulated processes: project downward from the laminae; articulate with inferior vertebra

LEFT LATERAL VIEW

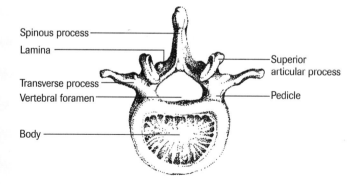

Spinous process

Transverse process

Superior articular process

Inferior articular process

SUPERIOR VIEW

Spinous process

Lamina

Transverse process

Vertebral foramen

Body

Superior articular process

Pedicle

Key characteristics of the thoracic vertebrae

- Located between the cervical and lumbar vertebrae
- Each articulates bilaterally with the ribs

Key characteristics of the lumbar vertebrae

- Lie between the thoracic vertebrae and the sacrum
- Are the largest and strongest vertebrae

Key characteristics of the sacrum

- Triangular bone formed by the fusion of five sacral vertebrae
- Lies between the hip bones

Key characteristics of the coccyx

- Triangular bone formed by the fusion of the four coccygeal vertebrae
- Articulates superiorly with the sacrum

Key facts about the bony thorax

- Consists of the thoracic vertebrae, 12 pairs of ribs, the sternum, and costal cartilages
- First seven pairs of ribs connect to the sternum by costal cartilages
- Remaining five pairs are false ribs
- The sternum joins the ribs anteriorly

- The bony connections between the body and the transverse processes are called *pedicles;* the bony connections between the transverse and spinous processes are called *laminae*
  - The *thoracic vertebrae* (designated T1 to T12) are located between the cervical and lumbar vertebrae
    - Each thoracic vertebra articulates bilaterally with the ribs
    - The first 10 have facets on the transverse processes that articulate with the *tubercles* of the ribs
  - The *lumbar vertebrae* (designated L1 to L5) lie between the thoracic vertebrae and the sacrum; they're the largest and strongest vertebrae
  - The *sacrum,* a triangular bone formed by the fusion of five sacral vertebrae, lies in the posterior portion of the pelvic girdle between the hip bones
  - The *coccyx,* a triangular bone formed by the fusion of the four coccygeal vertebrae, articulates superiorly with the sacrum
- As vertebrae articulate, alignment of the vertebral foramina forms the vertebral canal
- Several ligaments attach to the vertebrae
  - The anterior longitudinal ligament is a broad sheath of connective tissue along the anterior surface of the vertebral bodies
  - The posterior longitudinal ligament, narrower than the anterior one, lies along the posterior surface of the vertebral bodies inside the vertebral canal
  - Other ligaments—the flaval, interspinous, and supraspinous ligaments—attach in various ways to the spinous processes

● **Bony thorax**
- The bony thorax, or rib cage, forms a protective enclosure for the heart, lungs, and great vessels of the thoracic cavity
- It also supports the pectoral (shoulder) girdle and provides attachment points for various muscles
- The bony thorax consists of the thoracic vertebrae (posteriorly), the ribs (laterally), and the sternum and costal cartilages (anteriorly)
- The bony thorax includes 12 pairs of ribs
  - The first seven pairs (sometimes eight) connect to the sternum by costal cartilages; they're called *true ribs*
  - The remaining five pairs are called *false ribs*
    - The first three pairs of false ribs connect to the costal cartilages immediately above them
    - The last two pairs of false ribs, which don't connect to the costal cartilages, are called floating ribs
- The *sternum* is a flat bone that joins the ribs anteriorly to close the wall of the bony thorax

– It consists of the *manubrium* (triangular superior portion), *body* (middle and largest portion), and *xiphoid process* (inferior smaller portion)

– The manubrium has a superior depression called the *suprasternal notch*

APPENDICULAR SKELETON

● **Key concepts**
  • The *appendicular skeleton* (so named because its bones are appended to the axial skeleton) consists of the pectoral (shoulder) and pelvic girdles and the bones of the upper and lower limbs
  • Its 126 bones include the clavicle, scapula, upper limb bones, hip bones, and lower limb bones (see *Bones of the human skeleton,* page 83)
  • The upper limb bones attach to the shoulder girdle; the lower limb bones, to the pelvic girdle
    – The shoulder girdle consists of the clavicle (anteriorly) and scapula (posteriorly)
    – The pelvic girdle consists of the hip bones (*os coxae,* or innominate bones)

● **Shoulder girdle**
  • The *clavicle* (collar bone) is a slender, curved flat bone that forms the anterior portion of the shoulder girdle
    – At the medial end, the clavicle articulates with the manubrium portion of the sternum
    – At the distal end, it articulates with the scapula
  • The *scapula* (shoulder blade) is a triangular flat bone
    – Laterally, it contains a shallow cavity called the *glenoid fossa,* which articulates with the humerus of the arm to form the shoulder joint
    – Superiorly, the scapula has two prominent bony projections— the *coracoid process* in front and the *acromion process* in back
    – Posteriorly, the scapula attaches only to muscle, not to the thorax

● **Bones of the upper limbs**
  • The upper limbs consist of 30 bones each, including the humerus, ulna, radius, and hand bones
  • The *humerus* is the largest and longest bone of the upper arm
    – It articulates with the scapula medially
    – It also articulates with the radius and ulna distally (at the elbow)
  • The *ulna* is the longer of the two forearm bones
    – It articulates with the humerus to form the elbow joint

Key facts about the appendicular skeleton
  • Includes the clavicle, scapula, upper limb bones, hip bones, and lower limb bones
  • Upper limb bones attach to the shoulder girdle
  • Lower limb bones connect to the pelvic girdle

Key characteristics of the shoulder girdle
  • Formed anteriorly by the clavicle
  • Contains the scapula, which articulates with the humerus to form the shoulder joint

Key facts about bones of the upper limbs
  • Contain 30 bones each
  • Humerus: largest and longest bone of the upper arm
  • Ulna: longer forearm bone
  • Radius: shorter forearm bone
  • Hand bones include carpus, metacarpus, and phalanges

– It also articulates with the radius at the proximal and distal ends
– The *olecranon* and *coronoid processes* are located at the proximal end of the ulna
– The *styloid process* is found on the medial side of the distal head of the ulna
• The *radius* is the shorter of the two forearm bones
– Proximally, the upper concavity of the head of the radius articulates with the capitulum of the humerus
– Medially, the head articulates with the radial fossa of the ulna
– The radial tuberosity (protuberance) is a projection immediately below the proximal head
– Distally, the radius has a medial ulnar notch and a lateral styloid process
• *Hand bones* include the *carpus* (wrist), *metacarpus* (palm), and *phalanges* (digits or fingers)
– The eight carpals (short bones) of the wrist are joined tightly by ligaments, which limit them to gliding movements
– The *flexor retinaculum,* which forms the carpal tunnel for passage of the flexor tendons, maintains wrist concavity
– The five metacarpals radiate from the carpus to form the framework of the palm; beginning with the thumb (pollex), they're numbered one through five (instead of named)
– Each hand has 14 phalanges, or tapering bones
  · The thumb has only proximal and distal phalanges
  · The other four fingers have proximal, middle, and distal phalanges

● **Pelvic girdle**
• Formed by the hip bones, the *pelvic girdle* attaches the lower limbs to the axial skeleton
• In the front of the body, the hip bones articulate with each other; in the back of the body, they articulate with the sacrum
• Together with the sacrum, the pelvic girdle forms the bony pelvis
• At birth, each coxa contains three bones—the ilium, ischium, and pubis
– Although these bones fuse in the adult, the names are still used to describe the corresponding regions of the hip bones
– The pelvic girdle consists of paired coxal bones
• The *ilium* is a large, flaring bone located superiorly
– It forms the greater portion of the os coxa
– The *iliac crests* are the bony projections commonly called the *hips*
• The arc-shaped *ischium* forms the posteroinferior part of the os coxa; its inferior surface thickens to form the ischial tuberosity

Key characteristics of the pelvic girdle

• Formed by hip bones
• Attaches lower limbs to axial skeleton
• The pelvic girdle joins with sacrum to form bony pelvis
• Consists of the ilium, the ischium, and the pubis

- The *pubis* (pubic bone) forms the anterior part of the os coxa
  - It joins the ischium posterolaterally to form the *obturator foramen,* a large opening
  - The two pubic bones articulate anteriorly at the symphysis pubis
  - A deep, round socket (acetabulum) forms on the lateral surface of the os coxa; the acetabulum articulates with the head of the femur

- **Bones of the lower limbs**
  - The lower limbs consist of 30 bones each, including the femur, patella, tibia, fibula, and bones of the foot—the talus, calcaneus, cuboid, and navicular bones; the medial, intermediate, and lateral cuneiform; the five metatarsals; and the 14 phalanges
  - Because these bones support the weight of the entire body and endure great force, they're thicker and stronger than those of the upper limbs
  - The *femur* (thigh bone) is the longest, thickest, and strongest bone in the body
    - The ball-like proximal head of the femur articulates with the acetabulum of the pelvis
    - The greater trochanter is a bony projection located superolaterally to the neck of the femur; the lesser trochanter is located inferomedially
    - Distally, the femur ends in the lateral and medial condyles, which articulate with the tibia
  - The *patella* (kneecap) articulates with the anterior surface between the condyles
  - The shape of the leg comes from the tibia and fibula
    - The *tibia* is the leg's weight-bearing bone
      · Proximally, its medial and lateral condyles articulate with the femur
      · The large tibial tuberosity for attachment of the patellar ligament lies immediately below the condyles
      · Distally, the tibia articulates with the talus of the ankle
      · Medially, at the distal end, an inferior projection called the *medial malleolus* forms the medial bulge of the ankle
    - The *fibula* bears no weight
      · It articulates proximally and distally with the tibia
      · An inferior projection called the *lateral malleolus* lies at the distal end of the fibula
  - Foot bones include the *tarsals* (ankle), *metatarsals* (instep), and *phalanges* (toes)
    - The foot supports the body and acts as a lever during locomotion

Key facts about bones of the lower limbs

- Thicker and stronger than upper limbs
- Femur: longest, thickest, and strongest bone in the body
- Tibia: the leg's weight-bearing bone
- Fibula: bears no weight
- Foot bones include the tarsals, metatarsals, and phalanges

- The seven tarsals—the talus, calcaneus, cuboid, and navicular bones and the medial, intermediate, and lateral cuneiforms—correspond to the carpals in the wrist
- The five metatarsals are numbered one through five, beginning with the great toe (hallux)
- The 14 phalanges in the toes correspond to those in the fingers
  · The great toe has only two phalanges, proximal and distal
  · The other toes have proximal, middle, and distal phalanges

JOINTS

● **Key concepts**
- Also called *articulations, joints* are the junction points between two or more bones
- Usually composed of fibrous connective tissue and cartilage, joints permit movement
- Joints are classified according to function and structure
  - The degree of movement a joint allows determines its functional classification; thus, a joint may be a synarthrosis (an immovable joint), an amphiarthrosis (a slightly movable joint), or a diarthrosis (a freely movable joint)
    · The axial skeleton has mainly synarthrotic and amphiarthrotic joints
    · The appendicular skeleton has mostly diarthrotic joints, with some amphiarthrotic joints; most limb joints are diarthrotic
  - The type of material holding the joint bones together determines its structural classification; thus, a joint may be fibrous, cartilaginous, or synovial

● **Synarthroses**
- *Synarthroses* are immovable joints that fall into three types—sutures, gomphoses, and synchondroses
  - *Sutures* are fibrous joints with closely united opposing surfaces, such as the coronal suture
  - *Gomphoses* have a conical process inserted into a socketlike portion (such as teeth in the dental alveoli); like sutures, they allow no movement
  - *Synchondroses* usually are temporary joints in which the intervening hyaline cartilage converts to bone by adulthood; the epiphyseal plates of long bones are an example
- Fibrous connective tissue closely binds the articular surfaces of the two bones, allowing little or no movement

Key facts about joints

- Junction points between two or more bones
- Permit movement
- Classified according to function and structure

Key characteristics of synarthroses

- Immovable joints
- Consist of three types: sutures, gomphoses, and synchondroses
- Sutures and gomphoses allow no movement
- Synchondroses are temporary joints

● **Amphiarthroses**
- *Amphiarthroses* are joints in which cartilage connects one bone to another; they allow only slight movement
- They fall into two categories—syndesmoses and symphyses
  - *Syndesmoses* have intervening connective tissue that forms an interosseous membrane or ligament, such as the tibiofibular and radioulnar joints
  - *Symphyses* have an intervening pad of fibrocartilage; examples are the intervertebral joints, the symphysis pubis, and the joint between the manubrium and sternum

● **Diarthroses**
- *Diarthroses* are joints in which the contiguous bony surfaces are covered by articular cartilage and joined by ligaments lined with synovial membrane; they're freely movable
- Most joints of the upper and lower limbs are diarthroses
- Diarthrotic joints have five structural features
  - *Articular cartilage* (hyaline cartilage) covers and cushions the articulating ends of bones
  - The *joint cavity,* a potential space, separates the articulating surfaces of the two bones
  - The double-layered *articular capsule* has a heavier outer layer of fibrous tissue lined with a vascular synovial membrane
  - *Synovial fluid,* a viscid fluid produced by the synovial membrane, lubricates the joint
  - *Reinforcing ligaments,* consisting of fibrous connective tissue, connect bones within the joint and reinforce the joint capsule
- Diarthrotic joints fall into various categories based on their structure and the type of movement they allow
  - *Gliding joints* (plane or nonaxial joints) have flat or slightly curved articular surfaces
    · They allow gliding movements; however, they may not allow movement in all directions because these joints are bound by ligaments
    · Examples include the intercarpal and intertarsal joints of the hands and feet
  - *Hinge joints* (uniaxial joints) have a convex portion of one bone that fits into a concave portion of another
    · They can only flex and extend, like a metal hinge
    · Examples include the elbow and knee
  - *Pivot joints* (uniaxial joints) have a rounded portion of one bone that fits into a groove in another bone
    · They allow only uniaxial rotation of the first bone around the second

Key characteristics of amphiarthroses
- Joints in which cartilage connects one bone to another
- Allow slight movement

Key characteristics of diarthroses
- Freely movable joints
- Articular cartilage covers articulating ends of bones
- The joint cavity separates the articulating surfaces of the two bones
- The articular capsule has a heavier outer layer of fibrous tissue lined with a vascular synovial membrane
- Synovial fluid lubricates the joint
- Ligaments connect bones within the joint

Key characteristics of gliding joints
- Flat or slightly curved surface
- Allow gliding movements

Key characteristics of hinge joints
- Convex portion of one bone fits into concave portion of another
- Flex and extend

Key characteristics of pivot joints
- Rounded portion of one bone fits into groove of another
- Allows uniaxial rotation of first bone around second

Key characteristics of condyloid joints

- Oval surface on one bone fits into concavity in another
- Permit flexion, extension, abduction, adduction, and circumduction

Key characteristics of saddle joints

- Resemble condyloid joints
- Allow greater freedom of movement

Key characteristics of ball-and-socket joints

- Spherical head of one bone fits into a concave "socket" of another
- Allow the greatest freedom of motion

Key characteristics of bursae

- Flattened fibrous sacs lined with synovial membrane and filled with synovial fluid
- Decrease stress on nearby tissues by acting as cushions
- Tendon sheaths: elongated bursae wrapped around a tendon subjected to friction

Key characteristics of tendons

- Bands of fibrous connective tissue that attach muscles to bones
- Enable bones to move when skeletal muscles contract

Key characteristics of ligaments

- Bands of strong, flexible connective tissue that connect the articular ends of bones
- Provide stability
- May either limit or help movement

· The head of the radius, which rotates within a groove of the ulna, is an example

– *Condyloid joints* (biaxial or ellipsoidal joints) have an oval surface on one bone that fits into a concavity in another
  · They permit flexion, extension, abduction, adduction, and circumduction
  · The radiocarpal and metacarpophalangeal joints of the hand are examples

– *Saddle joints* (biaxial joints) resemble condyloid joints but allow greater freedom of movement; the carpometacarpal joints of the thumb are the only saddle joints in the body

– In a *ball-and-socket joint* (multiaxial joint), the spherical head of one bone fits into a concave "socket" of another
  · They allow the greatest freedom of motion of all diarthrotic joints
  · The shoulder and hip joints are the only ball-and-socket joints in the body

● **Joint contact and movement**

- Bursae, tendons, and ligaments hold the articular surfaces of the diarthroses in contact with each other; bursae and tendon sheaths prevent friction on adjacent structures during joint movement

  – *Bursae* are flattened fibrous sacs lined with synovial membrane and filled with synovial fluid; they decrease stress on nearby tissues by acting as cushions
    · They're found in areas where ligaments, muscles, skin, or tendons rub against bone
    · An example is the subacromial bursa beneath the coracoacromial ligament in the shoulder

  – *Tendon sheaths* are elongated bursae wrapped around a tendon that's subjected to friction; they occur at the wrist and ankle joints

  – *Tendons* are bands of fibrous connective tissue that attach muscles to bones; they enable bones to move when skeletal muscles contract

  – *Ligaments* are bands of strong, flexible, fibrous connective tissue that connect the articular ends of bones; they provide stability and may either limit or help movement

- Diarthroses permit 13 basic types of movement
  – *Flexion* decreases the joint angle
  – *Extension* increases the joint angle
  – *Hyperextension* increases the joint angle beyond the anatomic position
  – *Circumduction* moves the limb in a circle

– *Abduction* moves the limb away from midline

– *Adduction* moves the limb toward midline

– *Rotation* revolves the limb around a longitudinal axis, moving it toward midline (internal rotation) or away from midline (external rotation)

– *Supination* turns the palm upward

– *Pronation* turns the palm downward

– *Inversion* turns the plantar surface inward

– *Eversion* turns the plantar surface outward

– *Retraction* moves the jaw backward

– *Protraction* moves the jaw forward

• Injuries (such as sprains and strains) and disorders (such as arthritis and bursitis) can decrease joint movement

NCLEX CHECKS

It's never too soon to begin your NCLEX preparation. Now that you've reviewed this chapter, carefully read each of the following questions and choose the best answer. Then compare your responses with the correct answers.

1. The nurse is caring for a client with a fractured nose. Which statement would the nurse make to the client about the cartilage in the nose?

☐ **1.** "It receives a generous blood supply."
☐ **2.** "It protects body structures."
☐ **3.** "It's well-innervated."
☐ **4.** "It cushions and absorbs shock."

2. Which instruction would the nurse give to a client with osteoporosis?

☐ **1.** "Get plenty of rest."
☐ **2.** "Disregard pain because it signals bone growth."
☐ **3.** "Sleep on a firm mattress."
☐ **4.** "Avoid foods high in calcium and vitamin D."

3. The nurse is caring for a client with a fracture of a long bone. Which of the following is a long bone?

☐ **1.** Femur
☐ **2.** Patella
☐ **3.** Sternum
☐ **4.** Vertebrae

4. The nurse who's performing a physical assessment on a 16-year-old male client understands which statement is true about bone growth near the end of adolescence?

Types of movement of diarthroses

• Flexion
• Extension
• Hyperextension
• Circumduction
• Abduction
• Adduction
• Rotation
• Supination
• Pronation
• Inversion
• Eversion
• Retraction
• Protraction

TOP 10

Items to study for your next test on the skeletal system

1. Classification of bones
2. Structure and function of bones
3. Process of bone formation, remodeling, and resorption
4. Developmental considerations of bone formation and resorption
5. Types of cartilage
6. Bones of the axial skeleton
7. Bones of the appendicular skeleton
8. Functional classification of joints
9. Basic joint movements
10. Structure and function of bursae, tendons, and ligaments

☐ **1.** Bone breakdown exceeds formation, causing a gradual decrease in bone density.

☐ **2.** Bone continues to increase in length and thickness through adulthood.

☐ **3.** Following closure of the epiphyses, increases in bone length may still occur.

☐ **4.** Epiphyseal lines are converted to bone, preventing further increases in bone length.

5. The nurse is explaining bone remodeling to a postmenopausal client. Which statement would the nurse make to this client?

☐ **1.** "Taking less vitamin D will promote remodeling."

☐ **2.** "Taking more calcium will encourage remodeling."

☐ **3.** "Sex hormones have no influence on remodeling."

☐ **4.** "Heavy physical activity impairs remodeling."

6. The nurse is assessing the axial skeleton of a client with osteoporosis. Which bones are the nurse assessing?

☐ **1.** Vertebrae and humerus

☐ **2.** Clavicle and scapula

☐ **3.** Sternum and ribs

☐ **4.** Sacrum and femur

7. The nurse is assessing the arm of a client with a fracture of the ulna. Identify the bone that the nurse is assessing.

8. The nurse palpates crepitus in a client's knee. The knee is functionally classified as what type of joint?

☐ **1.** Synarthrosis

☐ **2.** Amphiarthrosis

☐ **3.** Diarthrosis

☐ **4.** Syndesmosis

9. A client tells the nurse that he's having pain in his elbow. The nurse understands that this is what type of diarthrotic joint?

☐ **1.** Gliding
☐ **2.** Hinge
☐ **3.** Pivot
☐ **4.** Condyloid

10. While performing range-of-motion exercises on a client, the nurse flexes the client's foot and explains that flexion:

☐ **1.** increases the joint angle beyond the anatomic position.
☐ **2.** increases the joint angle.
☐ **3.** doesn't change the joint angle.
☐ **4.** decreases the joint angle.

ANSWERS AND RATIONALES

1. CORRECT ANSWER: 4
Cartilage supports, cushions, and shapes body structures but doesn't protect body structures. Besides hyaline cartilage, which forms the nose, types of cartilage include fibrocartilage and elastic cartilage. Cartilage is avascular and isn't well-innervated.

2. CORRECT ANSWER: 3
Clients with osteoporosis should sleep on a firm mattress, perform regular weight-bearing exercise, and eat foods high in calcium and vitamin D. All clients should get plenty of rest, not just those with osteoporosis. The client should report any new pain, especially after trauma.

3. CORRECT ANSWER: 1
Long bones, whose length exceeds their width, include the femur, tibia, and fibula in the lower body; the clavicle, humerus, radius, and ulna in the upper body; and the metatarsals, metacarpals, and phalanges. Short bones, such as the patella, lack a long axis. Flat bones are thin and include the sternum, ribs, and most skull bones. Irregular bones don't fit the other classifications; they include the vertebrae, hip bones, and some skull bones.

4. CORRECT ANSWER: 4
Near the end of adolescence, the epiphyseal lines are converted into bone. After closure occurs, no further increase in bone length can occur. In old age, bone breakdown exceeds formation, leading to a decrease in bone density.

5. CORRECT ANSWER: 2
New bone tissue replaces old bone tissue in bone remodeling. Bone remodeling requires minerals (such as calcium and phosphorus), vitamins

(such as vitamin D), and hormones (such as sex and growth hormones). During remodeling, heavy physical activity and weight-bearing exercise promote bone strength and thickness.

6. CORRECT ANSWER: 3

The axial skeleton consists of the bones that form the longitudinal axis of the body and covers three major regions: the skull, vertebral column, and bony thorax. This includes the sternum, ribs, vertebrae, and sacrum. The appendicular skeleton consists of the pectoral and pelvic girdles and the bones of the upper and lower limbs. This includes the humerus, clavicle, scapula, and femur.

7. CORRECT ANSWER:

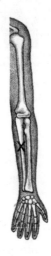

The ulna is the longer of the two bones in the forearm.

8. CORRECT ANSWER: 3

Joints may be classified according to function and structure. Functional classification depends on the degree of movement the joint allows. A diarthrosis, such as the knee, moves freely; a synarthrosis can't move; and an amphiarthrosis can move only slightly. A syndesmosis, such as the tibiofibular or radioulnar joint, is a type of amphiarthrosis with intervening connective tissue forming an interosseous membrane or ligament.

9. CORRECT ANSWER: 2

Diarthrotic joints fall into various categories based on their structure and the type of movement they allow. The elbow is a hinge joint in which the convex portion of one bone fits into a concave portion of another. A gliding joint has flat or slightly curved articular surfaces, such as the intercarpal and intertarsal joints of the hands and feet. A pivot joint has a rounded portion on one bone that fits into a groove in another bone, such as the head of the radius, which rotates within a groove of the ulna. In a condyloid joint, the oval surface of one bone fits into a concavity in another, such as the radiocarpal and metacarpophalangeal joints of the hand.

10. CORRECT ANSWER: 4
When the foot is flexed, the joint angle decreases. Hyperextension increases the joint angle beyond the anatomic position. Extension increases the joint angle.

8

Muscular system

After studying this chapter, you should be able to:

- Explain impulse transmission in muscle fibers.
- Discuss metabolism of muscle tissue.
- Compare the three types of muscle structure and function.
- Describe skeletal muscle attachment and points of insertion and origin.
- Identify muscles of the axial and appendicular skeleton and their functions.
- Explain contraction of the three types of muscles.

CHAPTER OVERVIEW

The muscular system animates the bones and joints of the skeletal system, which provide a framework for it. The skeletal muscles are responsible for every body movement. The cardiac and smooth muscles handle less visible motions, such as the pumping of the heart and the passage of urine and feces. Because the muscular system produces these vital actions, the nurse must understand its normal structures and functions to recognize the effects of problems in the muscular system. This chapter reviews muscle tissue; smooth, cardiac, and skeletal muscles; muscles of the axial and appendicular skeleton; and skeletal, cardiac, and smooth muscle contractions.

MUSCLE TISSUE

● **Key concepts**
- Muscle tissue accounts for roughly 40% of total body weight
- The three types of muscle tissue—smooth, cardiac, and skeletal—differ in cell structure, location, and function (see *Comparing muscle types*, page 102)
- Muscle tissue consists of fibers that contain the proteins actin and myosin
  - Myosin is the most abundant protein in muscle
  - Myosin and actin are responsible for muscle contraction
- Each muscle is innervated by sensory and motor neurons

● **Muscle functions**
- Muscle permits movement, maintains posture, and generates heat
  - The integrated function of muscles, bones, and joints produces body movements, such as walking and running
  - Skeletal muscle contractions maintain posture by holding body parts in postural positions
  - Muscles generate heat during contraction
- Muscle tissue has four special properties that help maintain homeostasis
  - *Excitability* allows a muscle to receive and respond to a stimulus so that the body can respond to internal and external environmental changes
  - *Contractility* allows a muscle to shorten when it receives a stimulus of sufficient strength
  - *Extensibility* allows a muscle to stretch
  - *Elasticity* allows a muscle to return to its original shape after contraction

● **Muscle fiber stimulation**
- Nerve impulses control smooth, cardiac, and skeletal muscles, although the different types of muscle receive and respond to stimulation in somewhat different ways
- Nerve fibers called *axons* transmit impulses from the central nervous system (CNS) to muscle fibers
- The axon terminates near a small depression on the surface of the muscle fiber called the *motor end plate;* a small gap called the *synapse* separates the axon terminal and motor end plate
- The motor end plate and the axon terminal together are called the *neuromuscular junction*

● **Nerve impulse transmission to muscle fibers**
- Vesicles in the axon terminal contain the neurotransmitter acetylcholine

---

Key facts about muscle tissue

- Makes up 40% total body weight
- Three types: smooth, cardiac, and skeletal
- Innervated by sensory and motor neurons

Key muscle functions

- Permits movement
- Maintains posture
- Generates heat
- Helps maintain homeostasis

Key facts about muscle fiber stimulation

- Nerve impulses control skeletal, cardiac, and smooth muscles
- Axons transmit impulses to muscle fibers from CNS
- Axon terminates at motor end plate
- Motor end plate and axon terminal are the neuromuscular junction

Comparing muscle types

Smooth, cardiac, and skeletal muscles differ in their location, appearance, striations, type of control, contraction speed, and function.

FEATURES	SMOOTH MUSCLE	CARDIAC MUSCLE	SKELETAL MUSCLE
Location	• Walls of hollow organs, blood vessels, skin, respiratory passages, and eyes	• Heart	• Attached to skeleton
Appearance	• Spindle-shaped fibers • Single, centrally located nucleus	• Cylindrical branched fibers • Single, centrally located nucleus • Intercalated disks that join the cells to one another	• Cylindrical fibers that may extend the entire length of a muscle • Multiple peripherally located nuclei
Striations	• Absent	• Present	• Present
Control	• Involuntary	• Involuntary	• Voluntary
Contraction speed	• Slow	• Moderate	• Fast
Function	• Food movement through the GI tract (peristalsis), urinary bladder emptying, uterine and tubal muscle contraction, regulation of blood vessel diameter, pupil size regulation, hair movement, and nipple erection	• Blood pumping	• Body movement

Key facts about nerve impulse transmission

- Vesicles in the axon terminal release acetylcholine to trigger muscle contraction
- Cholinesterase in the motor end plate breaks down acetylcholine to stop the contraction

– When a nerve impulse reaches the axon terminal, the vesicles release acetylcholine, which then diffuses across the synapse and attaches to receptors on the motor end plate
– Acetylcholine generates a depolarization wave, or impulse, which stimulates muscle fiber contraction
• The muscle membrane of the motor end plate contains the enzyme cholinesterase
– Cholinesterase rapidly breaks down the released acetylcholine into acetate and choline
– Acetylcholine breakdown prevents the nerve impulse from continuing to stimulate the skeletal muscle fiber and inducing a sustained contraction
• The axon terminal takes up choline, which then combines with acetate to form more acetylcholine

- The axon terminal vesicles store the acetylcholine until another impulse stimulates its release

● **Muscle metabolism**
- All muscle contractions require energy, which they can get from the breakdown of adenosine triphosphate (ATP) in muscle fiber
- As needed, skeletal muscle fibers can increase ATP production by the phosphagen, glycogen–lactic acid, and aerobic systems
  - The *phosphagen system* uses the breakdown of creatine phosphate for energy
  - The *glycogen–lactic acid system* breaks down muscle glycogen into glucose, which it metabolizes to generate ATP (energy) and pyruvic acid
  - The *aerobic system* oxidizes pyruvic acid into ATP, carbon dioxide, and water through cellular respiration
    · This process, called *aerobic metabolism* because it requires oxygen, is slower than glycolysis but provides more ATP
    · The body uses this system when muscle contractions last longer than about 30 seconds
- During vigorous exertion, the lungs and circulatory system may not be able to provide enough oxygen to muscles for aerobic metabolism; in such cases, muscle cells must get energy from anaerobic metabolism
  - *Anaerobic metabolism* breaks down muscle glycogen and blood glucose to lactic acid rather than pyruvic acid; it provides less ATP than aerobic metabolism, but it yields enough to sustain muscular activity
    · Some lactic acid accumulates in the muscles but most of it diffuses into the blood, which transports it to the liver
    · The liver reconverts lactic acid to glucose; the blood then transports the glucose back to the muscles, which reuse it for energy
  - With anaerobic metabolism, the muscles develop an oxygen debt that the body must repay through extra oxygen consumption after exertion stops
    · The person must breathe rapidly after exertion until the muscles obtain enough oxygen to restore them to their resting state
    · Elevated oxygen use after exercise is called *recovery oxygen consumption*
  - When oxygen supplies increase after exertion, the muscle fibers return to their normal resting state
    · Muscles resynthesize depleted muscle glycogen from glucose
    · Creatine phosphate is reformed

• Accumulated lactic acid in the muscle is reconverted to pyruvic acid and oxidized by the mitochondrial enzymes to carbon dioxide, water, and ATP

SMOOTH MUSCLE

● **Key concepts**
• Smooth-muscle tissue consists of elongated, spindle-shaped, nucleated fibers (cells); it lacks the striations (striped appearance) of cardiac and skeletal muscle
• Smooth muscle lines the visceral organs and urinary bladder and surrounds the blood vessels, bronchi, and various ducts
• Smooth-muscle contractions are involuntary, slow, and sustained; they occur sequentially as the nerve impulse spreads from one muscle fiber to the next

● **Types of smooth muscle**
• *Single-unit smooth muscle* has numerous gap junctions between adjacent fibers
 – *Gap junctions* occur in the heart and certain other smooth-muscle tissue containing electrically excitable tissue; the plasma membranes are situated close to each other, with hollow cylinders of protein linking the cells
 – Fibers in single-unit smooth muscle form a continuous network that contracts spontaneously in response to an appropriate stimulus
 – Contraction occurs in a wave over many adjacent fibers
 – Single-unit smooth muscle appears in the walls of the stomach, intestines, uterus, and bladder
• *Multiunit smooth muscle* consists of individual fibers, each with its own motor nerve ending; motor nerves carry impulses away from the CNS
 – Fibers in multiunit smooth muscle lack gap junctions
 – Stimulation of a multiunit smooth-muscle fiber causes contraction of that fiber only
 – Multiunit smooth-muscle tissue occurs in such structures as the walls of blood vessels and the muscles of the hair follicles and eyes (such as those of the iris)

CARDIAC MUSCLE

● **Key concepts**
• Cardiac muscle makes up most of the mass of the heart wall
• It consists of striated fibers

- – Fiber cells are short, branched, and shaped somewhat like quadrangles
  - – They have one or two centrally located nuclei
- Strong, thin bands called *intercalated disks* traverse the muscle fibers, separating them from each other
  - – These disks provide a low resistance for the flow of electric current through the heart
  - – They also strengthen the muscle and promote impulse conduction
- Cardiac muscle moves blood through the heart and into blood vessels
- Involuntary cardiac muscle contracts at a steady rate, regulated by an internal pacemaker
- Nerve fibers from the autonomic (involuntary) nervous system innervate cardiac muscle

Specialized fibers

- Specialized cardiac muscle fibers called *nodal tissues* make up the heart's conduction system
- They permit the rapid, rhythmic spread of a stimulus through cardiac muscle (for more details, see chapter 11, Cardiovascular system)

SKELETAL MUSCLE

Key concepts

- Skeletal muscle attaches to the skeleton and permits voluntary movements
- The human body contains approximately 700 skeletal muscles, which account for roughly 40% of body weight (see *Major skeletal muscles*, page 106)
- Skeletal muscles contract rapidly and vigorously for short periods
- Nerve fibers from the somatic (voluntary) nervous system innervate skeletal muscle
- The name of a skeletal muscle may come from its location, action, size, shape, attachment points, number of divisions, or direction of its fibers

Muscle structure

- Of all types of muscle tissue, skeletal muscle tissue has the longest fibers (see *Muscle structure up close,* page 107)
- Elongated and cylindrical, these fibers lie parallel to one another in bundles called *fasciculi*
  - – Skeletal muscle fibers are multinucleated and have distinct transverse striations
  - – A plasma membrane called a *sarcolemma* surrounds each fiber

Key facts about intercalated disks

- Traverse cardiac muscle fibers and separate them
- Provide low resistance for electric current flow through the heart
- Strengthen the heart and promote impulse conduction

Key characteristics of skeletal muscle

- Attached to the skeleton; consists of cylindrical fibers
- Allows body movement
- Contract rapidly and vigorously for short periods
- Voluntarily controlled

Key facts about skeletal muscle structure

- Have the longest fibers
- Fibers lie parallel in bundles called *fasciculi*
- Fibers consist of threadlike structures called *myofibrils*
- Sarcomeres are the functional units of the muscle

Major skeletal muscles

Anterior
- Sternocleidomastoid
- Pectoralis major
- Biceps brachii
- Rectus abdominus
- Abdominal oblique
- Brachioradialis
- Rectus femoris
- Sartorius
- Vastus lateralis
- Tibialis anterior

Posterior
- Trapezius
- Deltoid
- Triceps brachii
- Latissimus dorsi
- Gluteus medius
- Gluteus maximus
- Semimembranosus
- Biceps femoris
- Gastrocnemius
- Achilles tendon

Major skeletal muscles

The human body contains roughly 700 skeletal muscles. A muscle's name may reflect its size, shape, location, action, attachment points, number of divisions, or direction of its fibers. Skeletal muscles produce voluntary and reflex movements, generate body heat, and maintain posture. This illustration shows major muscles.

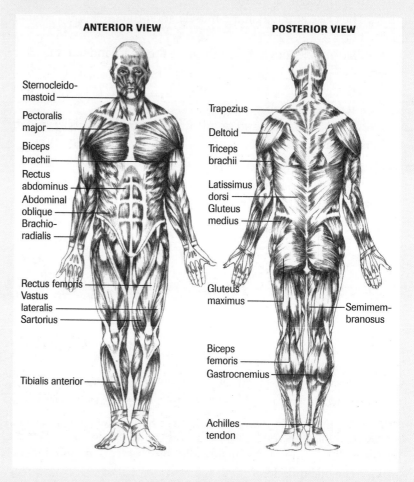

ANTERIOR VIEW

Sternocleido-
mastoid
Pectoralis
major
Biceps
brachii
Rectus
abdominus
Abdominal
oblique
Brachio-
radialis
Rectus femoris
Vastus
lateralis
Sartorius
Tibialis anterior

POSTERIOR VIEW

Trapezius
Deltoid
Triceps
brachii
Latissimus
dorsi
Gluteus
medius
Gluteus
maximus
Semimem-
branosus
Biceps
femoris
Gastrocnemius
Achilles
tendon

- Skeletal muscle fibers consist of threadlike structures called *myofibrils*
  - Myofibrils run lengthwise through the fiber
  - They're composed of thin and thick filaments that are stacked in compartments called *sarcomeres,* the functional units of skeletal muscle
    - Thin filaments are composed of actin; thick filaments are composed of myosin

Muscle structure up close

Skeletal muscle contains cell groups called *muscle fibers*. This illustration shows a typical skeletal muscle and its fiber constituents.

BOUND TOGETHER
The *perimysium*—a sheath of connective tissue—binds muscle fibers together into a fasciculus. The *epimysium* binds the fasciculi (bundles of muscle fibers) together; beyond the muscle, it becomes a tendon.

SURROUNDED
A *sarcolemma* (plasma membrane) surrounds each muscle fiber. Tiny myofibrils within the muscle fibers contain even finer fibers (myofilaments) containing *myosin* (thick filaments) and *actin* (thin filaments).

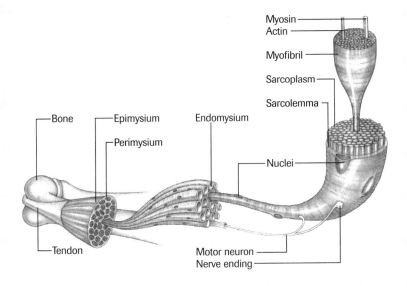

- Myosin
- Actin
- Myofibril
- Sarcoplasm
- Sarcolemma
- Bone
- Epimysium
- Endomysium
- Perimysium
- Nuclei
- Tendon
- Motor neuron
- Nerve ending

- During muscle contraction, thin and thick filaments slide over each other, reducing sarcomere length

● Skeletal muscle functions
- Skeletal muscle moves body parts or the body as a whole when acting in unison
  - Skeletal muscle produces movements by contracting; all movements of the body and its parts result from muscle contraction
  - Muscles shorten when they contract, pulling on the bones they're attached to
    - Muscle contraction that moves a body part away from the midline of the body is called *abduction*
    - Muscle contraction that moves a body part toward the midline of the body is called *adduction*

Key skeletal muscle functions
- Produces movement by contracting
- Abduction moves a body part away from the midline
- Adduction moves a body part toward the midline
- Most body heat results from skeletal muscle contractions

– Skeletal muscles are responsible for both voluntary and reflex movements
- Skeletal muscle contractions generate the most body heat because much of the body is composed of skeletal muscles
  – Cells release ATP to supply energy for muscle contraction; about 75% of this energy escapes as heat
  – Muscle fatigue occurs when a muscle can't regenerate ATP
    · This fatigue results from muscle overstimulation
    · It causes muscle contractions to become gradually weaker and eventually stop
- Skeletal muscles also maintain body posture; for instance, the combined contraction of skeletal muscles maintains an erect or seated posture

● **Muscle attachment**
- Most skeletal muscles attach to bones
  – During contraction, one of the bones to which the muscle attaches stays relatively stationary while the other is pulled in the opposite direction
  – The point where a muscle attaches to a stationary or less movable bone is called the *origin;* the point where it attaches to the more movable bone is called the *insertion* (see *Points of origin and insertion*)
- Muscles may attach to bones directly or indirectly
  – In a direct attachment, the *epimysium,* or fibrous sheath, of the muscle fuses to the periosteum of the bone
  – In an indirect attachment, the fascia extends past the muscle as a tendon or aponeurosis, which in turn attaches to bone; indirect attachments outnumber direct attachments

MUSCLES OF THE AXIAL SKELETON

● **Key concepts**
- Muscles of the axial skeleton include those of the head and neck, those that move the vertebral column, and the thoracic muscles responsible for respiration
- Abdominopelvic muscles are also sometimes categorized as muscles of the axial skeleton (in this text, they're included with muscles of the appendicular skeleton; see page 113)

● **Head and neck muscles**
- These muscles include those of the face, tongue, and neck and those that permit mastication, or chewing
- Fourteen muscles control facial expression
  – The *buccinator* compresses the cheek and pulls the corner of the mouth

---

Key facts about skeletal muscle attachment

- Most attach to bones
- Origin is point of attachment to stationary or less movable bone
- Insertion is point of attachment to movable bone
- Attachment may be direct or indirect

Key axial skeletal muscles

- Muscles of the head and neck
- Muscles that move the vertebral column
- Thoracic muscles used for respiration

Points of origin and insertion

This table lists the points of origin and insertion for the major skeletal muscles.

MUSCLE	ORIGIN	INSERTION
Biceps brachii	• Long head: scapula (supraglenoid tubercle) • Short head: scapula (coracoid process)	• Radius (tubercle)
Biceps femoris	• Long head: ischial tubercle • Short head: linea aspera	• Fibula (lateral surface of head) • Tibia (lateral condyle)
Brachialis	• Humerus (anterior surface of distal half)	• Ulna (coronoid process)
Brachioradialis	• Humerus (lateral supracondylar ridge)	• Radius (styloid process)
Buccinator	• Mandible (alveolar process) • Maxillary bone	• Orbicularis oris • Skin at mouth angle
Deltoid	• Clavicle (lateral third) • Acromion process • Scapula (spine)	• Humerus (deltoid tubercle)
Diaphragm	• Rib cage (inferior border) • Xiphoid process • Costal cartilages • Vertebrae (lumbar)	• Central tendon of diaphragm
External abdominal oblique	• Ribs (external surface of lower eight)	• Iliac crest (anterior half) • Linea alba
External intercostal muscles	• Ribs (inferior border) • Costal cartilages	• Next inferior rib (superior border)
Gastrocnemius	• Femur (medial and lateral condyles)	• Calcaneus (via Achilles tendon)
Gluteus maximus	• Ilium (posterior gluteal line) • Sacrum and coccyx (posterior surfaces)	• Femur (gluteal tubercle) • Iliotibial band
Infraspinatus	• Scapula (infraspinatus fossa)	• Humerus (greater tubercle)
Internal abdominal oblique	• Inguinal ligament • Iliac crest • Lumbodorsal fascia	• Linea alba • Pubic crest • Ribs (lower four)
Internal intercostal muscles	• Ribs (inner surface) • Costal cartilages	• Next inferior rib (superior border)
Latissimus dorsi	• Vertebrae (spinous processes of lower six thoracic and all lumbar) • Sacrum • Ilium (posterior crest)	• Humerus (medial margin of intertubercular groove)

(continued)

Points of origin and insertion *(continued)*

MUSCLE	ORIGIN	INSERTION
Levator scapulae	• Vertebrae (transverse processes of upper four cervical)	• Scapula (vertebral border, above spine)
Masseter	• Zygomatic arch	• Mandible (angle and ramus)
Medial pterygoid	• Sphenoid bone (lateral pterygoid plate) • Maxillary bone (tubercle)	• Mandible (inner surface)
Pectoralis major	• Clavicle (medial half) • Sternum • Ribs (costal cartilages of upper six) • External oblique (aponeurosis)	• Humerus (greater tubercle)
Plantaris	• Femur (lower surface, above lateral condyle)	• Calcaneus (via Achilles tendon)
Quadriceps femoris	• Rectus femoris: ilium (anterior inferior spine) • Vastus lateralis: femur (linea aspera, greater trochanter) • Vastus medialis: femur (linea aspera) • Vastus intermedius: femur (anterior surface of shaft)	• Tibia (via patella and patellar ligament)
Rectus abdominis	• Pubic crest	• Xiphoid process • Ribs (costal cartilages of fifth through seventh)
Rhomboideus major	• Vertebrae (spinous processes of second through fifth thoracic)	• Scapula (vertebral border, below spine)
Rhomboideus minor	• Vertebrae (spinous processes of seventh cervical and first thoracic)	• Scapula (vertebral border, at base of spine)
Sartorius	• Anterior superior iliac spine	• Tibia (proximal medial surface, below tubercle)
Scalene muscles	• Cervical vertebrae (transverse processes)	• Ribs (first and second)
Soleus	• Fibula (posterior surface of proximal third) • Tibia (middle third)	• Calcaneus (via Achilles tendon)
Sternocleidomastoid	• Sternum (manubrium) • Clavicle (medial portion)	• Temporal bone (mastoid process)
Supinator	• Humerus (lateral epicondyle)	• Radius (proximal end, lateral surface of shaft)
Supraspinatus	• Scapula (supraspinatus fossa)	• Humerus (greater tubercle)

Points of origin and insertion *(continued)*

MUSCLE	ORIGIN	INSERTION
Temporalis	• Temporal fossa	• Mandible (coronoid process and ramus)
Tibialis anterior	• Tibia (lateral condyle, proximal two-thirds of shaft) • Interosseous membrane	• Tarsal (first cuneiform) • Metatarsal (first)
Tibialis posterior	• Tibia (posterior surface) • Fibula (posterior surface) • Interosseous membrane (posterior surface)	• Navicular bone • All three cuneiforms • Cuboid bone • Second through fourth metatarsals
Transversus abdominis	• Inguinal ligament • Iliac crest • Lumbodorsal fascia • Ribs (costal cartilages of last six)	• Linea alba • Pubic crest
Trapezius	• Occipital bone • Ligamentum nuchae • Vertebrae (spinous processes of seventh cervical and all thoracic)	• Clavicle (lateral third) • Acromion process • Scapula (spine)
Triceps brachii	• Long head: scapula (infraglenoid tubercle) • Lateral head: humerus (posterior surface, above radial groove) • Medial head: humerus (posterior surface, below radial groove)	• Ulna (olecranon process)

– The *corrugator supercilii* draws the eyebrows together
– The *depressor anguli oris* pulls the mouth downward
– The *depressor labii inferioris* pulls the lower lip downward
– The *epicranius frontalis* raises the eyebrows and wrinkles the forehead skin
– The *epicranius occipitalis* draws the scalp backward
– The *levator labii superioris* raises the upper lip and opens the nostrils
– The *mentalis* raises the lower lip
– The *orbicularis oculi* closes the eyelids and tightens the forehead skin
– The *orbicularis oris* closes the lips
– The *platysma* depresses the jaw and tightens the skin of the neck
– The *procerus* wrinkles the skin between the eyebrows

Key characteristics of head and neck muscles

• Fourteen muscles used in facial expression
• Four muscles used in mastication
• Three muscles move the tongue
• One muscle flexes and rotates the head
• Eight muscles move the hyoid bone

– The *risorius* pulls the mouth backward

– The *zygomaticus major* raises the angle of the mouth

- Four muscles take part in mastication

  – The *temporalis* and the *masseter* close the jaws

  – The *pterygoideus medialis* closes the jaws and helps move them sideways

  – The *pterygoideus lateralis* opens the jaws and helps move them sideways

- The tongue has three skeletal muscles

  – The *genioglossus* protracts, retracts, and depresses the tongue

  – The *hyoglossus* depresses the tongue and draws its sides downward

  – The *styloglossus* retracts and elevates the tongue

- Neck muscles include the sternocleidomastoideus, suprahyoidei, and infrahyoidei

  – The *sternocleidomastoideus* flexes the vertebral column and rotates the head to the opposite direction

  – Four *suprahyoid* muscles move the hyoid bone (a single bone in the neck)

    · The *digastricus* raises the hyoid and helps open the jaws

    · The *stylohyoideus* raises the hyoid and pulls it backward

    · The *mylohyoideus* raises the hyoid and floor of the mouth

    · The *geniohyoideus* pulls the hyoid forward

  – The *infrahyoid* muscles also move the hyoid bone as well as the larynx

    · The *sternohyoideus* pulls the hyoid downward

    · The *sternothyroideus* pulls the larynx downward

    · The *thyrohyoideus* pulls the hyoid downward and raises the larynx

    · The *omohyoideus* pulls the hyoid downward

● Vertebral column muscles

- These muscles are located along the spine
- They move the vertebral column

  – The *semispinalis thoracis, semispinalis cervicis,* and *semispinalis capitis* are deep muscles that extend and rotate the vertebral column and head

  – The *multifidi* and *rotatores* extend and rotate the vertebral column

  – The *interspinales* extend the vertebral column

  – The *scalenus* muscles flex and rotate the neck and aid inhalation

  – The *intertransversarii* abduct the vertebral column

Key characteristics of vertebral column muscles

- Located along the spine
- Move the vertebral column
- Flex and rotate the neck

- The *splenius capitis* and *splenius cervicis* act together to extend the head and neck and act singly to abduct and rotate the head toward the same side
- The *erector spinae* muscles—the most prominent muscles that move the vertebral column—include a series of overlapping muscles
  - The *iliocostalis lumborum*, *iliocostalis thoracis*, and *iliocostalis cervicis* extend the vertebral column and bend it to one side
  - The *longissimus thoracis*, *longissimus cervicis*, and *longissimus capitis* extend the vertebral column and head, and rotate the head toward the same side
  - The *spinalis thoracis* and *spinalis cervicis* extend the vertebral column

● **Respiratory muscles**
- These muscles permit breathing
- This group includes five types of muscles
  - The *diaphragm* allows inspiration (inhalation) by pulling the central tendon of the diaphragm down and enlarging the thoracic cavity
  - The *intercostales externi* muscles elevate the ribs, aiding inspiration
  - The *intercostales interni* muscles draw the ribs together, aiding expiration (exhalation)
  - The *subcostales* muscles draw the ribs together, aiding expiration
  - The *transversus thoracis* draws the rib cage downward, aiding expiration

MUSCLES OF THE APPENDICULAR SKELETON

● **Key concepts**
- Muscles of the appendicular skeleton include those of the shoulder (pectoral) girdle, abdominopelvic cavity, and upper and lower limbs
- Although not typically considered part of the appendicular skeleton, abdominal muscles are included here because they're part of the abdominopelvic cavity

● **Shoulder girdle muscles**
- These muscles move the scapulae (shoulder blades)
- They include seven muscles
  - The *trapezius* elevates, depresses, rotates, adducts, and stabilizes the scapula
  - The *rhomboideus major* and *rhomboideus minor* adduct, stabilize, and rotate the scapula

**Key characteristics
of abdominopelvic
cavity muscles**

● Includes five muscles in abdominal wall
● Includes muscles that form the floor of the abdominopelvic cavity

**Key characteristics of
upper limb muscles**

● Classified according to the bones they move
● Also classified by whether they originate on the axial skeleton or the scapula
● Move bones of the arm, forearm, wrist, hands, and fingers

 – The *levator scapulae* elevates and adducts the scapula and bends the neck laterally
 – The *pectoralis minor* draws the scapula forward and downward
 – The *serratus anterior* stabilizes, abducts, and rotates the scapula upward and helps to abduct and raise the arm
 – The *subclavius* stabilizes and depresses the shoulder

● **Abdominopelvic cavity muscles**
 • These muscles include abdominal wall muscles and those that form the floor of the abdominopelvic cavity
 • The abdominal wall has five muscles
  – The *external abdominal oblique* and *internal abdominal oblique* muscles compress the abdominopelvic cavity and help flex and rotate the vertebral column
  – The *transversus abdominis* compresses the abdominopelvic cavity
  – The *rectus abdominis* compresses the abdominopelvic cavity and flexes the vertebral column
  – The *quadratus lumborum* pulls the thoracic cage toward the pelvis
 • Muscles that form the floor of the abdominopelvic cavity and support the pelvic viscera include the *levator ani* and *coccygeus*

● **Upper limb muscles**
 • These muscles are classified according to the bones they move, including bones of the arm, forearm, wrist, hands, and fingers
 • Further classification of muscles that move the upper arm (humerus) depends on whether they originate on the axial skeleton or the scapula
  – Two muscles originate on the axial skeleton
   · The *pectoralis major* flexes, adducts, and medially rotates the arm
   · The *latissimus dorsi* extends, adducts, and medially rotates the arm; it also pulls the shoulder downward
  – Seven muscles originate on the scapula
   · The *deltoideus* abducts, rotates, and extends the arm
   · The *supraspinatus* abducts and causes slight lateral rotation of the arm
   · The *infraspinatus* rotates and causes slight lateral adduction of the arm
   · The *subscapularis* medially rotates the arm
   · The *teres major* adducts, extends, and medially rotates the arm
   · The *teres minor* laterally rotates the arm
   · The *coracobrachialis* flexes and adducts the arm

- Five muscles move the forearm
  - The *biceps brachii, brachialis,* and *brachioradialis* flex the forearm
  - The *triceps brachii* and *anconeus* extend the forearm
- Muscles that move the wrist, hand, and fingers include anterior superficial muscles, anterior deep muscles, posterior superficial muscles, and posterior deep muscles; the hand also has several intrinsic muscles
  - Five muscles are classified as anterior superficial muscles
    - The *pronator teres* pronates the forearm (rotates it forward)
    - The *flexor carpi radialis* flexes the wrist and abducts the hand
    - The *palmaris longus* flexes the wrist
    - The *flexor carpi ulnaris* flexes the wrist and adducts the hand
    - The *flexor digitorum superficialis* flexes the wrist and fingers
  - Three muscles are classified as anterior deep muscles
    - The *flexor digitorum profundus* flexes the wrist and fingers
    - The *flexor pollicis longus* flexes the thumb and helps flex the wrist
    - The *pronator quadratus* pronates the hand
  - Five muscles are classified as posterior superficial muscles
    - The *extensor carpi radialis longus* and *brevis* extend the wrist and abduct the hand
    - The *extensor digitorum communis* extends the fingers and wrist
    - The *extensor digiti minimi* extends the little finger
    - The *extensor carpi ulnaris* extends the wrist and adducts the hand
  - Five muscles are classified as posterior deep muscles
    - The *supinator* supinates the forearm (rotates it backward)
    - The *abductor pollicis longus* abducts the thumb and hand
    - The *extensor pollicis brevis* extends the thumb
    - The *extensor pollicis longus* extends and abducts the thumb
    - The *extensor indicis* extends the index finger
  - Intrinsic muscles of the hand include the thenar, hypothenar, and midpalmar muscle groups
    - Thenar muscles include the *abductor pollicis brevis,* which abducts the thumb; *opponens pollicis,* which pulls the thumb in front of the palm; *flexor pollicis brevis,* which flexes and adducts the thumb; and *adductor pollicis,* which adducts the thumb
    - Hypothenar muscles include the *palmaris brevis,* which pulls the skin toward the middle of the palm; *abductor digiti minimi manus,* which abducts the little finger; *flexor digiti minimi brevis manus,* which flexes the little finger; and *opponens digiti minimi,* which moves the little finger in front of the palm

Five anterior superficial muscles of the hand

- Pronator teres
- Flexor carpi radialis
- Palmaris longus
- Flexor carpi ulnaris
- Flexor digitorum superficialis

Three anterior deep muscles of the hand

- Flexor digitorum profundus
- Flexor pollicis longus
- Pronator quadratus

Five posterior superficial muscles of the hand

- Extensor carpi radialis longus
- Extensor carpi radialis brevis
- Extensor digitorum communis
- Extensor digiti minimi
- Extensor carpi ulnaris

Five posterior deep muscles of the hand

- Supinator
- Abductor pollicis longus
- Extensor pollicis brevis
- Extensor pollicis longus
- Extensor indicis

· Midpalmar muscles include the *lumbricales manus*, which extend the interphalangeal joints and flex the metacarpophalangeal joints; *interossei dorsales manus*, which abduct the fingers; and *interossei palmares*, which adduct the fingers

● **Lower limb muscles**
• These muscles include the muscles that move the femur (thigh bone), the muscles that move the foot and toes, and the intrinsic muscles of the foot
• Several muscles move the femur
  – The *iliopsoas* (a compound muscle) flexes the thigh
  – The *gluteus maximus* extends and laterally rotates the thigh
  – The *gluteus medius* and *minimus* abduct and medially rotate the thigh
  – The *tensor fasciae latae* helps flex, abduct, and medially rotate the thigh
  – The *piriformis* laterally rotates and helps extend and abduct the thigh
  – The *obturator internus, obturator externus, gemellus superior, gemellus inferior,* and *quadratus femoris* laterally rotate the thigh
  – The *adductor magnus, adductor longus,* and *adductor brevis* adduct and laterally rotate the thigh
  – The *pectineus* adducts, flexes, and laterally rotates the thigh
  – The *gracilis* adducts the thigh and flexes the leg
  – The *sartorius* flexes the thigh and leg
  – The *quadriceps femoris* (a compound muscle) extends the leg and flexes the thigh
  – The hamstrings group—*biceps femoris, semitendinosus,* and *semimembranosus*—flexes the leg and extends the thigh
• Muscles that move the foot and toes include those of the anterior, lateral, and posterior compartments; the last category includes both superficial and deep muscles
  – The anterior compartment includes four muscles
    · The *tibialis anterior* flexes the foot backward and inverts it (turns it inward)
    · The *extensor hallucis longus* flexes the foot backward, inverts the foot, and extends the great toe
    · The *extensor digitorum longus* flexes the foot backward and everts it (turns it outward); it also extends the toes
    · The *peroneus tertius* flexes the foot backward and everts it
  – The lateral compartment includes the *peroneus longus* and *peroneus brevis,* which flex and evert the foot
  – Superficial muscles of the posterior compartment include the *gastrocnemius, soleus,* and *plantaris;* these muscles flex the leg and foot

Key characteristics of lower limb muscles

● Move the femur
● Move the foot and toes
● Move the intrinsic muscles of the feet

Four anterior compartment muscles of the foot

● Tibialis anterior
● Extensor hallucis longus
● Extensor digitorum longus
● Peroneus tertius

Two lateral compartment muscles of the foot

● Peroneus longus
● Peroneus brevis

- The posterior compartment includes four deep muscles
  - The *popliteus* flexes and medially rotates the leg
  - The *flexor hallucis longus* flexes the foot and great toe
  - The *flexor digitorum longus* flexes the foot and toes
  - The *tibialis posterior* flexes and inverts the foot
- Intrinsic foot muscles include one dorsal muscle and several plantar muscles, which are subdivided into superficial, second, third, and fourth layers
  - The dorsal muscle, the *extensor digitorum brevis,* extends the second through fifth toes
    The superficial layer of the plantar muscles includes three muscles
    - The *abductor hallucis* abducts the great toe
    - The *flexor digitorum brevis* flexes the second through fifth toes
    - The *abductor digiti minimi pedis* abducts the small toe
  - The second layer includes two muscles
    - The *quadratus plantae* helps flex the second through fifth toes
    - The *lumbricales pedis* flex the second through fifth toes
  - The third layer includes three muscles
    - The *flexor hallucis brevis* flexes the great toe
    - The *adductor hallucis* adducts the great toe
    - The *flexor digiti minimi brevis pedis* flexes the small toe
  - The fourth layer includes two muscles
    - The *interossei plantaris* adduct the toes toward the second toe
    - The *interossei dorsales pedis* abduct the toes from the second toe and medially and laterally move the second toe

SKELETAL MUSCLE CONTRACTION

Key concepts
- Muscle contraction occurs in three periods
  - During the *latent period,* nothing appears to happen
  - During the *contraction period,* the muscle fibers shorten
  - During the *relaxation period,* the muscle fibers lengthen
- Skeletal muscle contraction involves calcium ion transport and nerve impulse transmission; relaxation normally follows contraction

Innervation
- Under voluntary control, skeletal muscle contracts in response to impulses that motor nerves transmit from the CNS

Key facts about innervation of skeletal muscles

- Motor nerves transmit impulses from CNS to cause contraction
- Each muscle innervated by sensory neurons and at least one motor nerve
- Contraction governed by the all-or-none response
- Contraction strength depends on the number of motor units activated

Key facts about skeletal muscle contraction and relaxation

- Nerve impulse travels along sarcolemma to the transverse tubules, which transmit it to interior of the muscle fiber
- Sarcoplasmic reticulum then releases calcium ions
- Calcium ions diffuse into sarcoplasm and bind to troponin
- This allows myosin heads to bind to actin filaments, resulting in contraction
- When stimulation of motor unit stops, calcium ions separate from troponin
- Tropomyosin unbinds cross bridges, actin and myosin filaments separate, and muscle fibers lengthen

- Each skeletal muscle is innervated by sensory neurons and at least one motor nerve, which contains hundreds of fibers from motor neurons
  - Sensory (afferent) neurons receive impulses about the degree of muscle contraction and transmit them to the CNS; this allows proper coordination of muscle activity
  - Motor (efferent) neurons convey impulses from the CNS to the muscle, triggering muscle contraction
  - As axons from a motor nerve enter a muscle, each branch innervates a muscle fiber; collectively, the neuron and the innervated fibers are called a *motor unit*
- Muscle fiber contraction of a motor unit is governed by the *all-or-none response*
  - If the nerve impulse is intense enough to stimulate contraction, all the muscle fibers in the motor unit contract
  - If the impulse isn't intense enough to stimulate all the muscle fibers in the motor unit to contract, then none contract
- Contraction strength depends on the number of motor units activated
  - Weak contractions activate only a few motor units
  - Stronger contractions activate more motor units

● **Contraction and relaxation**
- When a nerve impulse stimulates the muscle fiber at the neuromuscular junction, the impulse travels along the sarcolemma to the transverse tubules (tubelike extensions of the sarcolemma), which transmit it into the interior of the muscle fiber
- The impulse causes the sarcoplasmic reticulum to release calcium ions
- Calcium ions diffuse into the sarcoplasm and bind to troponin on the threadlike structures around the actin filaments, changing the position of these structures; as a result, tropomyosin can no longer prevent actin and myosin from binding
- Myosin heads bind to the actin filaments, forming structures called *cross bridges* that pull the actin filaments toward the center of the sarcomeres; this results in muscle fiber shortening, or contraction
- When stimulation of the motor unit stops, calcium ions separate from troponin and are transported back into the sarcoplasmic reticulum
- The threadlike structures return to their original positions
- Tropomyosin unbinds the cross bridges, and actin and myosin filaments separate, causing the sarcomeres (and muscle fibers) to lengthen

Muscle tone

- Normal muscle isn't completely relaxed; it maintains a slight, sustained contractility called *muscle tone,* which is a reflex contraction in response to stretching
  - When a muscle stretches, receptors in muscles, joints, and tendons respond by sending impulses to the nervous system
    - These afferent impulses travel to the spinal cord and cause the discharge of motor impulses that make the muscle fibers contract
    - How much the muscle fibers stretch regulates how much reflex contraction occurs
    - Overstretching a muscle can cause a strain or other muscle injury (see *Teaching a patient with a strain or sprain*)
  - Motor neurons then transmit impulses to the muscle fibers, causing them to contract and resist the stretching force; this contraction of muscles with opposing action maintains muscle tone
    - Flexor muscles respond to the pull of extensor muscles by contracting slightly
    - Extensor muscles, in turn, respond to the pull of flexors, resulting in a slight state of tension in all muscle groups
- This continuous contraction of the head, neck, and back muscles maintains posture
- Muscle tone around joints also maintains joint stability

TIME-OUT FOR TEACHING

Teaching a patient with a strain or sprain

When teaching a patient with a strain or sprain, make sure you:
- explain the nature of the injury and its potential complications
- prepare him for diagnostic tests such as X-rays
- teach about RICE treatments: rest, ice, compression, and elevation
- describe how anti-inflammatory and analgesic drugs relieve swelling and pain
- discuss physical therapy for rehabilitation
- describe immobilization devices, such as elastic bandages, casts, and crutches
- discuss the possibility of surgery for severe sprains
- provide sources of information and support.

Key concepts of cardiac muscle contraction

- Contracts rhythmically to pump blood
- Sarcoplasmic reticulum isn't as prominent as in skeletal muscle
- Muscle cells interconnect to form branching networks

Key facts about cardiac muscle contraction and relaxation

- Similar to skeletal muscle cells in arrangement of actin and myosin and general mechanism of contraction and relaxation
- Contractions occur more slowly and last longer than skeletal muscle contractions
- Cardiac muscle cells have larger blood supply and more mitochondria
- Cardiac muscle fibers don't rely on anaerobic metabolism during increased activity
- Cardiac muscle fibers can generate impulses and contract even without nervous stimulation

CARDIAC MUSCLE CONTRACTION

● **Key concepts**
- In the heart, cardiac muscle contracts rhythmically to pump blood
- The sarcoplasmic reticulum of the cardiac muscle fiber isn't as prominent as that of skeletal muscle, and the T tubules aren't as closely associated with the sarcoplasmic reticulum
- Cardiac muscle cells interconnect to form branching networks

● **Contraction and relaxation**
- Cardiac muscle cells have the same arrangement of actin and myosin and employ the same general mechanism of contraction and relaxation as skeletal muscle cells; however, there are some differences, especially in how stimulation occurs
- Cardiac muscle contractions occur at a slower rate and last longer than skeletal muscle contractions because the T tubules and sarcoplasmic reticulum are farther apart in cardiac muscles, making nerve impulse transmission less efficient
- Cardiac muscle fibers have a more abundant blood supply and more mitochondria than skeletal muscle fibers
  - Cardiac muscle fibers obtain enough ATP for energy from aerobic metabolism of nutrients in the mitochondria
  - Unlike skeletal muscle fibers, cardiac fibers don't rely on anaerobic metabolism during increased activity and don't develop an oxygen deficit
- Cardiac muscle fibers aren't organized into motor units the way skeletal muscle fibers are
  - Interconnections called *intercalated disks* between the branching cardiac muscle fibers permit action potentials to pass from cell to cell
  - These muscle fibers function as an integrated unit
- The autonomic nervous system regulates cardiac rate and rhythm, but cardiac muscle fibers can generate impulses and contract rhythmically even when deprived of nervous stimulation
- During cardiac muscle contraction, electrocardiography can measure the electrical activity associated with depolarization of cardiac muscle

SMOOTH-MUSCLE CONTRACTION

● **Key concepts**
- The sarcoplasm of smooth-muscle fibers contains fewer actin and myosin filaments than that of skeletal muscle fibers; because

smooth-muscle filaments aren't organized into sarcomeres, the fibers don't look striated
- Smooth-muscle fibers don't have a well-developed sarcoplasmic reticulum; they also don't have a network of T tubules, but *cytoplasmic vacuoles* that connect with the surface of the fibers may serve the same function
- The sarcoplasm contains a network of *intermediate filaments* attached to cytoplasmic structures called *dense bodies;* actin filaments attach to dense bodies during contraction

● **Contraction and relaxation**
- Contraction and relaxation of smooth muscle works basically the same way as in skeletal muscle, with some variations
- Actin and myosin filaments slide together during contraction, pulling on the network of intermediate filaments and dense bodies; this shortens the smooth-muscle fibers
- Smooth muscle contracts and relaxes more slowly than skeletal muscle does
- Smooth-muscle contraction requires less energy than skeletal muscle contraction
- Smooth-muscle fibers receive motor impulses from the autonomic nervous system; they aren't under voluntary control

NCLEX CHECKS

It's never too soon to begin your NCLEX preparation. Now that you've reviewed this chapter, carefully read each of the following questions and choose the best answer. Then compare your responses with the correct answers.

1. The nurse is assessing a client's musculoskeletal system. Which type of muscle is voluntary?
- ☐ **1.** Cardiac
- ☐ **2.** Smooth
- ☐ **3.** Skeletal
- ☐ **4.** Epimysium

2. The nurse is providing discharge instruction to a client who sprained a leg muscle earlier in the day. Which statement would the nurse make to the client during the teaching session?
- ☐ **1.** "Exercise the affected leg."
- ☐ **2.** "Place a warm compress on the affected muscle."
- ☐ **3.** "Apply an elastic bandage to the affected leg."
- ☐ **4.** "Place the affected leg in a dependent position."

3. The nurse is teaching a client about developing an exercise program. In response to the client's questions, the nurse explains that lactic acid is caused by which type of metabolism?

☐ **1.** Phosphagen
☐ **2.** Anaerobic
☐ **3.** Aerobic
☐ **4.** Creatine phosphate

4. The nurse is assessing a client's bowel sounds. The nurse understands that the intestines consist of which type of muscle?

☐ **1.** Striated
☐ **2.** Skeletal
☐ **3.** Cardiac
☐ **4.** Smooth

5. The nurse is preparing to give a client an I.M. injection into the left vastus lateralis. Identify the area where the nurse will administer the injection.

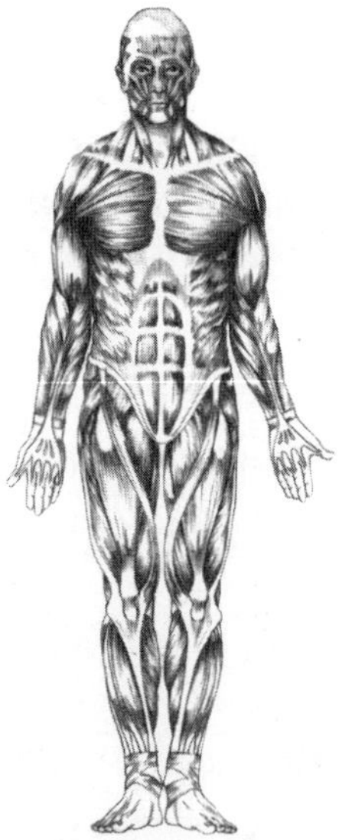

6. The nurse is teaching a client to perform range-of-motion exercises and instructs him to move his limb away from the midline of the body. This is called:

☐ **1.** abduction.
☐ **2.** adduction.
☐ **3.** flexion.
☐ **4.** extension.

7. The nurse is assessing a client with gastrocnemius pain. The nurse knows that which are the origin and insertion sites of this muscle, respectively?

☐ **1.** Scapula and humerus
☐ **2.** Femur and calcaneus
☐ **3.** Ribs and iliac crest
☐ **4.** Humerus and ulna

8. When the nurse asks the client to move his tongue during a neurologic assessment, which muscle is being assessed?
☐ **1.** Mentalis
☐ **2.** Temporalis
☐ **3.** Masseter
☐ **4.** Hypoglossus

9. The nurse extends the forearm of a client while performing passive range-of-motion exercises. The nurse knows that which muscle extends the forearm?
☐ **1.** Triceps brachii
☐ **2.** Biceps brachii
☐ **3.** Deltoideus
☐ **4.** Brachialis

10. The nurse is helping a client who has had a stroke gain independence with feeding. Which concept about nerve cells should the nurse keep in mind while helping the client with his exercises?
☐ **1.** Sensory neurons receive impulses from the muscles and transmit them to the CNS.
☐ **2.** Sensory neurons receive impulses from the CNS and transmit them to the muscles.
☐ **3.** Motor neurons transmit impulses from the muscle to the CNS, triggering contraction.
☐ **4.** Motor neurons transmit impulses from the CNS to the muscles, triggering relaxation.

ANSWERS AND RATIONALES

1. CORRECT ANSWER: 3
Skeletal muscle is voluntary, meaning it can be moved at will. Cardiac and smooth muscle can't be moved at will. Epimysium binds muscle bundles together.

2. CORRECT ANSWER: 3
Applying an elastic or compression bandage to a sprained muscle controls swelling. Treatment of a sprained muscle also includes resting the affected leg, applying ice, and elevating the leg.

3. CORRECT ANSWER: 2
During vigorous exercise, muscle cells derive energy through anaerobic metabolism, which breaks down muscle glycogen and blood glucose to

lactic acid rather than pyruvic acid. The phosphagen system uses the breakdown of creatine phosphate for energy. Aerobic metabolism oxidizes pyruvic acid into ATP, carbon dioxide, and water through cellular respiration.

4. CORRECT ANSWER: 4
Smooth muscle lines the visceral organs, including the intestines, urinary bladder, blood vessels, bronchi, and various ducts. Striated or skeletal muscle is found in muscle attached to the skeleton. Cardiac muscle is found in the heart.

5. CORRECT ANSWER:

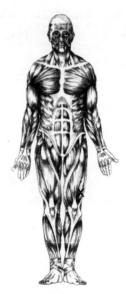

The vastus lateralis is located in the mid-left lateral portion of the thigh.

6. CORRECT ANSWER: 1
Movement of a body part away from the midline of the body is called *abduction*. Movement toward the midline of the body is called *adduction*. Flexion decreases a joint angle; extension increases the angle.

7. CORRECT ANSWER: 2
The origin of the gastrocnemius is the femur, and its insertion is the calcaneus. The origin of the infraspinatus is the scapula, and the insertion is the humerus. The origin of the external abdominal oblique is the ribs, and the insertion is the iliac crest. The origin of the brachialis is the humerus, and the insertion is the ulna.

8. CORRECT ANSWER: 4
The hypoglossus muscle depresses the tongue and draws its sides downward. The mentalis muscle raises the lower lip. The temporalis and masseter muscles close the jaws.

9. CORRECT ANSWER: 1

The triceps brachii and anconeus extend the forearm. The biceps brachii, brachialis, and brachioradialis flex the forearm. The deltoideus abducts, rotates, and extends the arm.

10. CORRECT ANSWER: 1

Each skeletal muscle is innervated by sensory neurons and at least one motor nerve, which contains hundreds of fibers from motor neurons. Sensory, or afferent, neurons receive impulses about muscle contraction and transmit them to the CNS, allowing coordination of muscle activity. Motor, or efferent, neurons convey impulses from the CNS to the muscle, triggering muscle contraction.

9

Nervous system

CHAPTER OVERVIEW

By serving as the body's control and communication center, the nervous system directs every body system and governs all movement, sensation, thought, and emotion. It senses internal and external changes, analyzes and stores this sensory information, makes decisions about it, and responds to it—all within a very brief time. To help patients maintain a properly functioning nervous system—vital to homeostasis—the nurse must understand the anatomy and physiology of the nervous system. This chapter reviews the basic principles of the nervous system, nervous tissue and cells, the synapse, the central and peripheral nervous systems, neurotransmission, and control centers.

BASIC PRINCIPLES

● **Key concepts**
  • The nervous system allows communication among different parts of the body and between the body and the external environment
  • Anatomically, the nervous system consists of the *central nervous system* (CNS), which includes the brain and spinal cord, and the *peripheral nervous system* (PNS), which includes all nervous tissue outside the CNS (the cranial and spinal nerves and the autonomic nervous system)
  • Functionally, the nervous system is divided into the *sensory (afferent) division,* which conveys impulses from the periphery to the CNS, and the *motor (efferent) division,* which conveys impulses from the CNS to the periphery

● **Function of nervous system**
  • The chief functions of the nervous system are to monitor, integrate, and respond to environmental stimuli
  • The nervous system carries out these functions in three general steps
    – Sensory receptors monitor changes inside and outside the body
    – The nervous system processes (integrates) the information gathered by sensory receptors
    – The nervous system activates the appropriate muscle or gland to respond to the sensory information
  • With the endocrine system, the nervous system also helps maintain homeostasis
    – The nervous and endocrine systems regulate certain aspects of the body's internal environment; for instance, the nervous system regulates heart rate, and the endocrine system produces epinephrine
    – Although the nervous system chiefly controls certain functions and the endocrine system controls others, the two generally work together; signals from either system affect functions in the other

NERVOUS TISSUE AND CELLS

● **Key concepts**
  • Nervous tissue consists of densely packed, intertwined nervous system cells
  • Nervous system cells fall into two categories—neurons (neural cells) and neuroglia (supporting cells)

Structure of a neuron

The main parts of a neuron are the *cell body* and its cytoplasmic processes—*axons* and *dendrites*. The cytoplasm of the cell body contains a large nucleus with a prominent nucleolus and delicate threads called *neurofibrils*. In a typical neuron, one axon and many dendrites extend from the cell body. The axon conducts nerve impulses away from the cell body; dendrites conduct impulses toward the cell body. The axon may vary from quite short to quite long (up to about 3′ [1 m]). A typical axon has terminal branches and is covered by a myelin sheath. Gaps called *nodes of Ranvier* separate segments of this sheath.

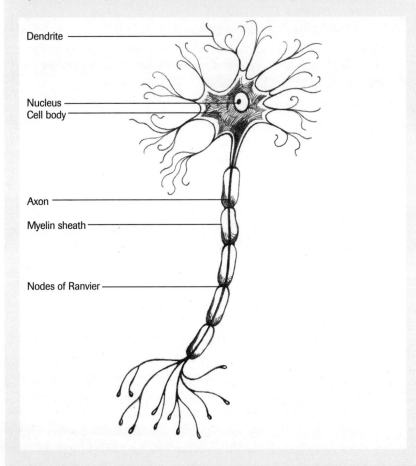

Dendrite

Nucleus
Cell body

Axon

Myelin sheath

Nodes of Ranvier

Key facts about neurons

- Specialized cells that conduct nerve impulses
- Each has a cell body and a nucleus
- Axons carry impulses away from the cell body
- Dendrites receive impulses and carry them toward cell body
- Myelin sheath wraps nerve fibers
- Can be classified by structure or function

● **Neurons**
- Neurons are highly specialized cells that conduct nerve impulses
- Each neuron has a *cell body* (perikaryon, or soma) and a large, spherical nucleus with a prominent nucleolus and abundant granular cytoplasm (see *Structure of a neuron*)
  - Most of the neuronal bodies are found in the CNS
  - A few are found in the PNS, clustered in structures called *ganglia*

- Cytoplasmic processes called *axons* and *dendrites* extend outward from the cell body
  - Typically, a neuron has only one axon, which carries impulses away from the cell body, and many short, thick, diffusely branched extensions called *dendrites,* which receive impulses from other cells and carry them toward the cell body
  - In the CNS, bundles of neuron processes (axons and dendrites) are called *tracts*; in the PNS, they're called *nerves*
- The *myelin sheath* is a white, fatty (phospholipid) segmented covering that wraps around nerve fibers (see *Teaching a patient with multiple sclerosis*)
  - Most axons in the PNS are myelinated (covered by a myelin sheath)
  - The CNS contains both myelinated and unmyelinated axons
    - Portions of the CNS containing myelinated axons are called *white matter*
    - Portions containing unmyelinated axons are called *gray matter*
  - In the PNS, a sheath of Schwann cells called the *neurilemma* envelops the myelin sheath; in the CNS, nerve fibers don't have a neurilemma
- Neurons can be classified by structure or function
  - Neurons are multipolar, bipolar, or unipolar in structure

---

 TIME-OUT FOR TEACHING

Teaching a patient with multiple sclerosis

Make sure you teach a patient with multiple sclerosis about:
- progressive demyelination, including signs and symptoms, complications, and treatments
- diagnostic tests, such as magnetic resonance imaging, electroencephalography, lumbar puncture, and evoked potential studies
- prescribed drugs, including names, indications, dosages, adverse effects, and special considerations
- the course of this chronic disease, including unpredictable exacerbations

- what can trigger an attack, including temperature extremes, stress, fatigue, and infections, and how to avoid these triggers
- maintaining independence and performing activities of daily living
- preventing constipation, including consuming roughage and plenty of fluids and regularly scheduling suppositories
- relieving urinary incontinence and retention, including Credé's maneuver and self-catheterization
- the need for daily exercise and rest periods to prevent fatigue
- other sources of information and support.

Key teaching topics for a patient with multiple sclerosis

- Describe signs and symptoms
- Review what can trigger an attack
- Explain diagnostic tests
- Review drugs and treatments
- Stress the importance of preventing constipation and urinary incontinence and the need for daily exercise with rest periods

- *Multipolar neurons*, the most common type, have one axon and several dendrites
- *Bipolar neurons* have one axon and one dendrite; they serve as receptor cells in special sense organs
- *Unipolar neurons* (pseudounipolar neurons) have a single process that divides into a proximal fiber (axon) and a distal fiber (dendrite)
  – Based on function, neurons are classified as sensory, motor, or association neurons
  - *Sensory (afferent) neurons* transmit impulses from sensory receptors in the skin or internal organs toward the CNS; the cell bodies of these unipolar neurons lie within sensory ganglia (special sense organs have bipolar neurons)
  - *Motor (efferent) neurons* carry impulses away from the CNS; except for some neurons in the autonomic system, motor neurons are multipolar, with cell bodies in the CNS
  - *Association (connecting) neurons* (or interneurons) convey impulses between motor and sensory neurons; the most common type, they're typically multipolar and confined to the CNS
- Sensory receptors (also called dendritic end organs) are modified dendritic endings of sensory neurons
  – These receptors are specialized to respond to environmental stimuli
  – They're described mainly by location, type of stimulus detected, or structure
  - *Exteroceptors,* located at or near the body surface, are sensitive to outside stimuli, such as touch, pressure, temperature, and sound
  - *Interoceptors,* or *visceroceptors,* respond to stimuli arising from the viscera (internal organs) and blood vessels
  - *Proprioceptors* respond to internal stimuli and alert the brain to body movements; they exist in skeletal muscles, tendons, joints, ligaments, connective tissue and, possibly, the inner ear (equilibrium receptors)
  - *Mechanoreceptors* respond to pressure, touch, sound, vibration, and tissue stretching in the lungs, blood vessels, and bladder
  - *Thermoreceptors,* typically found in the skin, respond to temperature changes
  - *Photoreceptors,* found in the retina, respond to light
  - *Chemoreceptors* respond to chemical stimuli, such as flavors, odors, and changes in blood gas levels

Types of sensory receptors

- Exteroceptors: sensitive to outside stimuli
- Interoceptors: respond to stimuli from the viscera
- Proprioceptors: respond to internal stimuli and alert the brain to body movements
- Mechanoreceptors: respond to pressure, touch, sound, vibration, and tissue stretching
- Thermoreceptors: respond to temperature changes
- Photoreceptors: respond to light
- Chemoreceptors: respond to chemical stimuli
- Nociceptors: sensitive to excessive heat and pressure, extreme cold, and chemicals released at inflammation sites
- Cutaneous receptors: occur in epithelial and connective tissue

· *Nociceptors* (pain receptors) are sensitive to excessive heat and pressure, extreme cold, and chemicals released at inflammation sites; most sensory receptors also function as nociceptors

· *Cutaneous receptors* typically occur in epithelial and connective tissue; most sensory receptors are also cutaneous receptors

● **Supporting cells**
  • Supporting cells have less specialized functions than neurons; unlike neurons, they don't conduct impulses, but they can reproduce
  • Supporting cells include astrocytes, microglia, oligodendrocytes, ependymal cells, Schwann cells, and satellite cells
    – *Astrocytes* attach to neurons and capillaries; these abundant cells help supply nutrients to neurons and control ions present around the neuron
    – *Microglia*, a special type of macrophage, protect the CNS against microorganisms and engulf dead neural tissue
    – *Oligodendrocytes* are small, branching cells; their cytoplasmic extensions wrap tightly around nerve fibers to form a myelin sheath
    – *Ependymal cells* are ciliated cells that line the CNS cavities of the brain and spinal cord; they beat their cilia to promote circulation of *cerebrospinal fluid* (CSF), a plasma-like fluid that bathes, cushions, and protects the brain and spinal cord
    – Phagocytic *Schwann cells* form myelin sheaths around nerve fibers; they're separated by gaps called *nodes of Ranvier*
    – *Satellite cells,* found in the PNS, may help maintain the chemical balance of neurons

SYNAPSE

● **Key concepts**
  • Electrical or chemical impulses move from one neuron to another across the *synapse*, or junction, between neurons
    – Most synapses exist between the axon of one neuron and the dendrites or cell body of another neuron
    – Some synapses occur between nerve endings and *effector cells* (gland cells or muscle cells)
  • Synapses allow nerve impulses to travel in only one direction

● **Electrical synapse**
  • An electrical synapse lets impulses move rapidly from one neuron to the next
  • Contact between adjacent cell membranes occurs

- Tissues, such as cardiac and smooth muscle, contain many electrical synapses, which allow rhythmic, sequential responses

● **Chemical synapse**
- A chemical synapse releases and receives *neurotransmitters*, chemicals that modify or trigger impulse transmission across the synapse
- When an impulse arrives, vesicles at the end of the axon empty the neurotransmitter into the synaptic gap
- The neurotransmitter crosses the gap and combines with receptors on the other neuron, which receive the impulse

CENTRAL NERVOUS SYSTEM

● **Key concepts**
- The CNS consists of the brain and spinal cord
- Bony enclosures (the skull and vertebrae), the membranous *meninges*, and the watery CSF protect the CNS

● **Brain**
- The brain has four main regions—the cerebrum, diencephalon, cerebellum, and brain stem (see *A close look at major brain structures*)
- The cerebrum and cerebellum have an outer cortex of gray matter (unmyelinated nerve fibers) surrounding a central core of white matter (myelinated nerve fibers); this pattern changes in the brain stem and spinal cord until, at the caudal (tail) end of the brain stem and throughout the spinal cord, white matter surrounds gray matter
- The *cerebrum* occupies the superior portion of the cranial cavity
  - The largest region of the brain, the cerebrum is divided into right and left hemispheres connected by nerve fibers
  - The cerebrum performs motor, sensory, and integrative functions
  - The wrinkles and folds of the cerebral surface—ridges of tissue (gyri), shallow grooves (sulci), and deeper grooves (fissures)—greatly increase its surface area
    · The *median longitudinal fissure* separates the hemispheres
    · The *transverse fissure* separates the hemispheres from the cerebellum
- The cerebrum surrounds the *diencephalon*
  - The diencephalon forms the central core of the forebrain and connects the cerebrum with the brain stem
  - It consists of the thalamus, hypothalamus, and epithalamus
    · The *thalamus* forms the superolateral walls of the third ventricle; it serves as a relay station for sensory information

Key facts about the brain

- Four main regions: cerebrum, diencephalon, cerebellum, and brain stem
- The cerebrum and cerebellum have an outer cortex of gray matter surrounding a central core of white matter
- From end of brain stem throughout the spinal cord, white matter surrounds gray matter

Key characteristics of the cerebrum

- Largest brain region
- Divided into right and left hemispheres
- Performs motor, sensory, and integrative functions
- Surface wrinkles and folds increase its surface area
- Diencephalon connects cerebrum to the brain stem; contains the thalamus, hypothalamus, and epithalamus

A close look at major brain structures

This illustration shows the two largest regions of the brain—the cerebrum and cerebellum (the other major regions include the diencephalon and brain stem). Several fissures divide the cerebrum into hemispheres and lobes:

- The *fissure of Sylvius,* or the lateral sulcus, separates the temporal lobe from the frontal and parietal lobes.
- The *fissure of Rolando,* or the central sulcus, separates the frontal lobes from the parietal lobe.
- The *parieto-occipital fissure* separates the occipital lobe from the two parietal lobes.

LOBE FUNCTIONS
Each lobe has a particular function:

- The *frontal lobe* influences personality, judgment, abstract reasoning, social behavior, language expression, and voluntary movement (in the motor portion).
- The *temporal lobe* controls hearing, language comprehension, and storage and recall of memories (although memories are stored throughout the entire brain).
- The *parietal lobe* interprets and integrates sensations, including pain, temperature, and touch. It also interprets size, shape, distance, and texture. The parietal lobe of the nondominant hemisphere is especially important for awareness of body shape.
- The *occipital lobe* functions mainly to interpret visual stimuli.

Major brain structures

- Frontal lobe: influences personality, social behavior, judgment, language expression, and voluntary movement
- Temporal lobe: controls hearing, language comprehension, and memory recall
- Parietal lobe: interprets sensations, size, shape, distance, and texture
- Occipital lobe: interprets visual stimuli

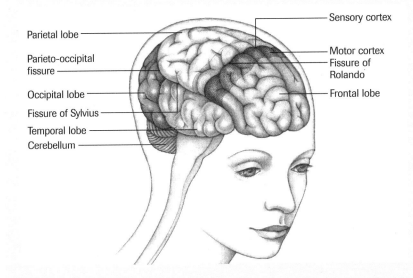

- The *hypothalamus* forms the base of the diencephalon and extends from the optic chiasm to the posterior margin of the mamillary bodies; it regulates the autonomic nervous system
- The *epithalamus,* located dorsally, forms the floor of the third ventricle
  - It contains an external projection called the *pineal gland*
  - Internally, a mass of capillaries called the *choroid plexus* produces CSF

Key characteristics of the cerebellum

- Second largest brain region
- Consists of two lateral hemi-spheres, each divided into three lobes
- Regulates and coordinates all complex motor activities

Key characteristics of the brain stem

- Situated between the cerebrum and the spinal cord
- Major structures include the midbrain, pons, and medulla ob-longata

Key characteristics of brain ventricles

- Right and left lateral ventricles communicate with the third ventricle through the foramen of Monro
- Cerebral aqueduct connects third and fourth ventricles
- Fourth ventricle connects with central canal of the spinal cord
- CSF forms in ventricles

- The *cerebellum,* the second largest region of the brain, is posterior and inferior to the cerebrum; it's attached to the pons
  - It consists of two lateral hemispheres, divided into three lobes each
  - The cerebellum has an outer cortex of gray matter and an inner core of white matter
  - The cerebellum regulates and coordinates all complex motor activities
- The *brain stem* lies immediately inferior to the cerebrum, just anterior to the cerebellum
  - It's situated between the cerebrum and spinal cord
  - Major structures include the midbrain, pons, and medulla oblongata
    - The *midbrain,* situated between the diencephalon superiorly and the pons inferiorly, consists of two bundles of nerve tracts called the *cerebral peduncles*
    - The *pons* lies between the midbrain and medulla oblongata, forming part of the anterior wall of the fourth ventricle
    - The *medulla oblongata,* the most inferior portion of the brain stem, joins the spinal cord at the level of the *foramen magnum,* an opening in the occipital portion of the skull
    - The brain stem has three general functions
      - It produces the rigid, autonomic behaviors necessary for survival; for instance, it increases heart rate
      - It provides pathways for nerve fibers between higher and lower neural centers
      - It serves as the origin for 10 of the 12 pairs of cranial nerves
- The brain also contains four *ventricles,* or small cavities
  - The right and left lateral ventricles are embedded in the right and left cerebral hemispheres, respectively; they communicate with the narrow third ventricle in the diencephalon by a small opening called the *interventricular foramen (foramen of Monro)*
  - The cerebral aqueduct, which crosses the midbrain, connects the third and fourth ventricles
  - The fourth ventricle connects with the central canal of the spinal cord
    - It lies dorsal to the pons and medulla and ventral to the cerebellum
    - Three openings (or apertures) connect the fourth ventricle and subarachnoid space (the fluid-filled area around the brain)
  - The ventricles serve as a site of CSF formation

Spinal cord

- An oval-shaped cylinder that lies within the spinal cavity, the *spinal cord* extends from the medulla to the first or second lumbar vertebra and is protected by the vertebral column (see *Spinal cord and spinal nerves*)

Spinal cord and spinal nerves

A cylindrical structure in the vertebral canal, the spinal cord extends from the foramen magnum at the base of the skull to the upper lumbar region of the vertebral column. Along with the brain, it constitutes the central nervous system. The spinal cord conducts nerve impulses to and from the brain and controls reflexes. Its inner core consists of gray matter (unmyelinated nerve fibers); its outer core consists of white matter (myelinated nerve fibers). Thirty-one pairs of spinal nerves arise from the cord. As this illustration shows, these nerves are designated (from top to bottom) as C1 through S5, plus the coccygeal nerve. At the inferior end of the cord, nerve roots cluster in the cauda equina.

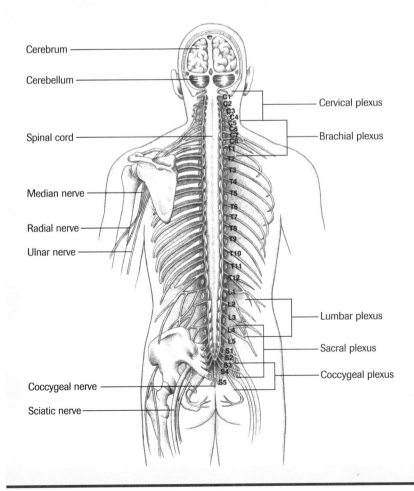

Key spinal cord structures

- Dorsal horn
- White matter
- Gray matter
- Ventral horn
- Posterior root
- Sensory neuron dendrite
- Posterior root ganglion
- Spinal nerve
- Motor neuron axon
- Anterior root

A look inside the spinal cord

This cross section of the spinal cord shows an H-shaped mass of gray matter divided into horns, which consist primarily of neuron cell bodies. Cell bodies in the posterior, or dorsal, horn primarily relay information. Cell bodies in the anterior, or ventral, horn provide voluntary or reflex motor activity.

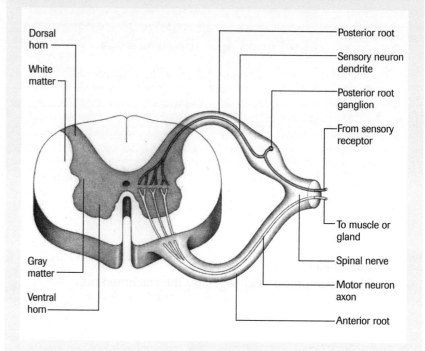

- The cord has a butterfly-shaped inner core of gray matter and an outer layer of white matter (see *A look inside the spinal cord*)
  - Bilateral posterior projections of gray matter, called *posterior (dorsal) horns,* contain sensory neurons
  - Bilateral anterior projections of gray matter, called *anterior (ventral) horns,* contain motor nerves
- The spinal cord provides pathways for nerve impulses to and from the brain and performs sensory, motor, and reflex functions
  - Bundles of sensory (afferent) nerve fibers in the cord, called *ascending tracts,* conduct impulses up the cord to the brain
  - Bundles of motor (efferent) nerve fibers, called *descending tracts,* conduct impulses down the cord from the brain
  - The gray matter of the spinal cord contains reflex centers for spinal reflexes
- Thirty-one pairs of spinal nerves arise from the cord and exit the vertebral column through openings called *foramina*

- The *cauda equina,* a collection of nerve roots at the inferior end of the cord, travels through the vertebral canal; typically, it exits the cord between the 12th thoracic and 3rd lumbar vertebrae

● **Meninges**
- Three connective tissue membranes called the *meninges* cover the brain and spinal cord
- The meninges protect the brain and spinal cord, enclose the venous sinuses, contain CSF, and form partitions within the skull
- The outer meningeal membrane is called the *dura mater* ("tough mother"), or pachymeninx
  - The portion of the dura mater that covers the brain has two layers; the portion that covers the spinal cord has only one layer
  - The two layers that cover the brain are fused except where they enclose the dural sinuses (which collect venous blood from the brain and convey it to the internal jugular veins of the neck)
  - The dura mater forms septa (partitions) that anchor the brain to the skull in four locations
- The middle meningeal membrane, called the *arachnoid* ("resembling a spider's web"), is a loose covering
  - The narrow *subdural space* separates the arachnoid from the dura mater
  - The *subarachnoid space* separates the arachnoid from the innermost meningeal layer; it contains CSF and all major arteries and veins of the brain
  - The *arachnoid villi* protrude through the dura mater into the dural sinuses
- The *pia mater* ("gentle mother") is the innermost meningeal layer
  - This transparent layer contains blood vessels and reticular and elastic fibers
  - It adheres to the outer surface of the brain and spinal cord
  - Collectively, the arachnoid and pia mater are called the *leptomeninges*

● **Cerebrospinal fluid**
- The clear, colorless CSF cushions the CNS, protecting it from damage; it's similar in composition to blood plasma
- CSF forms continuously in clusters of capillaries called *choroid plexuses,* found in the roof of each ventricle
- It flows through the ventricles, exits through openings in the roof of the fourth ventricle, and circulates around the brain and spinal cord
  - The *arachnoid villi* absorb CSF into the venous sinuses
  - Veins on the surface of the brain also directly absorb CSF

Key facts about the meninges

- Covers the brain and spinal cord
- Consists of three layers: dura mater, arachnoid, and pia mater

Key facts about cerebrospinal fluid

- Cushions the CNS
- Produced continuously by choroid plexus
- Flows through the ventricles and circulates around the brain and spinal cord
- Rates of production and absorption balance so volume and pressure remain constant

- Normally, the rates of CSF production and absorption balance so the CSF volume remains constant and the CSF pressure remains normal

PERIPHERAL NERVOUS SYSTEM

● Key concepts
- The PNS consists of all nervous tissue (nerves and ganglia) outside the CNS
- It provides the link between the CNS and body functions through continuous nerves and nerve tracts
- The PNS includes 12 pairs of cranial nerves and 31 pairs of spinal nerves
- Its two major divisions, the autonomic and somatic nervous systems, control different functions

● Cranial nerves
- These paired nerves arise from the undersurface of the brain and exit the skull through the foramina
- The first two pairs of nerves originate in the forebrain; the remaining 10 pairs, in the brain stem
- Cranial nerves are described by type (sensory or motor) and function; starting with the most anterior nerve, they're designated by Roman numerals and by name (see *Cranial nerve functions*)
- The cranial nerves transmit motor (efferent) and sensory (afferent) messages between the brain or brain stem and the head and neck.

● Spinal nerves
- The 31 pairs of spinal nerves originate in the spinal cord and exit through the vertebrae (see *Spinal cord and spinal nerves,* page 135)
  - They include eight cervical, 12 thoracic, five lumbar, and five sacral pairs and one pair of coccygeal nerves
  - They're designated according to the level of the vertebral column where they emerge; for instance, T1 refers to the first spinal nerve exiting from the thoracic segment of the vertebral column
- Each spinal nerve contains a dorsal (sensory, or afferent) root and a ventral (motor, or efferent) root
  - Cell bodies of afferent fibers lie outside the spinal cord in the dorsal root ganglion
  - Cell bodies of efferent fibers lie within the ventral gray column of the cord
- Spinal nerves divide into branches called *rami; ventral rami* exit the anterior portion of the spine, and *dorsal rami* exit the posterior portion

Key facts about the peripheral nervous system
- Consists of all nervous tissue outside the CNS
- Links the CNS and body functions
- Two major divisions: autonomic and somatic

Key characteristics of cranial nerves
- Described by type and function
- Designated by Roman numerals and by name
- Transmit motor and sensory messages between the brain or brain stem and the head and neck

Key characteristics of spinal nerves
- Each contains a dorsal root and a ventral root
- Divide into branches called *rami*
- Damage to a spinal nerve can lead to paralysis or loss of sensation in the area supplied by the nerve

Cranial nerve functions

The 12 cranial nerves perform a wide range of sensory and motor functions, as described here.

NERVE NUMBER AND NAME	TYPE	FUNCTION
I (olfactory)	Sensory	• Provides a sense of smell
II (optic)	Sensory	• Provides vision
III (oculomotor)	Motor	• Moves the eyes and raises the eyelids • Adjusts the amount of light entering the eyes and focuses the lenses • Provides a sense of eye muscle movement
IV (trochlear)	Motor	• Moves the eyes • Provides eye muscle movement
V (trigeminal)	Motor and sensory	• Moves the muscles of mastication and those in the floor of the mouth • Provides sensory input from the eye surface, tear glands, upper eyelids, forehead, and scalp • Provides sensory input from the upper teeth, gingivae, and lip; palate lining; and facial skin • Provides sensory input from the lower teeth, gingivae, and lip; scalp; and skin over the jaw
VI (abducens)	Motor	• Moves the eyes • Provides eye muscle movement
VII (facial)	Motor and sensory	• Allows facial expression • Innervates tear and salivary glands • Provides a sense of taste to the anterior tongue
VIII (vestibulo-cochlear [acoustic])	Sensory	• Provides a sense of hearing • Provides a sense of equilibrium
IX (glosso-pharyngeal)	Motor and sensory	• Allows swallowing by controlling pharynx muscles • Innervates salivary glands • Provides a sense of taste to the posterior tongue • Provides sensory input from the pharynx, tonsils, and carotid arteries
X (vagus)	Motor and sensory	• Allows speech and swallowing by controlling pharynx muscles • Innervates muscles of the heart and smooth muscles of thoracic and abdominal organs • Provides sensory input from the pharynx, larynx, esophagus, and thoracic and abdominal organs
XI (spinal accessory)	Motor	• Allows movement of the soft palate, pharynx, and larynx • Allows movement of the neck and back
XII (hypoglossal)	Motor	• Allows tongue movement

Cranial nerve functions

- Olfactory (CN I): smell
- Optic (CN II): vision
- Oculomotor (CN III): most eye movement, pupillary constriction, upper eyelid elevation
- Trochlear (CN IV): Down and in eye movement
- Trigeminal (CN V): chewing, corneal reflex, face and scalp sensations
- Abducens (CN VI): lateral eye movement
- Facial (CN VII): expressions in the forehead, eye, and mouth; taste
- Vestibulocochlear (acoustic) (CN VIII): hearing and balance
- Glossopharyngeal (CN IX): swallowing, salivating, and taste
- Vagus (CN X): swallowing; gag reflex; talking; sensations of the throat, larynx, and abdominal viscera; activities of the thoracic and abdominal viscera
- Spinal accessory (CN XI): shoulder movement and head rotation
- Hypoglossal (CN XII): tongue movement

– The ventral rami of the first four cervical nerves form the *cervical plexus;* this plexus connects with cranial nerves XI and XII, phrenic nerves, and the skin and muscles of the head, neck, and upper part of the shoulders

– The ventral rami of spinal nerves C5 to C8 and T1 (with contributions from C4 and T2) form the *brachial plexus;* this plexus provides the entire nerve supply to the arms and several neck and shoulder muscles

– The ventral rami of spinal nerves L1 to L4 form the *lumbar plexus,* which supplies the anterolateral abdominal wall, external genitals, and part of the legs

– The ventral rami of spinal nerves L4 to L5 and S1 to S4 form the *sacral plexus,* which supplies the buttocks, perineum, and legs

• Damage to a spinal nerve can lead to muscular paralysis or loss of sensation in the area supplied by the nerve

– Most spinal nerves innervate specific areas of the skin called *dermatomes*

– Testing each dermatome helps determine which spinal nerve has been affected

● **Autonomic nervous system**

• The *autonomic nervous system* (ANS) controls involuntary (or automatic) body functions, such as the activity of cardiac muscle, smooth muscle, and glandular epithelial tissue; although it consists entirely of motor nerves, sensory neurons participate in its function

• It has two subdivisions—the sympathetic and parasympathetic systems

– The two systems are anatomically and functionally distinct

– Although the two systems generally serve the same organs, they counterbalance each other; each system can inhibit the organs excited by the other (see *Responses to autonomic nervous system stimulation*)

• The *sympathetic system* originates from the lateral horns of the first thoracic through first lumbar segments of the spinal cord

– It helps the body cope with events in the external environment

– It functions mainly during stress, triggering the *fight-or-flight response* (increased heart and respiratory rate; cold, sweaty palms; and pupil dilation)

• The *parasympathetic system* consists of the vagus nerve, which originates in the medulla of the brain stem, and spinal nerves originating in the sacral region of the spinal cord

– It activates the GI system

– It also supports restorative, resting body functions through such actions as replenishing fluid and electrolytes

---

Key facts about the autonomic nervous system

● Controls involuntary body functions
● Divided into the sympathetic and parasympathetic systems

Key characteristics of the sympathetic nervous system

● Originates from the lateral horns of the first thoracic through first lumbar segments of the spinal cord
● Functions mainly during stress, triggering the fight-or-flight response

---

Key characteristics of the parasympathetic nervous system

● Consists of the vagus nerve and spinal nerves
● Activates the GI system
● Supports restorative, resting body functions

Responses to autonomic nervous system stimulation

The parasympathetic and sympathetic divisions of the autonomic nervous system innervate most effector organs. These divisions usually produce opposite responses, as shown in the following examples.

EFFECTOR ORGANS	PARASYMPATHETIC RESPONSES	SYMPATHETIC RESPONSES
Eye • Radial muscle of iris • Sphincter muscle of iris	• None • Contraction for near vision	• Contraction (mydriasis) • None
Heart	• Decreased rate and contractility	• Increased rate and contractility
Lung • (bronchial muscle)	• Contraction	• Relaxation
Stomach • Motility and tone • Sphincters	• Increased • Relaxation	• Decreased (usually) • Contraction (usually)
Intestine • Motility and tone • Sphincters	• Increased • Relaxation	• Decreased • Contraction
Urinary bladder • Bladder muscle • Trigone and sphincter	• Contraction • Relaxation	• Relaxation • Contraction
Skin • Erector pilli • Sweat glands	• None • Generalized secretion	• Contraction • Slight localized secretion
Adrenal medulla	• None	• Secretion of epinephrine and norepinephrine
Liver	• None	• Glycogenolysis
Pancreas • (acini)	• Increased secretion	• Decreased secretion
Adipose tissue	• None	• Lipolysis
Juxtaglomerular cells	• None	• Increased renin secretion

• The arrangement of neurons in the ANS differs from that in the somatic nervous system (see *Neuron pathways in the peripheral nervous system,* pages 142 and 143)

● **Somatic nervous system**
  • The somatic nervous system consists of motor and sensory nerves
  • It controls skeletal muscles (those under voluntary or conscious control)

(Text continues on page 144.)

Key facts about the somatic nervous system
• Consists of motor and sensory nerves
• Controls skeletal muscles under voluntary control

GO WITH THE FLOW

Neuron pathways in the peripheral nervous system

The peripheral nervous system consists of the autonomic nervous system (ANS), which has parasympathetic and sympathetic divisions, and the somatic nervous system. Each of these systems has different neuron pathways, as described below.

ANS pathways consist of two neurons: one neuron extends from the central nervous system (CNS) to a ganglion (preganglionic neuron); the other extends from the ganglion to the effector organ or gland (postganglionic neuron). Somatic nervous system pathways consist of only one neuron.

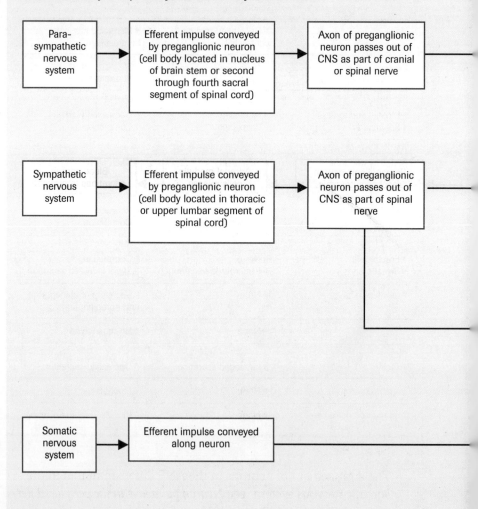

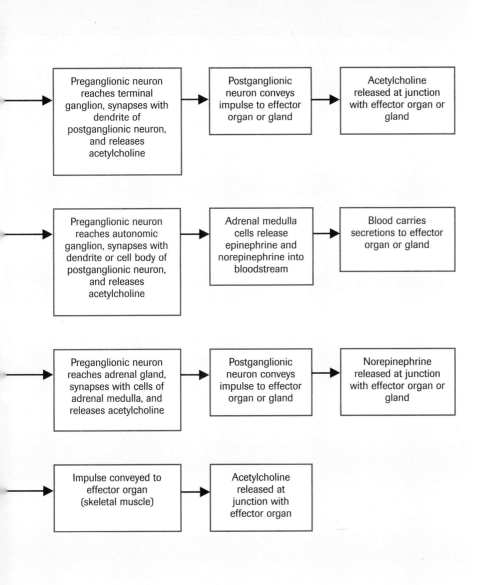

- The somatic nervous system produces a motor response through efferent fibers from the CNS, which transmit impulses to the skin and skeletal muscles

NEUROTRANSMISSION

● **Key concepts**
- *Neurotransmission* is the conduction of impulses throughout the nervous system; it occurs through the actions of neurons, which detect and transmit stimuli as electrochemical impulses (see *How neurotransmission occurs*)
- Electrical transmission occurs within the nerve fiber
  - Each neuron has an *electrical potential* (resting membrane potential) caused by different concentrations of sodium and potassium ions on each side of the membrane; normally, the neuron is *polarized* (positive outside and negative inside)
  - Stimulation of a nerve alters membrane permeability, allowing sodium to enter and causing the membrane to *depolarize* (positive inside and negative outside)
  - The spread of increased permeability and electrical current along the membrane is a nerve impulse
- Chemical transmission occurs between two neurons or between a neuron and a muscle
  - When the impulse reaches the end of a neuron, a *neurotransmitter* (a chemical essential for neurotransmission) is released, which causes the impulse to cross the synapse
  - When the next neuron receives the impulse, a *neuropeptide* (a chemical that regulates or modulates neurotransmitters) breaks down the neurotransmitter to prevent sustained impulse transmission
- Sensory impulses ultimately reach the brain for interpretation; the brain transmits motor impulses to the muscles or other effector - organs

● **Transmission within nerve fibers**
- During the electrical state of *polarization,* the nerve fiber doesn't transmit an impulse
  - The exterior of the nerve fiber is positively charged; the interior is negatively charged
  - The voltage difference between the exterior and interior of the nerve fiber is approximately –70 millivolts (the minus sign indicates that the interior of the cells is negatively charged)
  - This voltage difference, or resting membrane potential, results from the unequal distribution of sodium ions (Na^+) and potassium ions (K^+) on the two sides of the cell membrane

How neurotransmission occurs

Neurons receive and transmit stimuli by electrochemical messages. Dendrites on the neuron receive an impulse sent by other cells and conduct it toward the cell body. The axon then conducts the impulse away from the cell.

When the impulse reaches the end of the axon, it stimulates synaptic vesicles in the presynaptic axon terminal. A neurotransmitter substance is then released into the synaptic cleft between neurons. This substance diffuses across the synaptic cleft and binds to special receptors on the postsynaptic membrane. This stimulates or inhibits stimulation of the postsynaptic neuron.

SENSORY (AFFERENT) NEURON   **MOTOR (EFFERENT) NEURON**

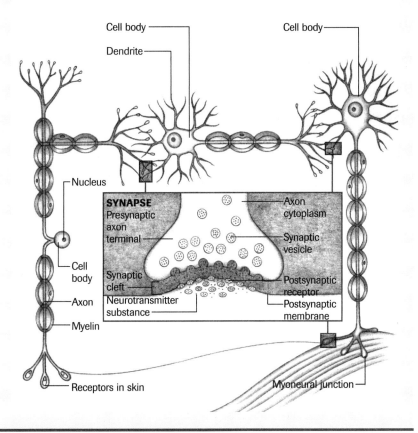

- An active transport mechanism called the *sodium-potassium pump* transports potassium ions in through the membrane and simultaneously transports sodium ions out
- The pump carries in approximately two potassium ions for every three sodium ions carried out, causing a relative excess of positively charged ions on the exterior of the membrane
- In the electrical state of *depolarization,* the nerve fiber's resting membrane potential moves toward zero

Key facts about transmission within nerve fibers

- During polarization, the nerve fiber doesn't transmit an impulse
- The sodium-potassium pump transports ions through the membrane, resulting in an excess of positively charged ions on the exterior
- Stimulation changes membrane permeability, and sodium ions flow into the nerve fiber, enhancing depolarization
- After depolarization, the interior of the nerve fiber has a positive charge relative to the exterior
- In unmyelinated nerve fibers, the impulse progresses without interruption
- In myelinated nerve fibers, the wave of depolarization jumps between gaps in the myelin sheath, making depolarization faster

– Stimulation causes a change in membrane permeability in the stimulated area; positively charged sodium ions flow into the nerve fiber, enhancing depolarization
– Any stimulus strong enough to depolarize the membrane and initiate a nerve impulse will cause the depolarization wave, or impulse, to travel along the nerve fiber
– The membrane potential changes to zero and then reverses, with the interior of the nerve fiber having a positive charge relative to the exterior; this rapid change in the resting membrane is called an *action potential*
  - The reversed polarity causes the membrane permeability to change again
    - Sodium ions are prevented from entering, while potassium ions are allowed to exit
    - This quickly returns the nerve fiber to its original polarity, with the interior negatively charged compared with the outside
  - Before the original polarization returns, however, the voltage difference between the area of reversed polarity and the adjacent polarized area of the membrane causes a current flow
    - This current flow depolarizes the adjacent area of the membrane; the action potential occurs there, causing a current flow to the next polarized area
    - The process continues along the entire length of the membrane, causing a depolarization wave that travels along the nerve fiber
    - As the nerve impulse travels in a depolarization wave, the previously depolarized area becomes repolarized and its resting membrane potential is restored
– In an unmyelinated nerve fiber, the impulse progresses without interruption along the entire length of the nerve fiber
– In a myelinated nerve fiber, impulse conduction is similar but influenced by the myelin sheath
  - The wave of depolarization "jumps" between the gaps in the myelin sheaths, bypassing the myelin-covered segments of the nerve fiber between the nodes of Ranvier
  - This transmission process, called *saltatory conduction*, occurs much more rapidly than the progressive depolarization wave that moves along an unmyelinated nerve fiber
– After nerve impulse transmission, a brief interval called the *refractory period* occurs; during this period, the nerve fiber can't respond and transmit another impulse until its membrane repolarizes

● **Transmission across synapses**
- Chemicals that stimulate neurons transmit nerve impulses across synapses from neuron to neuron
- Although organized in chains, neurons don't directly touch each other
  - Synapses separate the neurons
  - At the synapse, the axon terminal of the presynaptic neuron (the one transmitting the impulse) is close to the cell body or dendrite of the postsynaptic neuron (the next neuron in the chain) or to the muscle or organ it innervates
- When the nerve impulse reaches the presynaptic axon terminal, it stimulates vesicles there to release a neurotransmitter
  - The neurotransmitter diffuses across the synapse and binds to receptors on the membrane of the postsynaptic neuron; this changes the permeability of the postsynaptic neuron, which initiates membrane depolarization and impulse transmission
  - The neurotransmitter released from the axon terminals is quickly inactivated by various mechanisms to prevent a sustained response
- Each type of neuron releases its own specific type of neurotransmitter
- Because neurotransmitters are released only from axon terminals, transmission across a synapse can take place only from an axon to a dendrite, to the cell body of the next neuron, or to a muscle or other effector organ
- Some neurons release *inhibitory neurotransmitters,* which inhibit—rather than stimulate—impulse transmission
  - An inhibitory neurotransmitter causes the membrane of the postsynaptic neuron to become more permeable to potassium and chloride (Cl⁻) ions, without affecting the permeability to sodium
  - Potassium ions diffuse out and chloride ions diffuse in, increasing the negative charge of the postsynaptic neuron membrane
  - When this occurs, the membrane depolarizes less readily, which inhibits impulse transmission

● **CNS neurotransmitters**
- Neurotransmitters are essential for neurotransmission in the CNS; other substances may also be involved
  - Neuropeptides—molecules composed of short chains of amino acids that usually appear in the axon terminals at synapses—modify or regulate neurotransmitter activity
  - Other substances (such as the amino acids glycine, glutamic acid, and aspartic acid) may play a role in neurotransmission

Key facts about transmission across synapses
- Synapses separate neurons
- When the nerve impulse reaches the presynaptic axon terminal, it stimulates vesicles to release a neurotransmitter
- Each type of neuron releases its own specific neurotransmitter
- Some neurons release inhibitory neurotransmitters, which inhibit impulse transmission

Key facts about CNS neurotransmitters
- Neurotransmitters are essential for neurotransmission in the CNS
- Neuropeptides regulate or modulate the actions of neurotransmitters
- All neurotransmitters, neuropeptides, and related substances must be inactivated after release to limit their duration of activity

147

CNS neurotransmitters

- Acetylcholine
- Norepinephrine
- Dopamine
- Serotonin
- GABA

Key characteristics of acetylcholine

- Stored in synaptic vesicles called *cholinergic neurons*
- Release triggered by nerve stimulation
- Inactivated by cholinesterase

Key characteristics of norepinephrine

- One of a group of neurotransmitters called *catacholamines*
- Released from most postganglionic neurons
- Inactivated by reuptake and the enzymes COMT and MAO

- All neurotransmitters, neuropeptides, and related substances must be inactivated after release to limit their duration of activity
- The chief CNS neurotransmitters include acetylcholine, norepinephrine, dopamine, serotonin, and gamma-aminobutyric acid (GABA)
  - *Acetylcholine* is stored in the synaptic vesicles of certain neurons called *cholinergic neurons*; these neurons include all preganglionic neurons of the sympathetic and parasympathetic nervous systems, all postganglionic parasympathetic neurons, and postganglionic neurons that innervate sweat glands and some blood vessels
    - Nerve stimulation triggers the release of acetylcholine, which then activates postganglionic neurons
    - The enzyme *cholinesterase* rapidly inactivates acetylcholine, breaking it down into acetate and choline
      - Some acetate diffuses away and is used by cells for energy
      - Axon terminals take up the choline, which then combines with acetate to form more acetylcholine
      - Synaptic vesicles store this acetylcholine for later release in response to further nerve stimulation
  - *Norepinephrine* is stored in the synaptic vesicles of *adrenergic neurons,* which include most postganglionic neurons of the sympathetic nervous system
    - One of a group of neurotransmitters collectively called *catecholamines,* norepinephrine is released from the axon terminals of most postganglionic neurons
    - Norepinephrine is inactivated in two ways
      - The synaptic vesicles in the axon terminals take some norepinephrine back in; this is called *reuptake*
      - The enzymes catechol O-methyltransferase (COMT) and monoamine oxidase (MAO) inactivate the rest
  - *Dopamine,* a precursor of norepinephrine, is also a catecholamine (see *Teaching a patient with Parkinson's disease*)
    - After release from axon terminals, dopamine stimulates postsynaptic neurons
    - It's inactivated in the same two ways as norepinephrine
  - *Serotonin* is a derivative of the amino acid tryptophan
    - It's stored in the synaptic vesicles of axon terminals
    - Nerve stimulation triggers the release of serotonin, which in turn stimulates postsynaptic neurons
    - Reuptake and enzymatic (MAO) breakdown inactivate serotonin

TIME-OUT FOR TEACHING

Teaching a patient with Parkinson's disease

Make sure you teach a patient with Parkinson's disease:
- about the progressive nature of the disease
- what diagnostic tests to expect to rule out other disorders
- which complications require immediate medical attention
- what drugs may be prescribed, including names, indications, dosages, adverse effects, and special considerations (such as dietary restrictions and the need to stand up slowly when taking levodopa)
- the importance of maintaining activities, including range-of-motion exercises, activities of daily living, and walking
- muscle relaxation techniques, such as baths and massage
- ways to prevent pressure ulcers and contractures
- safety measures to help prevent accidents
- aspiration precautions
- where to find sources of information and support.

- – *GABA*, an inhibitory neurotransmitter produced from the amino acid glutamic acid, is inactivated by enzymatic breakdown
- Closely related to neurotransmitters, neuropeptides are chains of amino acids (peptides) that regulate or modulate the actions of neurotransmitters
  - – A neuropeptide called *substance P*, found in sensory nerves and in the spinal cord, aids in the transmission of pain sensations to the brain
  - – Other neuropeptides, such as enkephalins, endorphins, and dynorphins, inhibit the perception of pain impulses transmitted to the brain

● ANS neurotransmitters
- *Acetylcholine* is a key neurotransmitter in the ANS
  - – It's released from the axons of preganglionic neurons connected with the ANS, including all preganglionic neurons, postganglionic parasympathetic neurons, and postganglionic sympathetic neurons that innervate sweat glands and cause vasodilation in certain blood vessels in skeletal muscle (sympathetic vasodilator nerves)
  - – Acetylcholine stimulates postganglionic neurons, which in turn release acetylcholine or the neurotransmitter norepinephrine from their axons

– As a postganglionic neurotransmitter, it also activates effector organs

– Cholinesterase rapidly breaks down acetylcholine, preventing a sustained response

- *Norepinephrine*, another key neurotransmitter in the ANS, is related to epinephrine, which is produced by the adrenal medulla

  – Most postganglionic sympathetic neurons release norepinephrine

  – After norepinephrine is released from nerve endings, some is inactivated by reuptake into axons and some by the action of COMT and MAO

  – Because norepinephrine inactivation doesn't occur as rapidly as acetylcholine inactivation, the effects of sympathetic stimulation persist longer than the effects of parasympathetic stimulation

  – Sympathetic stimulation also triggers the release of epinephrine and norepinephrine from the adrenal medulla, which augments the effects of the norepinephrine produced by postganglionic sympathetic neurons

- Neurotransmitter receptors are found in effector organs

  – Acetylcholine released from postganglionic autonomic nerve endings produces its effect by combining with specific receptors on effector organs called *cholinergic receptors*

  – When released from the postganglionic sympathetic neurons, norepinephrine produces its effects by combining with specific receptors on effector organs called *adrenergic receptors*

    · Adrenergic receptors are divided into *alpha* and *beta receptors*

      - Alpha receptors contain two subgroups: $alpha_1$ and $alpha_2$

      - Beta receptors also contain two subgroups: $beta_1$ and $beta_2$

    · Most effector organs contain either alpha or beta receptors; some contain both

      - Organs that contain beta receptors commonly contain $beta_1$ and $beta_2$ receptors, but usually one type predominates

      - Blood vessel walls contain $alpha_1$ receptors, which cause vasoconstriction and tend to dominate over the counterbalancing effects of $alpha_2$ receptors, located primarily in terminals of postganglionic sympathetic neurons

    · Usually, norepinephrine stimulates alpha-adrenergic receptors

    · Epinephrine stimulates $alpha_1$, $alpha_2$, $beta_1$, and $beta_2$ receptors

---

Key characteristics of adrenergic receptors

- Divided into alpha and beta receptors
- Alpha receptors contain $alpha_1$ and $alpha_2$
- Beta receptors contain $beta_1$ and $beta_2$
- Organs contain $beta_1$ and $beta_2$ receptors
- Blood vessels contain $alpha_1$ receptors

· Alpha and beta receptors respond differently to adrenergic stimulation
  - Stimulation of $alpha_1$ receptors produces contraction (vasoconstriction) of the smooth-muscle walls of blood vessels
  - Stimulation of $alpha_2$ receptors produces the opposite effect by inhibiting norepinephrine release from sympathetic nerve endings
  - Stimulation of $beta_1$ receptors, which predominate in cardiac muscle, causes the heart to beat faster and more forcefully
  - Stimulation of $beta_2$ receptors, which predominate in the smooth muscle of bronchial walls and blood vessels, dilates bronchi and relaxes blood vessels

CONTROL CENTERS

● **Key concepts**
  • The control centers for most nervous system functions are located in the brain
  • The cerebrum, cerebellum, diencephalon, and brain stem control specialized groups of functions
  • The brain modulates the spinal cord, which is primarily a reflex response center
  • Most simple reflexes result from neurotransmission through the reflex arc—a three-neuron chain composed of sensory, connecting, and motor neurons

● **Cerebrum**
  • The cerebrum, which controls all advanced mental activities, is divided into two hemispheres
    – The *corpus callosum,* a connecting bridge of nerve fibers, joins the hemispheres
    – Large fissures divide the two hemispheres into the frontal, parietal, temporal, and occipital lobes
  • The *cerebral cortex,* which covers the surface of each hemisphere, is composed of gray matter containing the cell bodies of neurons and white matter containing their myelinated nerve fibers
  • Masses of gray matter called *basal ganglia* are found deep within each cerebral hemisphere; basal ganglia form part of the *extrapyramidal system,* which controls the coordination of muscle groups that function together to perform voluntary motion
  • The *internal capsule* is white matter, consisting of bundles of nerve fibers, that passes through the basal ganglia, carrying sensory and motor impulses to and from the cerebral cortex

Key facts about control centers

● The cerebrum, cerebellum, diencephalon, and brain stem control specialized groups of functions
● The brain modulates the spinal cord, which is primarily a reflex response center
● Most simple reflexes result from neurotransmission through the reflex arc

Key facts about the cerebrum

● Controls all advanced mental activities
● Divided into two hemispheres, which are connected by the corpus callosum
● The cerebral cortex covers the surface of each hemisphere
● Inside each hemisphere are basal ganglia, which control the coordination of muscle groups
● Functional areas of the cortex relate to specialized functions

- Parts of the cortex called *functional areas* are related to specialized functions; however, because these areas are extensively interconnected, functions aren't sharply separated
  - The *motor area* controls voluntary motor activity
    - The area contains neurons that control specific body parts
      - Neurons in the upper part of the motor area control muscles in the lower part of the body
      - Neurons in the lower part of the area control muscles in the head, neck, and upper part of the body
    - The number of neurons supplying a muscle depends on the type of movement it performs
      - Muscles capable of fine movements, such as finger muscles, have large areas of cortical representation
      - Muscles capable only of relatively gross movements, such as large limb and back muscles, are represented with smaller areas
  - The *sensory area* receives sensory impulses
    - Upper part of the sensory cortex receives impulses from the lower part of the body
    - Lower part of the sensory cortex receives impulses from the upper part of the body
- Each cerebral hemisphere receives sensory impulses from, or supplies motor impulses to, the opposite side of the body because almost all the *fiber tracts* (bundles of nerve fibers carrying impulses) cross to the opposite side of the brain, brain stem, or spinal cord as they ascend or descend the CNS
- Cortical areas associated with vision are located in the occipital lobe; those associated with hearing are located in the temporal lobes
- Motor areas related to speech are located in the frontal lobes; cortical areas related to olfactory sensations are on the undersurface of the temporal lobes
- Other cortical areas surrounding the primary areas (directly affecting a specific function) are called *association areas;* although they're concerned with the same types of functions as the primary areas, they're more involved with interpretation, learning, and memory
- The frontal areas primarily involve personality and judgment

● **Cerebellum**
- The cerebellum receives sensory impulses from muscles, joints, and tendons that convey a sense of position; it also receives impulses from the inner ear that involve balance and equilibrium
- Cerebellar motor impulses regulate muscle groups that coordinate position and balance

Key facts about the cerebellum

- Cerebellar motor impulses regulate muscle groups that coordinate position and balance
- Bundles of fibers called the *cerebellar peduncles* connect the cerebellum to the brain stem

- Bundles of fibers called the *cerebellar peduncles* connect the cerebellum to the brain stem
  - Cerebellar peduncles transmit nerve impulses to the spinal cord, medulla, and brain
  - The peduncles transmit impulses from the cerebellum to the thalamus for eventual transmission to the cortex

● **Diencephalon and brain stem**
  - The diencephalon connects to the top of the brain stem and contains the slitlike third ventricle
    - The thalamus, which forms the lateral walls of the third ventricle, contains relay stations that receive sensory impulses and transmit them to the cortex
    - The hypothalamus contains neurons that control hormone output from the endocrine glands and regulate the activity of the ANS; these neurons control such basic body functions as temperature regulation, food and water intake, and sexual behavior
  - The brain stem is divided into the midbrain, pons, and medulla
    - The *midbrain* contains cell bodies of cranial nerves and large nerve fiber bundles that convey impulses to and from the cerebral hemispheres
    - The *pons* is a transverse bridge of fibers that connects the brain stem to the cerebellum; the pons also contains fiber tracts extending to and from the cerebral hemispheres, neurons of several of the cranial nerves, and neurons involved with spontaneous respiratory movements
    - The *medulla* is the lowest part of the brain stem; it forms the floor of the fourth ventricle, which is partially covered by the cerebellum
      · The medulla contains nerve cell bodies of cranial nerves and nerve fiber bundles, which relay impulses to higher and lower levels in the nervous system
      · The medulla also serves as an autonomic reflex center to maintain homeostasis; it contains the cardiac center (which adjusts the force and rate of myocardial contractions), respiratory center (which regulates breathing depth and rate), and vasomotor center (which regulates blood pressure)

● **Spinal cord**
  - The major reflex center in the CNS, the spinal cord mediates most reflexes
  - *Reflexes* are automatic actions, such as a knee jerk in response to a tap on the patellar tendon
    - Hyperactive reflexes may result from a disease or injury of certain descending motor tracts

Common types of skeletal muscle reflexes

- Stretch reflex
- Flexor reflex
- Crossed-extensor reflex

– Hypoactive reflexes may indicate degeneration or damage of the sensory or motor nerves
- Three common types of somatic (skeletal muscle) reflexes are the *stretch reflex* (involving two neurons and one synapse), the *flexor reflex* (involving sensory, motor, and connecting neurons and more than one synapse), and the *crossed-extensor reflex* (involving the flexor reflex and a contralateral reflex arc)
- Most simple reflexes result from nerve impulse transmission through a three-neuron chain between sensory, connecting, and motor neurons; these neurons form the *reflex arc* (see *The reflex arc*)
  – The sensory (afferent) neuron carries the impulse into the spinal cord through the dorsal root to the connecting neuron in the posterior horn of the spinal cord gray matter
  – The connecting neuron relays the impulse to a motor neuron in the anterior horn of the gray matter

The reflex arc

A simple reflex arc requires a sensory (afferent) neuron and a motor (efferent) neuron as well as a connecting neuron in the spinal cord.

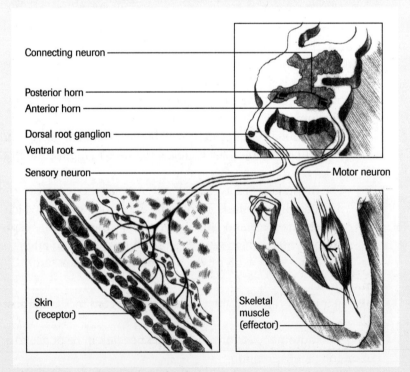

– The motor neuron sends out a motor (efferent) impulse via an axon in the ventral root of the spinal cord; this impulse causes muscle contraction

– Although described in terms of a three-neuron chain, many sensory, connecting, and motor neurons are involved in a reflex arc

– In many reflexes, impulses initiated by sensory neurons are also relayed up and down the spinal cord by connecting neurons, causing a coordinated response from many different groups of motor neurons

• Different types of reflexes may occur

– A person may be aware of some reflex responses because the cortex receives both the stimulus that initiates the reflex and the perception of the response; for example, a person can perceive the automatic patellar reflex

– Some reflexes, such as those that regulate heart rate and blood pressure, function automatically; a person isn't aware of the reflex control of these functions

– Conscious effort allows control of some reflexes, such as the urination and defecation reflexes

– A person may learn *conditioned reflexes* (conditioned responses), such as salivation at the sight or smell of food, as a result of past associations

NCLEX CHECKS

It's never too soon to begin your NCLEX preparation. Now that you've reviewed this chapter, carefully read each of the following questions and choose the best answer. Then compare your responses with the correct answers.

1. The nurse performing a neurologic assessment should understand that the CNS includes which of the following?
- ☐ **1.** Spinal cord and cranial nerves
- ☐ **2.** Brain and spinal cord
- ☐ **3.** Sympathetic and parasympathetic nervous systems
- ☐ **4.** Cranial nerves and spinal nerves

2. A client with a potential head injury is brought to the hospital after falling off a roof. The nurse explains to the client and his family that the brain is protected from shock and infection by which structures?
- ☐ **1.** Bones, the meninges, and CSF
- ☐ **2.** Gray matter, bones, and the ventricles
- ☐ **3.** Fissures, CSF, and white matter
- ☐ **4.** Axons, neurons, and meninges

TOP 10

Items to study for your next test on the nervous system

1. Four main regions of the brain
2. Major functions of the nervous system
3. Structure and function of the central and peripheral nervous systems
4. Structure and function of a neuron
5. Chemical and electrical synapses
6. Sensory and motor functions of the cranial nerves
7. Comparison of the autonomic and somatic nervous systems
8. Process of neurotransmission
9. Reflexes and the reflex arc
10. Teaching tips for patients with Parkinson's disease or multiple sclerosis

3. While performing a cranial nerve assessment, the nurse must keep in mind that the cranial nerves transmit sensory and motor messages between which structures?

☐ **1.** Spine and body dermatomes
☐ **2.** Brain and the head and neck
☐ **3.** Viscera and the brain
☐ **4.** Brain and skeletal muscles

4. The nurse is assessing a client with a tumor in the brain stem. The nurse should expect alterations in which functions? Select all that apply.

☐ **1.** Motor function
☐ **2.** Sensory function
☐ **3.** Respiratory function
☐ **4.** Cardiac function
☐ **5.** Thermoregulation
☐ **6.** Reflexes

5. The nurse is teaching a client and his family about multiple sclerosis. The nurse tells the client to perform which action to avoid triggering an attack?

☐ **1.** "Use air conditioning to keep your home cold."
☐ **2.** "Avoid rest naps during the day."
☐ **3.** "Practice relaxation to reduce stress."
☐ **4.** "Wear heavy clothing to stay warm."

6. The nurse understands that which is the most common type of neuron with one axon and several dendrites?

☐ **1.** Unipolar
☐ **2.** Pseudounipolar
☐ **3.** Bipolar
☐ **4.** Multipolar

7. The nurse is checking a client's balance. Which sensory receptor is the nurse assessing?

☐ **1.** Proprioceptors
☐ **2.** Exteroceptors
☐ **3.** Nociceptors
☐ **4.** Interoceptors

8. During a hearing examination, the nurse is assessing which cranial nerve?

☐ **1.** Olfactory
☐ **2.** Optic
☐ **3.** Abducens
☐ **4.** Vestibulocochlear

9. The nurse explains to a client that stress stimulates the sympathetic nervous system to produce which response?
- ☐ **1.** Decreased heart rate
- ☐ **2.** Constricted pupils
- ☐ **3.** Increased respiratory rate
- ☐ **4.** Hot, flushed skin

10. The nurse is giving the client an alpha$_1$-adrenergic blocker to reduce his high blood pressure. The nurse explains to the client that alpha$_1$ receptors produce which effect?
- ☐ **1.** Vasoconstriction
- ☐ **2.** Vasodilation
- ☐ **3.** Tachycardia
- ☐ **4.** Bronchodilation

ANSWERS AND RATIONALES

1. CORRECT ANSWER: 2
The two main divisions of the nervous system are the CNS, which includes the brain and spinal cord, and the PNS, which consists of the cranial nerves, spinal nerves, and autonomic nervous system.

2. CORRECT ANSWER: 1
Bones (skull and vertebral column), the meninges, and CSF protect the brain from shock and infection. Gray matter consists of unmyelinated axons; white matter is made of myelinated axons. Ventricles are cavities in the brain where CSF is formed. Fissures are deep grooves in the cerebrum that increase its surface area. Axons carry impulses away from a cell body. Neurons are highly specialized cells that conduct nerve impulses.

3. CORRECT ANSWER: 2
The 12 pairs of cranial nerves transmit motor (efferent) and sensory (afferent) messages between the brain or brain stem and the head and neck.

4. CORRECT ANSWER: 3, 4, 6
The brain stem consists of the pons, medulla, and midbrain. The pons helps regulate respiration. The medulla controls cardiac, respiratory, and vasomotor functions. The midbrain serves as a reflex center. The cerebrum performs motor, sensory, and integrative functions. It's also the center of intellect, language, memory, and consciousness. The diencephalon consists of the thalamus (which relays sensory information), the hypothalamus (which regulates the ANS), and the epithalamus (which produces CSF). The cerebellum coordinates complex motor activities.

5. CORRECT ANSWER: 3

To avoid triggering a multiple sclerosis attack, the client should avoid stress, extremes of temperature, and fatigue. The client should also take steps to avoid illness and infection, which can trigger an attack. Extremes of temperature, such as occurs with air-conditioner use, can trigger an attack; likewise, dressing too warmly may also trigger an attack.

6. CORRECT ANSWER: 4

Neurons are multipolar, bipolar, or unipolar (pseudounipolar). Multipolar neurons, the most common type, have one axon and several dendrites. Unipolar neurons have a single process that divides into a proximal fiber (axon) and a distal fiber (dendrite). Bipolar neurons have one axon and one dendrite and serve as receptor cells in special sense organs.

7. CORRECT ANSWER: 1

Proprioceptors respond to internal stimuli and alert the brain to body movements. They're found in skeletal muscle, tendons, joints and, possibly, the inner ear. Exteroceptors, located at or near the body surface, are sensitive to outside stimuli, such as touch, pressure, temperature, and sound. Nociceptors (pain receptors) respond to excessive heat and pressure, extreme cold, and chemicals released at inflammation sites. Interoceptors respond to stimuli arising from the internal organs and blood vessels.

8. CORRECT ANSWER: 4

The vestibulocochlear (acoustic) nerve (cranial nerve VIII) is a sensory nerve that provides a sense of hearing and equilibrium. The olfactory nerve (cranial nerve I) is a sensory nerve that controls the sense of smell. The optic nerve (cranial nerve II) is a sensory nerve that controls vision. The abducens nerve (cranial nerve VI) is a motor nerve that moves the eyes.

9. CORRECT ANSWER: 3

The sympathetic nervous system helps the body cope with stress by triggering the fight-or-flight response, causing increased heart and respiratory rates; cold, sweaty palms; and pupil dilation.

10. CORRECT ANSWER: 1

Stimulation of $alpha_1$ receptors produces vasoconstriction of the smooth muscle of blood vessels. An $alpha_1$ receptor blocker lowers blood pressure by blocking this response, leading to vasodilation. Stimulation of $alpha_2$ receptors produces vasodilation. Stimulation of $beta_1$ receptors produces tachycardia. Stimulation of $beta_2$ receptors causes relaxation of the bronchial walls, leading to bronchodilation.

10

Sensory system

LEARNING OBJECTIVES

After studying this chapter, you should be able to:

- Describe the structures and functions of the eyes.
- Explain light refraction, image formation, and visual pathways.
- Explain structures and functions of the external, middle, and inner ear.
- Discuss the processes of sound wave transmission and equilibrium.
- Describe the structures and functions of the nose.
- Identify the structure and function of the taste buds.
- Identify the types of general senses and their structures and functions.

CHAPTER OVERVIEW

Through the sensory system, the body perceives and reacts to its environment. This system provides the senses of sight, sound, balance, smell, taste, touch, pressure, temperature, and pain. Without these protective senses, the body would constantly be in danger. To help safeguard patients' health, the nurse must understand the structures and functions of the sensory system. This chapter reviews sensory system divisions, the eyes and vision, the ears and hearing, equilibrium maintenance, the nose and smell, the taste buds and taste, and the general senses.

Key facts about sensory system divisions

- Divided into special senses and general senses
- Special senses have receptors in relatively small area of body
- General senses have receptors throughout the body

Key special senses

- Vision
- Hearing
- Equilibrium
- Smell
- Taste

Key general senses

- Touch
- Pressure
- Temperature
- Pain

Key facts about the eyes and vision

- The eyes collect light waves and transmit as nerve impulses to the brain
- The eye is composed of three layers of tissue and a lens
- The iris divides the space between the cornea and lens into the anterior and posterior chambers

SENSORY SYSTEM DIVISIONS

● **Key concepts**
- The sensory system may be divided into the *special senses*—vision, hearing, equilibrium, smell, and taste—and the *general senses*—touch, pressure, temperature, and pain
- Special senses have receptors in complex organs in a relatively small area of the body; general senses have receptors throughout the body
- When stimulated, receptors generate nerve impulses, which sensory neurons carry to the central nervous system (CNS); the brain then processes this information and makes a suitable response

● **Special senses**
- The senses of vision, hearing, equilibrium, smell, and taste have receptors in specific areas of the body
  - Vision receptors are in the retina of the eye
  - Hearing receptors are found in the inner ear
  - Equilibrium receptors exist in the ear
  - Smell receptors are in the upper nose
  - Taste receptors are found in the tongue
- The sensory organ of hearing plays two roles, maintaining the senses of hearing and equilibrium

● **General senses**
- General senses include touch, pressure, temperature, and pain
- Receptors for these senses are distributed widely in the skin and other body tissues
  - Because the number of receptors for each sense varies greatly, not all parts of the body have equal sensitivity
  - The fingertips and tip of the tongue, for example, are much more sensitive than the back of the neck

EYES AND VISION

● **Key concepts**
- The eyes, the sensory organs for vision, collect light waves and transmit them as nerve impulses along the visual pathways to the brain, which translates them into images
- The eye is a complex structure composed of three layers of tissue—the cornea and sclera, a middle choroid coat, and an inner retina—and a lens
- The iris divides the space between the cornea and lens into the anterior and posterior chambers
- The eyes normally form a clear retinal image of an object 20′ (6.1 m) away; they must make several changes to adapt for near vision

- *Binocular vision* contributes to depth perception (the ability to judge relative distances of objects)

● **Structures**
  - The eye is a spherical structure that measures about 1" (2.5 cm) in diameter; it contains 70% of the body's sensory receptors (see *Looking at intraocular structures,* page 162)
  - Accessory structures of the eye include the eyebrows, eyelids, conjunctiva, lacrimal glands, and eye muscles (superior, inferior, lateral, and medial rectus muscles and superior and inferior oblique muscles)
    - The *conjunctiva,* a thin vascular membrane that lines the inner surface of the eyelids and sclera, is attached to the sclerocorneal junction but doesn't extend over the cornea
    - Lacrimal glands discharge fluid secretions to moisten the conjunctiva; the fluid collects in the lacrimal ducts, which have openings on the ridges of the eyelids near the nose, and discharges into the nose (see *A close look at tears,* page 163)
    - The paired eye muscles work together to perform eye movement
  - The outermost layer (fibrous tunic) of the eye's three layers contains the sclera and cornea
    - The *sclera* represents the bulk of the fibrous tunic
      · It's composed of opaque, white, dense connective tissue
      · Posteriorly, the sclera is continuous with the dura mater of the brain; anteriorly, it's continuous with the cornea
    - The *cornea* is a convex, transparent structure that bulges where it joins the sclera
      · An internal layer (endothelium) and an external layer (epithelium) of epithelial tissue cover the cornea
      · The cornea refracts light (bends light waves)
  - The middle layer (uvea or vascular tunic) has three regions—the choroid, ciliary body, and iris
    - The *choroid* is a highly vascular coat that surrounds most of the eye
      · Posteriorly, it stops at the point where the optic nerve exits the eye
      · Anteriorly, it's continuous with the ciliary body
    - The *ciliary body,* a thick ring of smooth muscle, encircles the lens and helps maintain its shape
    - The *iris* is the most anterior portion of the uvea
      · This is the colored portion of the eye
      · Shaped like a flat doughnut, it's continuous with the ciliary body

Key structures of the eye
- The eye contains 70% of the body's sensory receptors
- Accessory structures include the eyebrows, eyelids, conjunctiva, lacrimal glands, and eye muscles
- Outermost layer of the eye's three layers contains the sclera and cornea
- Middle layer has three regions—the choroid, ciliary body, and iris
- Innermost layer is the retina

Looking at intraocular structures

Some intraocular structures, such as the sclera, cornea, iris, pupil, and anterior chamber, are visible to the naked eye. Others, such as the retina, are visible only with an ophthalmoscope. These illustrations show the major structures within the eye.

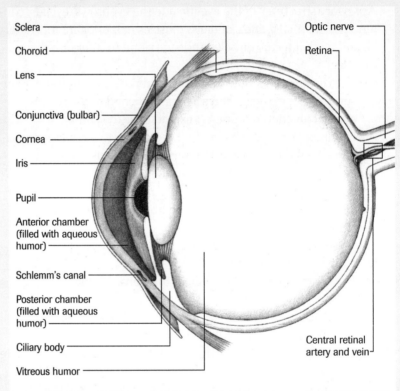

Sclera
Choroid
Lens
Conjunctiva (bulbar)
Cornea
Iris
Pupil
Anterior chamber (filled with aqueous humor)
Schlemm's canal
Posterior chamber (filled with aqueous humor)
Ciliary body
Vitreous humor
Optic nerve
Retina
Central retinal artery and vein

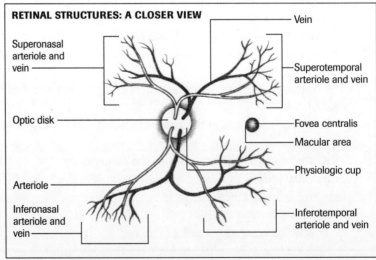

RETINAL STRUCTURES: A CLOSER VIEW

Vein
Superonasal arteriole and vein
Superotemporal arteriole and vein
Optic disk
Fovea centralis
Macular area
Physiologic cup
Arteriole
Inferonasal arteriole and vein
Inferotemporal arteriole and vein

A close look at tears

Tears begin in the lacrimal gland and drain through the nasolacrimal duct into the nose.

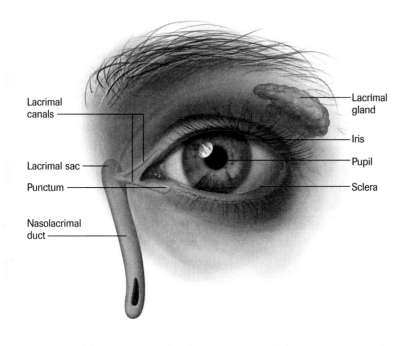

Lacrimal canals — Lacrimal gland — Iris — Lacrimal sac — Pupil — Punctum — Sclera — Nasolacrimal duct

Key characteristics of the retina

- Innermost layer
- Contains rods and cones that process images
- Nerve fibers from the retina converge to form the optic nerve

- The innermost layer (sensory tunic) of the eye is the *retina* (see *Teaching a patient with retinal detachment,* page 164)
    - Its outer, pigmented layer lies adjacent to the choroid
    - Its inner, transparent neural layer contains *photoreceptors* (rods and cones) that process external images
    - Nerve fibers from the retina converge to form the *optic nerve,* which penetrates the posterior surface of the sclera
- The *lens* is a transparent, encapsulated, biconvex structure
    - It attaches to the ciliary muscle by suspensory ligaments
    - Contraction or relaxation of the ciliary muscles varies the tension on the suspensory ligament, which in turn adjusts the thickness of the lens and lets the eye focus for near and far vision
- The eye is divided into anterior and posterior cavities
    - The *anterior cavity* contains an anterior and a posterior chamber
        - The *anterior chamber* is bounded anteriorly by the cornea and posteriorly by the iris and lens

Key characteristics of the lens

- The lens is transparent, encapsulated, and biconvex
- Adjusts its thickness to focus for near and far vision

Key teaching topics for a patient with retinal detachment

- Explain signs and symptoms
- List risk factors
- Describe treatments
- Review postoperative care

Key facts about aqueous humor formation and circulation

- Lymphlike fluid secreted by the epithelium of the ciliary bodies
- Aqueous humor secretion normally balances absorption
- This keeps pressure in anterior chamber stable at 20 to 25 mm Hg

TIME-OUT FOR TEACHING

Teaching a patient with retinal detachment

Make sure you teach a patient with retinal detachment:
- the disease process of retinal tear and detachment
- signs and symptoms that require immediate attention (such as vision loss)
- the risk factors for retinal detachment, such as aging and trauma
- what treatments (such as bed rest) and procedures (such as cryotherapy, laser therapy, and scleral buckling) to expect
- postoperative care and activity restrictions
- how to instill eyedrops.

- The *posterior chamber* is bounded by the iris, ciliary body, and lens
  - The anterior and posterior chambers contain *aqueous humor*, a clear, watery fluid similar in composition to blood plasma
    – The posterior cavity, located dorsal to the lens, contains the *vitreous humor*, a thick, clear, gelatinous fluid

● **Aqueous humor formation and circulation**
- Aqueous humor is a lymphlike fluid secreted by the epithelium of the ciliary bodies
- After the fluid flows into the posterior chamber of the eye, it passes through the pupil into the anterior chamber; it's absorbed into *Schlemm's canal*, a ring-shaped canal that encircles the eyeball at the sclerocorneal junction
- The porous portion of the eyeball between the anterior chamber and Schlemm's canal contains a network of channels called the *trabecular meshwork* that leads to the canal
  – Aqueous humor flows through the trabecular meshwork into Schlemm's canal
  – The fluid then enters the veins that drain blood from the eyeball
- Normally, aqueous humor secretion balances its absorption and the pressure in the anterior chamber remains relatively constant at about 20 to 25 mm Hg (about one-fifth of systemic arterial pressure); elevated intraocular pressure may lead to vision loss when the pressure is transmitted to the vitreous humor, where it damages retinal neurons

Light refraction

- Light rays that enter a transparent medium at an oblique angle to the surface are refracted as they pass into another medium of different density, such as from air to glass or from air to the eye
- The degree of refraction depends on two factors: the angle of the light rays and the difference in the refractive indices (measures of the density of the media) of the two media through which the light rays pass
  - The more oblique the angle of the light rays, the greater the refraction
  - The greater the difference in the refractive indices, the greater the refraction; for example, light rays passing from air (with a refractive index of 1) to glass (with a refractive index of 1.4) bend more than rays passing from water (refractive index of 1.33) to glass because the difference between the refractive indices of air and glass is greater
- The cornea is an efficient refracting medium because its refractive index (1.33) is significantly higher than air's index (1) and light rays travel through air before striking the cornea
- Lens curvature can also refract light rays; the greater the curvature, the more it causes light rays to refract
  - Concave lenses (those curved inward), such as the type used to correct nearsightedness, cause light rays to diverge
  - Convex lenses (those curved outward), such as the cornea and lens of the eye, cause light rays to converge
- Parallel rays from an object more than 20' (6.1 m) away that strike a convex lens come into focus at the *focal point* (principal focus); the distance from the lens to its focal point is the *focal length* of the lens
- The converging power of a convex lens is expressed in *diopters;* the reciprocal of the focal length of the lens is expressed in meters
  - A lens with a focal length of 1 m (3.3') has a strength of 1 diopter
  - A lens with a focal length of 50 cm (1.6') has a strength of 2 diopters because the reciprocal of $\frac{1}{2}$ is $\frac{2}{1}$, or 2
- The refractive power of a concave lens can't be expressed in focal length because this lens causes light rays to diverge instead of converge at a focal point
  - Refraction power of a concave lens is determined by its ability to counteract the converging power of a convex lens; its power is expressed by a minus sign
  - A concave lens that counteracts the converging power of a 0.5 diopter lens has a refractive power of -0.5 diopters

Key facts about image formation

- Light waves pass through the cornea, aqueous humor, lens, and vitreous humor before striking retina
- Rods and cones are receptor cells of the retina
- Rods are sensitive to low levels of light but can't distinguish color
- Cones are less sensitive to light and provide daylight color vision
- Cones respond to red, green, and blue light

Key facts about visual pathways

- Image forms on the retina when light stimulates rods and cones
- Each half of the retina receives visual input from the opposite visual field
- Two optic nerves converge at the base of the brain to form the optic chiasma

● Image formation

- The eye has a refractive power of about 60 diopters
  - The cornea performs most of the refraction because it's a convex lens with a high refractive index (1.33)
  - The lens itself has much less refractive power than the cornea because the media surrounding the lens (aqueous and vitreous humors) have almost the same refractive index as the cornea
  - The lens can change its focal length and can bring images into sharp focus on the retina through *accommodation*
- After passing through the cornea, aqueous humor, lens, and vitreous humor, light waves hit the retina
- Receptor cells of the retina (rods and cones) contain a photosensitive visual pigment (rhodopsin) that decomposes on light exposure, stimulating an impulse that's conveyed to the brain
  - *Rods* are the most numerous photoreceptors
    - They're concentrated at the periphery of the retina
    - Although sensitive to low levels of illumination, rods can't discriminate color
  - Rods don't function in bright light because it decomposes most of their rhodopsin, explaining why a person can't see well for a short time after moving from bright light into darkness; rhodopsin reforms and the rods start functioning again after a short period of darkness
  - *Cones* are less sensitive to light than rods
    - They're concentrated in the retina's center
    - Cones provide daylight color vision
  - Cones come in three types that respond to red, green, or blue light
    - Stimulation of various receptor combinations transmits impulses that the brain interprets as color
    - Color blindness occurs when one or more types of cones are absent or defective
- Images form in the eye in much the same way they form in an autofocus camera (see *Image perception and formation*)
  - The image on the retina is inverted
  - The brain reverses the image and perceives the object right side up

● Visual pathways

- An image forms on the retina when light stimulates the rods and cones
- Each half of the retina receives visual input from the opposite visual field, with the right half of each retina receiving input from the left visual field, and the left half, from the right visual field

GO WITH THE FLOW

Image perception and formation

The structures of the eye perform a series of steps that allow image perception and formation, as described and illustrated here.

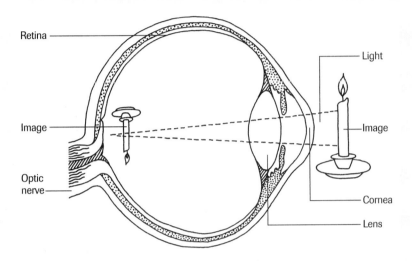

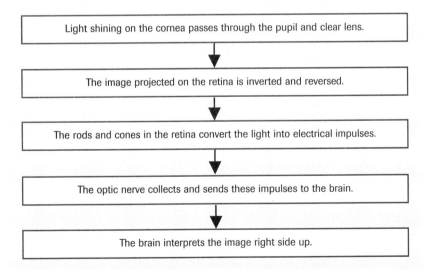

Light shining on the cornea passes through the pupil and clear lens.

↓

The image projected on the retina is inverted and reversed.

↓

The rods and cones in the retina convert the light into electrical impulses.

↓

The optic nerve collects and sends these impulses to the brain.

↓

The brain interprets the image right side up.

- Two optic nerves converge at the base of the brain to form the *optic chiasma*
  - The nerve fibers continue behind the chiasma, forming the *optic tracts*

- These tracts connect to neurons in the brain stem, which convey visual impulses to the occipital cortex by means of fiber tracts called the *optic radiations*
- Nerve fibers from the medial halves of both optic nerves cross in the optic chiasma, and fibers from the lateral halves of the optic nerves continue into the optic tracts without crossing

Near vision

- In an eye with normal refractive power, the retina forms a clear image of an object 20′ (6.1 m) away
- Viewing of objects closer than 20′ from the eye (near vision) requires three automatic changes: accommodation, pupillary constriction, and eye convergence
- *Accommodation* (adjustment of the refractory power of the lens) depends on the elasticity of the lens, which is surrounded by a strong capsule attached to suspensory ligaments
  - When the eye is at rest, suspensory ligaments hold the lens under tension, compressing and flattening it
  - During accommodation, the ciliary muscles contract, pulling the suspensory ligaments forward and relaxing their tension on the lens capsule; this makes the lens bulge and become more convex
  - Accommodation increases the refractive power of the eye, necessary for near vision
- *Pupillary constriction* blocks light rays that normally pass through the lens periphery; such rays are refracted more than those passing through the center because the refractive index of the periphery (1.36) is slightly different from that of the center (1.42)
  - Blocking these rays increases the sharpness of the image because all the rays focus more sharply on the retina
  - The pupils also constrict in response to bright light to protect the eyes
- *Convergence* allows an individual to see an object close up with both eyes without seeing double because the two images are focused on corresponding points on the two retinas

Binocular vision

- *Binocular vision* (single vision with two eyes) permits depth or distance perception and creates a larger field of vision
- During convergence, when the image falls at corresponding points on both retinas, each eye views the object from a slightly different angle
- The two slightly different images are relayed to the brain, which synthesizes (fuses) them into a single image; this conveys an impression of depth that the separate retinal images lack

Key characteristics of near vision

- Viewing objects closer than 20′ from the eye is near vision
- Near vision requires three automatic changes: accommodation, pupillary constriction, and eye convergence
- Accommodation depends on elasticity of the lens

Key characteristics of binocular vision

- Binocular vision permits depth or distance perception
- Each eye views the object from a slightly different angle
- The brain fuses this into a single image

EARS AND HEARING

● **Key concepts**
- Ears, the sensory organs for hearing, gather sound waves and transmit them as nerve impulses to the brain; the brain interprets these impulses as hearing
- The auditory apparatus consists of the external, middle, and inner ear (see *Ear structures,* page 170)
  - External ear collects sound
  - Middle ear conducts sound
  - Inner ear contains structures that transmit sound waves and maintain equilibrium

● **Ear structures**
- The ear contains various structures involved in hearing and maintaining equilibrium
- These include the external (outer), middle, and inner ear
- The *external ear* consists of the auricle (pinna) and the external auditory canal
  - The *auricle* is composed of elastic cartilage covered by thin skin; its outer rim is called the *helix*
  - The *external auditory canal,* a narrow chamber about 1″ (2.5 cm) long, connects the auricle with the tympanic membrane
    - The outer portion of the canal is framed by elastic cartilage; the inner portion lies within the temporal bone
    - The skin that lines the external auditory canal contains ceruminous glands; these modified apocrine sweat glands secrete a brown earwax called *cerumen*
- The *middle ear,* or tympanic cavity, is a mucosa-lined structure within the petrous (hard) portion of the temporal bone
  - It's bounded distally by the eardrum (tympanic membrane) and medially by the oval and round windows
    - The *oval window* is a small opening in the wall between the middle and inner ears into which the footpiece of the stapes fits; it transmits vibrations to the inner ear
    - The *round window,* also an opening in the wall between the middle and inner ears, is enclosed by a membrane called the *secondary tympanic membrane;* like the oval window, it transmits vibrations to the inner ear
  - The *eustachian tube* joins the middle ear with the nasopharynx
  - The middle ear contains three small ossicles (bones) called the *malleus* (hammer), *incus* (anvil), and *stapes* (stirrup)
    - The malleus attaches to the tympanic membrane
    - The stapes attaches to the oval window

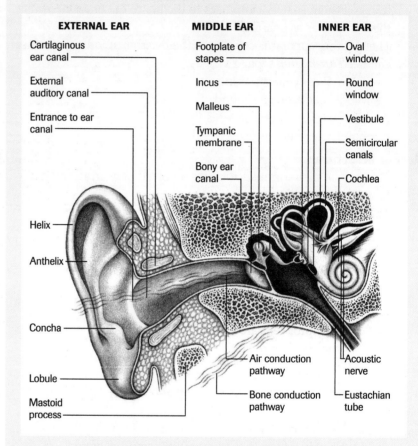

Ear structures

The ear is the organ of hearing. The structures of its three sections—external, middle, and inner—are illustrated below.

EXTERNAL EAR

Cartilaginous ear canal

External auditory canal

Entrance to ear canal

Helix

Anthelix

Concha

Lobule

Mastoid process

MIDDLE EAR

Footplate of stapes

Incus

Malleus

Tympanic membrane

Bony ear canal

Air conduction pathway

Bone conduction pathway

INNER EAR

Oval window

Round window

Vestibule

Semicircular canals

Cochlea

Acoustic nerve

Eustachian tube

Key characteristics of the inner ear

- Located in the temporal bone
- Vestibule serves as an entrance to the inner ear
- Three semicircular canals project from the back of the vestibule
- The cochlea extends from the anterior part of the vestibule

· The incus, located between the malleus and stapes, articulates with these structures during transmission of vibratory motion from the eardrum to the fluid of the inner ear; the vibration excites receptor nerve endings in the inner ear
· Two small muscles attached to the ossicles contract automatically in response to loud noises, dampening the ossicle vibrations that are normally transmitted to the inner ear and protecting the inner ear structures from damage
• The *inner ear*, or osseous (bony) labyrinth, is located in the temporal bone; it consists of the vestibule, semicircular canals, and cochlea
  – The *vestibule* is the central portion; it serves as the entrance to the inner ear and houses the saccule and utricle

- It's posterior to the cochlea and anterior to the semicircular canals
- Laterally, it contains the oval and round windows
- The *saccule* and *utricle* are membranous sacs suspended in a fluid called *perilymph* (similar to cerebrospinal fluid); they sense gravity changes and linear and angular acceleration

  – The three *semicircular canals* project from the posterior aspect of the vestibule
  - Each canal is oriented in one of three planes—superior, posterior, or lateral (horizontal)
  - The *semicircular duct*, which traverses the canals, is continuous with the utricle anteriorly
  - The *crista ampullaris*, located at the end of each canal, contains hair cells and supporting cells; it's stimulated by sudden movements or changes in the rate or direction of movement

  – The *cochlea* is a spiraling, bony cone that extends from the anterior part of the vestibule
  - The *cochlear duct*, located inside the cochlea, is a triangular, membranous structure that houses the *organ of Corti*; this organ contains auditory receptor cells (hair cells), supporting cells, and nerve fibers
    - Receptor cells are embedded in the basilar membrane of the cochlear duct; their free surfaces project into the endolymph of the duct
    - A gelatinous membrane called the *tectorial membrane* overhangs and touches these hair cells; stimulation of these cells causes sound wave transmission
  - The cochlear cavity has three chambers—the *scala vestibuli* and *scala tympani* (which are continuous with each other at the apex and contain perilymph) and the *scala media* (which contains endolymph, a substance similar to intracellular fluid)

Sound wave transmission

- Hearing requires sound wave reception and conduction to the organ of Corti, where waves are converted into nerve impulses; nerve impulses then travel to the auditory area in the cerebral cortex
- Sound waves may arise from any vibration source, such as the vocal cords or a musical instrument
- Sound waves differ in pitch, which reflects the number of cycles (vibrations) per second (CPS); the higher the pitch, the greater the number of CPS
  – The human ear can detect tones as low as 30 CPS and as high as 20,000 CPS

Key facts about sound wave transmission

- Sound waves are converted to nerve impulses at the organ of Corti
- Nerve impulses travel to the auditory center of the cerebral cortex
- Air conduction: external ear funnels sound waves toward the tympanic membrane, which vibrates
- Bone conduction: sound waves pass through the bones of the skull, causing the perilymph and basilar membrane to vibrate

– Ears are most sensitive to sounds ranging from 500 to 4,000 CPS
• Sound waves may travel to the inner ear by vibrations of the tympanic membrane and ossicles (air conduction) or by vibrations of the skull (bone conduction); these skull vibrations bypass the tympanic membrane and ossicles
• In *air conduction*, the external ear funnels sound waves into the ear canal, where they strike the tympanic membrane, causing it to vibrate
  – These vibrations are transmitted through the middle ear to the oval window, which is covered by the footplate of the stapes
    · Because the tympanic membrane has a surface area 20 times greater than that of the oval window, sound waves are concentrated and amplified at the footplate
  – Footplate vibrations travel to the perilymph of the vestibular canal and then into the perilymph of the tympanic canal
  – Each inward movement of the oval window causes a corresponding outward movement of the round window at the base of the tympanic canal, causing waves in the perilymph
  – Perilymph vibrations in the vestibular and tympanic canals set up corresponding vibrations in the basilar membrane of the cochlea duct
    · Basilar membrane vibrations cause the processes of the hair cells in contact with the tectorial membrane to bend, which stimulates these cells; the cells stimulate neurons that synapse on the hair cells
    · Sounds of different frequencies cause vibrations in different parts of the basilar membrane, which stimulate hair cells in different parts of the organ of Corti
  – The cochlear branch of the vestibulocochlear (acoustic) nerve (cranial nerve VIII) collects nerve impulses initiated by stimulated hair cells and transmits them to the brain
• In *bone conduction*, sound waves pass through the bones of the skull and cause perilymph and basilar membrane vibrations, which activate the hair cells in the same way they're activated in air conduction
• Weber's test and the Rinne test evaluate sound conduction; both tests use a tuning fork
  – In Weber's test, a vibrating tuning fork is placed on the patient's forehead at the midline; a patient with conductive hearing loss (loss due to interference with external or middle ear structures) hears sound on the affected side by bone conduction; a patient with sensorineural hearing loss (loss due to damage to inner ear structures, cranial nerve VIII, or temporal lobe) hears sound on the unaffected side

Types of sound conduction

• Air: sound waves in ear canal cause tympanic membrane to vibrate, activating hair cells
• Bone: sound waves pass through skull bones, causing membrane vibrations that activate hair cells

Tests to evaluate sound conduction

• Weber's test: vibrating tuning fork on patient's forehead
• Rinne test: vibrating tuning fork on patient's mastoid process

TIME-OUT FOR TEACHING

Teaching a patient with a hearing loss

When teaching a patient with a hearing loss, make sure you:
- explain sound and hearing loss measurement
- describe the type and possible cause of his hearing loss (conductive, sensorineural, or mixed)
- list common ototoxic substances and their effects on hearing
- prepare him as necessary for Weber's test, the Rinne test, and other diagnostic tests
- describe cerumen removal from the ears
- discuss possible hearing aid use
- prepare him for surgical options, if appropriate, such as stapedectomy and cochlear implant
- discuss hearing loss prevention, including the use of hearing protectors
- give tips to family members to help them communicate with a hearing-impaired person
- provide sources of information and support.

- In the Rinne test, a vibrating tuning fork is placed on the mastoid process; a patient with conductive hearing loss hears sound longer through bone conduction than air conduction, whereas a patient with sensorineural hearing loss hears sound longer through air conduction than bone conduction but in an abnormal ratio
- Patients with either type of hearing loss require education (see *Teaching a patient with a hearing loss*)

● **Sound perception and localization**
- The auditory center in the cerebral cortex interprets the pitch of a sound based on the part of the organ of Corti stimulated by vibrations
- Differences in loudness result from variations in hair cell stimulation; loud sounds stimulate more hair cells, which generate more impulses than soft sounds
- The brain interprets the direction of sound based on slight differences in the arrival time and intensity of the sound in each ear

MAINTAINING EQUILIBRIUM

● **Key concepts**
- The sense of *equilibrium*, or balance, is vital for maintaining stability during movement or at rest
- The vestibular apparatus of the inner ear controls the sense of equilibrium and position

---

Key teaching topics for a patient with hearing loss
- Review possible causes
- Explain Weber's test and the Rinne test
- Discuss hearing aid use
- Provide tips for prevention and effective communication

Key facts about sound perception and localization
- The part of the organ of Corti stimulated determines the pitch of the sound heard
- Number of hair cells stimulated determines loudness
- Perceived direction of sound is determined by arrival time and intensity of the sound

Key facts about equilibrium
- Vestibular apparatus controls sense of equilibrium and position
- The membranous semicircular canals respond to motion
- The utricle and saccule convey a sense of head position
- Loss of equilibrium may result from a nervous system disorder or an ear disorder

● **Structures**
- The *vestibular apparatus* consists of the membranous semicircular canals, which respond to motion, and the *utricle* and the *saccule*, which respond to position changes
- The three tubes of the semicircular canals are connected to the utricle; each tube lies at right angles to the other two
    - One end of each semicircular canal expands slightly where it joins the utricle and contains groups of specialized receptors called *hair cells* as well as supporting cells
        · These hair cells are similar to those in the organ of Corti
        · They're covered by gelatinous material called *cupula*
        · Endolymph movement in the semicircular canals during body movement stimulates them
    - These hair cells transmit nerve impulses over the vestibular branch of the vestibulocochlear (acoustic) nerve to the medulla, where they're interpreted as motion; impulses also travel to the cerebellum, where they initiate reflex movements of body and eye muscles
- The utricle and saccule convey a sense of head position to the brain by sending impulses to the cerebellum through the vestibulocochlear (acoustic) nerve
    - The utricle and saccule are filled with endolymph and contain hair cells; the free ends of the hair cells are embedded in a mass of gelatinous material, which contains calcium carbonate crystals called *otoliths*
    - Gravity presses on the otoliths and the cilia of the hair cells, stimulating nerve impulses that the brain interprets as the normal head position
    - During head movement, the weight of the otoliths shifts and the cilia bend, transmitting nerve impulses that the brain perceives as a change in head position
    - The impulses also initiate automatic reflex reactions that restore the head to its normal position

● **Equilibrium disorders**
- Loss of equilibrium may result from a nervous system disorder, such as acoustic neuroma or multiple sclerosis
- Ear disorders, such as labyrinthitis or Ménière's disease, can also cause a loss of equilibrium

NOSE AND SMELL

● **Key concepts**
- *Olfactory receptors* are specialized neurons with dendrites modified to respond to odors

Key facts about the nose and smell

- Olfactory receptors in the roof of the nasal cavity relay impulses responsible for smell
- Cavity also contains pain receptors, which respond to chemicals
- Air must pass through the nose to stimulate receptors
- Olfactory receptors have a life-span of 60 days

• Located in the roof of the nasal cavity, these receptors relay impulses to the olfactory bulbs in the cranial cavity, which transmit impulses to the cortical neurons that perceive odor

● **Nose structures**
• The nose contains olfactory (smell) receptors, located in the mucosal epithelium that lines the upper part of the nasal cavity
• This cavity also contains pain receptors; because pain receptors respond to chemicals (such as ammonia), they're sometimes confused with olfactory receptors
• Olfactory receptors are bipolar neurons
    – Each olfactory receptor has a dendrite that terminates in several long cilia called *olfactory hairs*
    – Olfactory hairs convey mucus, secreted by the mucosa, back to the nasopharynx
• Olfactory receptors have a life span of 60 days

● **Sensation of smell**
• Air must pass through the nose to stimulate the olfactory receptors
• A person can't smell if mucus, polyps, or other substances block the nostrils because no air can enter the nose to stimulate the olfactory receptors
• Olfactory receptors are sensitive to very low concentrations of odors, but they rapidly adapt to odors
    – After smelling an odor for a short time, a person no longer perceives it as intensely
    – This loss of odor sensitivity results from reduced responsiveness of the olfactory receptors and diminished perception of the odor in the olfactory portion of the cerebral cortex
    – The cerebral cortex stores memories of odors; after smelling an odor once, a person can recognize the odor readily if it occurs again

TASTE BUDS AND TASTE

● **Key concepts**
• Taste receptors are located in the taste buds in the mouth
• Taste buds are oval bodies that contain three types of epithelial cells—supporting, taste receptor, and basal cells
• Cranial nerves VII (facial), IX (glossopharyngeal), and X (vagus) conduct taste sensations to the brain, which perceives taste

● **Mouth structures**
• The tongue has the greatest concentration of taste receptors, but they also exist in the soft palate and throat

Key facts about taste buds and taste

• Taste receptors are on the tongue, soft palate, and throat
• Each taste of sweet, sour, bitter, and salt has its own receptor
• Substance must be in saliva solution for taste to occur

- The mouth has four types of taste receptors; each type can sense one of four basic tastes: sweet, sour, bitter, and salt
  - Tip of the tongue perceives sweet tastes
  - Sides of the tongue detect sour tastes
  - Back of the tongue detects bitter tastes
  - Tip and sides of the tongue perceive salty tastes

Taste sensation
- For taste to occur, substances must be in solution in saliva
- Taste perception results from both taste bud stimulation and olfactory receptor stimulation from the air passage through the nose
- Smell, texture, and temperature contribute to the perception of taste
- If the sense of smell isn't functioning properly—for example, if a person has a congested nose because of a cold—taste perception may be diminished or unusual

GENERAL SENSES

Key concepts
- General senses include touch, pressure, temperature, and pain
- Receptors for these senses are distributed widely throughout the skin and other body tissues
- Because the number of receptors for each general sense varies widely, body parts aren't equally sensitive to stimulation

Touch and pressure
- Receptors for these sensations lie in nerve endings around hair follicles and in the papillary layer of the skin
- When stimulated, these receptors transmit a nerve impulse along the cranial nerve to the brain, or along a spinal nerve to the spinal cord and then to the brain
- In the brain, the general sensory area located behind the central fissure interprets these impulses as touch or pressure

Temperature
- Cold receptors lie near the surface of the skin
- Heat receptors lie deep in the skin
- When stimulated, these receptors transmit a nerve impulse by the same transmission route as that of touch and pressure receptors
- The brain perceives and interprets these impulses similar to the way it does for touch and pressure

Pain
- Pain receptors are located throughout the body in the skin, muscles, tendons, and joints

Key characteristics of touch and pressure receptors
- Located in nerve endings around hair follicles and in papillary layer of the skin
- Transmit an impulse along the cranial or spinal nerve to the brain

Key characteristics of temperature receptors
- Cold receptors lie near skin surface
- Heat receptors lie deep in skin

- Pain serves a protective function by alerting a person to withdraw from a harmful stimulus; loss of the ability to feel pain makes a person more vulnerable to injury
- Pain impulses travel along myelinated and unmyelinated nerve fibers by the same transmission route as the other general senses
  - The brain perceives impulses conducted rapidly by myelinated fibers as sharp pain
  - The brain perceives impulses conducted more slowly by unmyelinated fibers as dull, aching pain
- Different types of pain result from stimulation of different areas
  - Pain in the skin, subcutaneous tissues, muscles, bones, and joints is called *somatic pain*
  - Pain in the internal organs (from distention, smooth-muscle spasm, or inadequate blood supply) is called *visceral pain*
  - Internal organ pain that seems to come from the body surface at a distant site is called *referred pain;* for example, a person may feel the pain of a myocardial infarction (MI) in the neck
    · Referred pain occurs because pain impulses from receptors in an internal organ enter the same part of the spinal cord as impulses from somatic pain receptors on the body's surface
    · The pain impulses then pass along pain pathways in the spinal cord to the brain
    · The brain misinterprets these sensations as coming from the pain receptors on the body surface rather than from those in the internal organ

NCLEX CHECKS

It's never too soon to begin your NCLEX preparation. Now that you've reviewed this chapter, carefully read each of the following questions and choose the best answer. Then compare your responses with the correct answers.

1. When caring for a client with a detached retina, the nurse explains that the visual receptors of the retina are composed of which structures?
- ☐ **1.** Pupils and lens
- ☐ **2.** Conjunctiva and lacrimal glands
- ☐ **3.** Vitreous humor and aqueous humor
- ☐ **4.** Rods and cones

2. The nurse is examining a client's external ear. Which structures is the nurse examining?
- ☐ **1.** Vestibule, cochlea, and semicircular canals
- ☐ **2.** Tympanic membrane, oval window, and round window
- ☐ **3.** Auricle and external auditory canal
- ☐ **4.** Malleus, incus, and stapes

Key characteristics of pain receptors

- Located in skin, muscles, tendons, and joints
- Pain helps protect against harm
- Different types of pain result from stimulation of different areas

TOP 10

Items to study for your next test on the sensory system

1. Structures of the eye
2. Aqueous humor formation and circulation
3. Light refraction and image formation
4. Visual pathways
5. Structures of the ear
6. Comparison of bone and air conduction
7. Structures of the nose related to sense of smell
8. Taste sensation
9. Location and function of general sense receptors
10. Teaching tips for patients with retinal detachment or hearing loss

3. When an elderly client comes to the clinic complaining of hearing loss, the nurse performs Weber's test to assess his ability to hear. Which actions would the nurse perform? Select all that apply.

- ☐ **1.** Place a vibrating tuning fork on the mastoid process.
- ☐ **2.** Place a vibrating tuning fork on the midline of the forehead.
- ☐ **3.** Ask the client on which side he hears the sound.
- ☐ **4.** Ask the client how long he hears the sound.
- ☐ **5.** Ask the client to identify when he hears a whispered voice.
- ☐ **6.** Examine the tympanic membrane with an otoscope.

4. When assessing a client's vision, the nurse should keep which fact in mind?

- ☐ **1.** The right half of each retina receives input from the right visual field.
- ☐ **2.** The left half of each retina receives input from the right visual field.
- ☐ **3.** The right optic tract contains nerve fibers from the left half of each retina.
- ☐ **4.** The left optic tract contains nerve fibers from the right half of each retina.

5. During an eye examination, a client asks the nurse why he can see a near object without seeing double. What does the nurse explain that this is called?

- ☐ **1.** Accommodation
- ☐ **2.** Pupillary constriction
- ☐ **3.** Convergence
- ☐ **4.** Binocular vision

6. During the admission history, a client tells the nurse that he has equilibrium problems. The nurse understands that this most likely involves which structure?

- ☐ **1.** Oval window
- ☐ **2.** Ossicles
- ☐ **3.** Organ of Corti
- ☐ **4.** Semicircular canals

7. A client with a nasal polyp tells the nurse that he can't smell odors. The nurse explains that he can't detect odors because the polyp has:

- ☐ **1.** blocked air from entering the nose.
- ☐ **2.** blocked the olfactory receptors.
- ☐ **3.** reduced the odor sensitivity of the olfactory receptors.
- ☐ **4.** reduced the effectiveness of olfactory hairs.

8. Which cranial nerves would the nurse test to assess the client's ability to perceive taste?

☐ **1.** VII, IX, X
☐ **2.** I, IV, V
☐ **3.** II, III, XII
☐ **4.** VI, VIII, XI

9. If a client has a lesion on the tip of his tongue, the nurse knows that which taste sensation will most likely be affected?

☐ **1.** Salty
☐ **2.** Bitter
☐ **3.** Sour
☐ **4.** Sweet

10. A client arrives in the emergency department with chest pain. When the nurse asks whether the pain is radiating to the shoulder, neck, or jaw, which type of pain is being assessed?

☐ **1.** Somatic
☐ **2.** Visceral
☐ **3.** Referred
☐ **4.** Sharp

ANSWERS AND RATIONALES

1. CORRECT ANSWER: 4

Photoreceptor neurons called *rods* and *cones* compose the visual receptors of the retina. The lens adjusts to focus for near and far vision. The pupil is a circular opening in the iris through which light passes. The conjunctiva is the thin vascular membrane that lines the inner surface of the eyelids and sclera. The lacrimal glands discharge fluid secretions to moisten the conjunctiva. The vitreous humor is a thick, gelatinous fluid in the posterior cavity. The aqueous humor is a clear, watery fluid found in the anterior and posterior chambers.

2. CORRECT ANSWER: 3

The auricle and external auditory canal are part of the external ear. The vestibule, cochlea, and semicircular canals are in the inner ear. The tympanic membrane, oval window, and round window are structures of the middle ear. The malleus, incus, and stapes are found in the middle ear.

3. CORRECT ANSWER: 1, 3

The nurse performs Weber's test by placing a vibrating tuning fork on the midline of the client's forehead. The nurse then asks the client on which side he hears sound. A person with conductive hearing loss hears sound on the affected side by bone conduction; someone with a sensorineural hearing loss hears sound on the unaffected side. During the Rinne test, the nurse would place a vibrating tuning fork on the mastoid process and ask the client how long he hears the sound. A person with conductive hearing loss hears sound longer through bone conduction than air conduction; someone with sensorineural hearing loss hears sound longer through air conduction than bone conduction but in an abnormal ratio. A whispered test and an otoscopic examination aren't part of Weber's test.

4. CORRECT ANSWER: 2

Each half of the retina receives visual input from the opposite visual field so that the right half of each retina receives input from the left visual field and the left half of each retina receives input from the right visual field. Each half of the retina receives an image of objects from the visual field on the opposite side. As a result, the right optic tract contains nerve fibers from the right half of each retina and the left optic tract contains nerve fibers from the left half of each retina.

5. CORRECT ANSWER: 3

Convergence allows a person to see an object up close with both eyes without seeing double because the two images are focused on corresponding points on the two retinas. Accommodation increases the refractive power of the eye, which is necessary for near vision. Pupillary constriction blocks light rays that normally pass through the lens periphery; such rays are refracted more than those passing through the center because the refractive index at the periphery is slightly different than that at the center. Blocking these rays increases the sharpness of the image because all rays are focused more sharply on the retina. Binocular vision permits depth perception and creates a larger field of vision.

6. CORRECT ANSWER: 4

The vestibular apparatus of the inner ear controls the sense of equilibrium and position. The vestibular apparatus consists of the semicircular canals, which respond to motion, as well as the utricle and the saccule, which respond to position changes. The oval window is a small opening in the wall between the middle and inner ears that the footpiece of the stapes fits into; it transmits vibrations to the inner ear. The middle ear contains three small ossicles: the malleus, incus, and stapes. Sound waves travel to the tympanic membrane, setting up vibrations that are transmitted through the ossicles to the oval window. The organ of Corti, in the inner ear, contains auditory receptor cells (hair cells), supporting cells, and nerve fibers.

7. CORRECT ANSWER: 1

The client can't detect odors if polyps block his nostrils because no air can enter his nose to stimulate the olfactory receptors. Reduced odor sensitivity occurs after smelling an odor for a short time. This loss of odor sensitivity results from reduced responsiveness of the olfactory receptors and diminished perception of the odor in the olfactory portion of the cerebral cortex. Olfactory hairs don't play a role in the sensation of smell; they convey mucus secreted by the mucosa to the nasopharynx.

8. CORRECT ANSWER: 1
Cranial nerves VII (facial), IX (glossopharyngeal), and X (vagus) conduct taste sensation to the brain. Cranial nerve VII is also involved in expressions of the forehead, eye, and mouth. Cranial nerve IX also provides swallowing and salivation. Cranial nerve X also controls swallowing, the gag reflex, talking, activities of the thoracic and abdominal viscera, and the sensations of the throat, larynx, and abdominal viscera. Cranial nerve I provides a sense of smell; II provides vision; III provides eye movement, papillary constriction, and upper eyelid elevation; V is involved with chewing, corneal reflex, and face and scalp sensations; VI provides lateral eye movement; VIII provides hearing and equilibrium; XI provides shoulder movement and head rotation; and XII provides tongue movement.

9. CORRECT ANSWER: 4
Sweet tastes are perceived on the tip of the tongue. The tip and sides of the tongue perceive salty tastes. The back of the tongue perceives bitter tastes. The sides of the tongue perceive sour tastes.

10. CORRECT ANSWER: 3
Internal organ pain that seems to come from the body surface at a distant site is called referred pain—for example, a client may feel the pain of an MI in the neck, shoulder, or jaw. Pain in the skin, subcutaneous tissues, muscles, bones, and joints is called somatic pain. Pain in the internal organs is called visceral pain. Sharp pain is perceived when impulses are conducted rapidly by myelinated fibers.

Cardiovascular system

LEARNING OBJECTIVES

After studying this chapter, you should be able to:

- Identify the structures and functions of the heart.
- Describe the events of the cardiac cycle.
- Explain the cardiac conduction system.
- Describe the three types of blood vessels.
- Trace the flow of blood through the heart and the systemic and pulmonary circulatory systems of the adult and fetus.
- Understand blood pressure and cardiac output and the factors that affect them.
- Explain factors that affect fluid movement between the capillaries and the interstitium.

CHAPTER OVERVIEW

In the cardiovascular system, the heart pumps constantly refreshed blood through thousands of miles of blood vessels, delivering nutrients to cells and removing their wastes. To provide comprehensive cardiovascular care, the nurse must recognize the structures of the heart and blood vessels as well as understand the cardiac cycle, cardiac conduction system, various types of circulation, and the regulation of blood pressure and cardiac output. This chapter reviews heart structures, the cardiac cycle, electrical conduction, blood vessels, circulation, blood pressure and its regulation, cardiac output, and fluid movement between the capillaries and interstitium.

CARDIOVASCULAR OVERVIEW

- **Key concepts**
  - Sometimes called the *circulatory system,* the cardiovascular system consists of the heart, blood vessels, and lymphatics
  - It works to bring necessary oxygen and nutrients to the body's cells, remove metabolic waste products, and carry hormones from one body part to another
- **Cardiac structures**
  - Major structures include the heart and blood vessels
  - The heart pumps blood through the blood vessels
  - Blood vessels include arteries, arterioles, capillaries, venules, and veins
- **Cardiovascular system functions**
  - The *cardiovascular system* moves blood and oxygen throughout the body
  - It helps maintain proper body pH and electrolyte composition and regulate body temperature

HEART STRUCTURE

- **Key concepts**
  - The heart is a hollow, fist-size, muscular organ located slightly to the left of the body's midline in the mediastinum, between the second rib and fifth intercostal space
  - A physiologic pump, the heart moves the body's entire volume of blood to and from lungs (*pulmonary circulation*) and to and from tissues (*systemic circulation*)
  - It acts as two separate pumps
    - The right side acts as a pulmonary pump, moving blood into the lungs
    - The left side acts as a systemic pump, moving blood to the rest of the body
- **Pericardium**
  - The *pericardium* is a fibroserous sac that encases the heart (see *Layers of the heart and pericardium,* page 184)
  - It has two portions
    - The fibrous pericardium is the outer portion

Key structures of the cardiovascular system

- Heart
- Arteries
- Arterioles
- Capillaries
- Venules
- Veins
- Lymphatics

Key facts about the heart

- Acts as a pump, moving the body's entire volume of blood
- Right side moves blood into the lungs
- Left side moves blood to the rest of the body

Key characteristics of the pericardium

- Fibroserous sac that encases the heart
- Fibrous pericardium is outer portion
- Serous pericardium is inner portion
- Pericardial space separates parietal and visceral layers of serous pericardium

Layers of the heart and pericardium

The heart wall and its surrounding pericardial sac consist of several layers, as shown here.

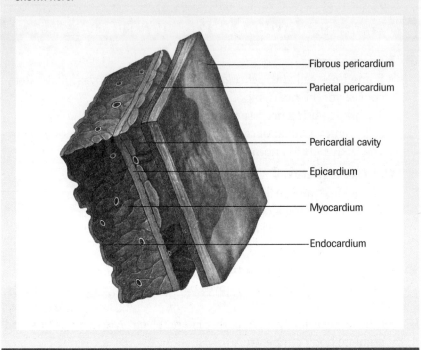

- Fibrous pericardium
- Parietal pericardium
- Pericardial cavity
- Epicardium
- Myocardium
- Endocardium

Key heart wall structures

- Epicardium: outer layer
- Myocardium: middle layer
- Endocardium: innermost layer

- Composed of tough, white, fibrous tissue, it fits loosely around the heart and is relatively inelastic
- It protects the underlying serous membrane and heart
  - The thin, smooth *serous pericardium* is the inner portion; it's composed of two layers
    - The *parietal layer* lines the inside of the fibrous pericardium
    - The *visceral layer* (epicardium) adheres to heart's outer surface
- The *pericardial space* separates parietal and visceral layers of serous pericardium; it contains serous fluid, which lubricates surface layers and aids heart movement during contraction
- *Pericarditis* (inflammation of the pericardium) typically stems from infection, connective tissue disorders, or radiation therapy
  - Inflammation causes loss of fluid from the pericardial space
  - This lets the heart muscle rub against the pericardium as it beats, causing a friction rub

● **Heart wall**
- The heart wall has three distinct tissue layers
- The *epicardium* is the outer layer

- It's composed of a sheet of squamous epithelial cells overlying connective tissue
- It's the visceral layer of the pericardium
- The *myocardium* is the middle layer
  - This muscular layer makes up the bulk of the heart wall
  - Thick and contractile, the myocardium has unique striated muscle fibers that cause the heart to contract
- The *endocardium* is the innermost layer
  - It consists of endothelial tissue
  - Small blood vessels and several bundles of smooth muscle also compose this layer

● **Heart chambers**
- The heart has two upper and two lower chambers (see *Structures and vessels of the heart*)
- Upper chambers are the *left atrium* and *right atrium*
  - Atria are separated by the *interatrial septum*
  - They receive blood returning to the heart
  - They pump blood only to lower chambers of the heart

Structures and vessels of the heart

This illustration shows a cross-sectional view of the heart's structures.

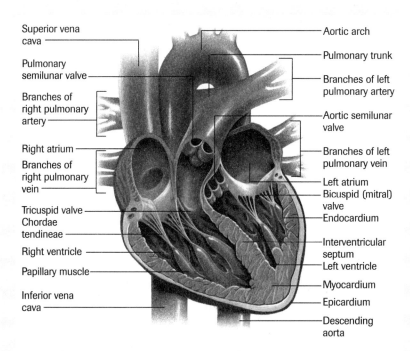

Superior vena cava
Pulmonary semilunar valve
Branches of right pulmonary artery
Right atrium
Branches of right pulmonary vein
Tricuspid valve
Chordae tendineae
Right ventricle
Papillary muscle
Inferior vena cava

Aortic arch
Pulmonary trunk
Branches of left pulmonary artery
Aortic semilunar valve
Branches of left pulmonary vein
Left atrium
Bicuspid (mitral) valve
Endocardium
Interventricular septum
Left ventricle
Myocardium
Epicardium
Descending aorta

- Lower chambers are the *left ventricle* and *right ventricle*
  - Ventricles are separated by the interventricular septum
  - They're larger and thicker-walled than atria; the left ventricle has thicker walls than the right ventricle
  - Composed of highly developed musculature, they receive blood from atria
  - Right ventricle pumps blood to and from lungs
  - Left ventricle pumps blood through all other vessels of the body
- Valves separate cardiac chambers from the bases of the aorta and pulmonary artery; they permit blood to flow in one direction only— away from the heart
- Each side of the heart pumps blood through a different branch of the circulatory system
  - Right atrium and ventricle pump blood through the pulmonary circulation
  - Left atrium and ventricle pump blood through the systemic circulation
  - The muscular walls of the left ventricle are thicker than those of the right ventricle because it pumps blood through the systemic circulation at a much higher pressure than that of the pulmonary circulation
- Right and left coronary arteries supply blood to the heart muscle; these arteries arise separately from the part of the aortic wall that's attached to the cusps of the aortic semilunar valves
- The cardiac conduction system sends impulses through the heart muscle to cause synchronized contractions of atria and ventricles, which pump blood throughout the body

CARDIAC CYCLE

● **Key concepts**
- Impulses generated by the conduction system cause synchronized contractions of atria and ventricles (see *Events in the cardiac cycle*)
- Each cardiac contraction (systole) is followed by a period of relaxation (diastole); atria and ventricles dilate during their respective diastoles
  - Atria and ventricles contract and relax in sequence
    · *Atrial systole* refers to atrial muscle contraction; *atrial diastole* refers to relaxation
    · *Ventricular systole* refers to ventricular muscle contraction; *ventricular diastole* refers to relaxation
  - When used without reference to a specific cardiac chamber, the terms systole and diastole refer to ventricular systole and diastole

Key facts about the cardiac cycle

- The conduction system generates impulses, causing the atria and ventricles to contract
- Each cardiac contraction (systole) is followed by a period of relaxation (diastole)

Events in the cardiac cycle

The cardiac cycle consists of the following five events.

1. ISOVOLUMETRIC VENTRICULAR CONTRACTION–In response to ventricular depolarization, tension in the ventricles increases. This rise in pressure within the ventricles leads to closure of the mitral and tricuspid valves. The pulmonic and aortic valves stay closed during the entire phase.

2. VENTRICULAR EJECTION– When ventricular pressure exceeds aortic and pulmonary arterial pressure, the aortic and pulmonic valves open and the ventricles eject blood.

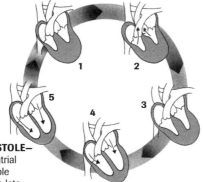

3. ISOVOLUMETRIC RELAXATION– When ventricular pressure falls below the pressure in the aorta and pulmonary artery, the aortic and pulmonic valves close. All valves are closed during this phase. Atrial diastole occurs as blood fills the atria.

4. VENTRICULAR FILLING– Atrial pressure exceeds ventricular pressure, which causes the mitral and tricuspid valves to open. Blood then flows passively into the ventricles. About 70% of ventricular filling takes place during this phase.

5. ATRIAL SYSTOLE– Known as the atrial kick, atrial systole (coinciding with late ventricular diastole) supplies the ventricles with the remaining 30% of the blood for each heartbeat.

– Events occurring during a single systole and diastole of atria and ventricles make up the cardiac cycle
- Actions during the cardiac cycle cause certain characteristic heart sounds and a palpable pulse

● **Systole and diastole**
- When atria contract, ventricles relax
  – Atrioventricular (AV) valves (valves between atrial and ventricular chambers) open during atrial systole
  – Atria eject blood into the ventricles through open AV valves
- When atria relax, ventricles contract
  – Ventricular contraction exerts pressure on the blood in the ventricles, increasing the intraventricular pressure
  – Rising pressure forces the AV valves to close, preventing blood from flowing backward into the atria
  – For a short time after AV valves close, intraventricular pressure isn't high enough to force the *semilunar valves* (valves between

Key characteristics of heart valves

- AV valves reside between the atria and ventricles
- AV valves open during atrial contraction
- AV valves close to prevent back-flow of blood into the atria
- Semilunar valves are between the ventricles and the aorta and pulmonary artery
- Semilunar valves open during ventricular contraction
- After contraction, semilunar valves close

Key facts about heart sounds

- Vibrations from AV valve closure cause an S_1
- Vibrations from the semilunar valve closure cause an S_2

the heart and the aorta and pulmonary artery) open; during this time, ventricles are completely closed chambers

  – Continued ventricular contraction increases intraventricular pressure until it exceeds the pressure of blood in the aorta and pulmonary artery

  – Increased intraventricular pressure forces open semilunar valves and ejects blood from ventricles

- While ventricles contract, venous blood from the systemic and pulmonary circulations flows into the relaxed atria

  – Blood stays in the atria because the AV valves are closed during ventricular systole

  – As blood fills the atria, intra-atrial pressure rises slightly

- Pressure in the aorta and pulmonary artery peaks during ventricular systole as ventricles eject blood, which distends these vessels

- After expelling blood, ventricles relax

  – Blood ejected from ventricles into the aorta and pulmonary artery loses its forward momentum caused by the force of ventricular contraction

    • Loss of momentum causes blood to flow back toward ventricles

    • Blood fills the cup-shaped cusps of semilunar valves, forcing the valves shut and preventing blood from refluxing into the ventricles; this maintains high pressure in the aorta and pulmonary artery

    • Stretched walls of the aorta and pulmonary artery return to their former dimensions by the end of ventricular diastole; this elastic recoil compresses the blood and maintains pressure on it, causing it to continue moving through blood vessels in intervals between ventricular contractions

  – Ventricular pressure falls during ventricular diastole; eventually, it falls below intra-atrial pressure

    • When this happens, AV valves open, allowing accumulated blood in the atria to flow into the ventricles

    • Such pressure changes also occur in the right ventricle and pulmonary artery, but with much lower pressures than in the left ventricle and aorta

- Events of the cardiac cycle repeat with each heartbeat

● Heart sounds

- Each cardiac cycle, or heartbeat, has characteristic heart sounds (*lubdub* followed by a pause)

- Placing an ear or a stethoscope against the chest allows these sounds to be heard

  – The *lub* results from vibrations caused by AV valve closure during ventricular systole; this produces the first heart sound (S_1) (see *Why we hear an S_1*)

Why we hear an S$_1$

The first heart sound (S$_1$) is linked with closure of the mitral and tricuspid valves (shown here) as well as with vibration of the ventricle walls as a result of increasing pressure.

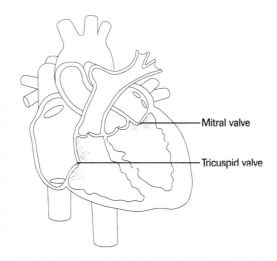

Mitral valve

Tricuspid valve

– The *dub* results from vibrations caused by semilunar valve closure during ventricular diastole; this produces the second heart sound (S$_2$) (see *Why we hear an S$_2$*)
– The pause is the interval between successive cardiac contractions

● **Pulse**
  • For a normally contracting heart, pulse assessment allows heart rate measurement; the *pulse rate* is typically assessed in a large artery

Why we hear an S$_2$

The second heart sound (S$_2$) is linked with closure of the pulmonic and aortic valves (shown here).

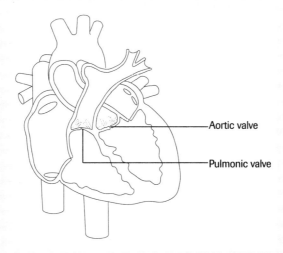

Aortic valve

Pulmonic valve

Key characteristics of the pulse

- Ventricular ejection causes a shock wave, producing a pulse
- The pulse rate is assessed by palpating a large artery

Key facts about cardiac electrical conduction

- Certain cardiac muscle cells are specialized to conduct electrical impulses
- Muscle fibers are polarized: positive charges outside balance negative charges inside
- Electrical impulse causes fibers to depolarize, resulting in contraction

Key components of the conduction system

- SA node: the heart's pacemaker
- AV node: electrical bridge between atria and ventricles
- Bundle of His: spreads an impulse from the AV node down the interventricular septum
- Purkinje fibers: connect the branches of the bundle of His to the ventricular walls

- The pulse is produced by a shock wave from ventricular ejection of blood into the aorta; this shock wave is transmitted through the walls of large arteries, like the vibrations transmitted along a metal pipe struck by a hammer
- The pulse rate is assessed by palpating an artery lying near the body's surface over a bone or other firm tissue and counting the number of pulsations felt in 1 minute

CARDIAC ELECTRICAL CONDUCTION

Key concepts
- The conduction system controls the heartbeat
- It consists of various structures composed of cardiac muscle cells specialized to conduct electrical impulses
- Cardiac muscle fibers are polarized; positive charges outside the fibers are balanced by negative charges inside
- The electrical impulse that causes heart contraction (systole) spreads as a wave through the cardiac muscle; it causes activated areas of the fibers to accumulate negative charges on the outside and positive charges on the inside (depolarization)
- During diastole, cell membranes repolarize, with positive charges on cell surfaces restored and cell interiors again accumulating negative charges

Conduction system
- The heart contains a specialized system of nodal tissue for generating and conducting impulses that cause rhythmic contractions
- The conduction system consists of nodal tissue that contains few myofibrils
- Four main components make up the conduction system: the sinoatrial (SA) node and internodal tracts, AV node, bundle of His, and Purkinje fibers
  – The *SA node* is located in the posterior wall of the right atrium near the opening of the superior vena cava
    · It serves as the heart's pacemaker
    · It initiates depolarization waves that set the pace of cardiac contraction (*sinus rhythm*)
    · Rhythmic impulses are conducted to the AV node by small bundles of fibers called *internodal tracts*
  – The *AV node* is located in the lower right interatrial septum, near the tricuspid valve (one of the AV valves)
    · It acts as an electrical bridge between atria and ventricles, receiving and passing on impulses from the SA node
    · Impulses slow in the AV node, allowing atria to contract and ventricles to fill with blood

· From the AV node, depolarization waves pass rapidly to the AV bundle (bundle of His), bundle branches, and Purkinje fibers, a network of muscle fibers spreading through the ventricular myocardium

– The *Bundle of His* originates in the AV node and divides into right and left bundle branches

· Branches extend down right and left sides of the interventricular septum

· The impulse from the AV node continues through the bundle of His to the right and left bundle branches, ensuring excitation of AV septal cells

– *Purkinje fibers* connect the right and left bundle branches to the papillary muscles and lateral walls of ventricles; fibers are more elaborate in the left ventricle than in the right

· The impulse moves through the Purkinje fibers, eventually reaching ventricular muscles

· Ventricular muscle stimulation begins in the intraventricular septum and moves downward, causing ventricular depolarization and contraction (see *Cardiac conduction route*)

Cardiac conduction route

In the cardiac conduction system, the impulse begins in the sinoatrial (SA) node, travels through the heart chambers, and reaches ventricular muscle. This illustration traces the conduction route through these cardiac structures.

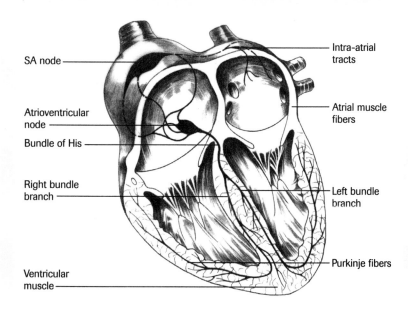

SA node

Atrioventricular node

Bundle of His

Right bundle branch

Ventricular muscle

Intra-atrial tracts

Atrial muscle fibers

Left bundle branch

Purkinje fibers

Key components of an ECG tracing

- P wave: reflects initial depolarizing wave in atrial systole
- QRS complex: reflects impulse transmission leading to ventricular systole
- T wave: reflects ventricular repolarization during diastole
- PR interval: reflects the time from the beginning of the P wave to the beginning of the QRS complex
- ST segment: reflects the time from the end of the S wave to the beginning of the T wave

Characteristic PQRST patterns

Electrocardiogram wave patterns are identified by letters; each waveform corresponds to specific electrical events in the cardiac cycle.
- The P wave reflects the initial wave of depolarization associated with atrial systole.
- The Q, R, and S waves (collectively called the QRS complex) reflect impulse transmission through the right and left bundles into the terminal branches, leading to ventricular systole.
- The T wave indicates ventricular repolarization during diastole.
- The PR interval (the time from the beginning of the P wave to the beginning of the QRS complex) represents the time needed for an impulse to pass from the atria to the ventricles through the bundle of His.
- The ST segment (the time from the end of the S wave to the beginning of the T wave) represents the time between the end of the spread of the impulse through the ventricle and repolarization of the ventricle.

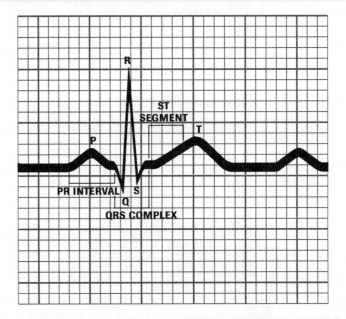

ECG tracings
- The *electrocardiogram (ECG)* traces serial changes in electrical conduction associated with depolarization and repolarization of cardiac muscle fibers
- Changes are recorded as a series of positive and negative deflections, commonly called *waveforms,* which produce characteristic patterns (see *Characteristic PQRST patterns*)

TIME-OUT FOR TEACHING

Teaching a patient with an arrhythmia

When teaching a patient with an arrhythmia, make sure you:
- explain normal cardiac conduction
- describe his specific arrhythmia
- discuss diagnostic tests he might undergo, such as an electrocardiogram and electrolyte levels
- instruct him about appropriate activities such as regular moderate exercise
- help him understand dietary changes, such as increasing potassium intake and moderating alcohol and caffeine use
- describe medications such as antiarrhythmic drugs
- prepare him as necessary for treatments, such as pacemaker implantation or electrocardioversion
- provide guidelines as needed on how to use and maintain a pacemaker or automatic implantable cardioverter-defibrillator
- show him how to take his pulse
- provide sources of information and support.

- An ECG can detect arrhythmias (abnormal heart rate or rhythm), which result from any disruption of normal conduction (see *Teaching a patient with an arrhythmia*)

BLOOD VESSELS

● **Key concepts**
  - *Blood vessels* are tubules that convey blood between the heart and every functioning cell in the body
  - Three main types include arteries, veins, and capillaries
    - *Arteries* give rise to smaller vessels called *arterioles*
    - *Veins* give rise to smaller vessels called *venules*
    - Arterioles and venules decrease in size to become *capillaries*

● **Arteries**
  - These large vessels carry blood from the heart to lungs and tissues
  - Their three-layered walls are thicker than those of veins and capillaries
    - The *tunica adventitia* is the outer wall layer
    - The *tunica media* is the thick middle layer
    - The *tunica intima* is the inner layer
  - Large arteries close to the heart are called *elastic arteries* because their tunica media contains more elastic fibers than those of other arteries

- Medium and small arteries branching from large arteries are called *muscular arteries*
  – The tunica media of these arteries contains more smooth-muscle and fewer elastic fibers than those of large arteries
  – These arteries are also called *distributing arteries* because they distribute blood to various organs
- Arteries have low vascular resistance to blood flow; mean arterial pressure (average of diastolic and systolic pressures) remains around 100 mm Hg
- *Arterioles,* the smallest arteries, lie between arteries and capillaries
  – Walls consist mainly of muscle; they have the same three layers as arteries but are smaller in diameter
  – Contraction of arteriolar muscle helps control the flow of blood into capillaries
  – Arterioles have lower intravascular pressure than arteries; mean pressure is about 85 mm Hg

● **Veins**
- The body's largest vessels, *veins* transport blood from lungs and tissues to the heart
- Walls are composed of a tunica adventitia, tunica media, and tunica intima, like arteries; however, the vein's tunica media is much thinner than that of an artery
- Veins have valves composed of tunica intima that prevent backflow of blood away from the heart
- The superior and inferior venae cavae are the main tributaries that collect venous blood for return to the heart
- Mean venous pressure is less than 15 mm Hg
- *Venules,* the smallest veins, carry blood from capillaries to veins
  – The smallest venules have only a tunica intima and tunica adventitia
  – In some larger venules, the tunica media contains spiraling smooth-muscle fibers
  – Blood pressure is only about 15 mm Hg when blood begins to return to the heart

● **Capillaries**
- Microscopic vessels, *capillaries* connect arterioles with venules to form a network throughout the body
- Walls are extremely thin, consisting only of tunica intima
  – In some cases, they consist of only a single endothelial cell
  – Capillary walls serve as the exchange site for various substances between blood and tissue cells
- Vascular resistance to blood flow is very low in capillaries; mean pressure is about 35 mm Hg

Key characteristics of veins
- Veins transport blood from the lungs and tissues to the heart
- Veins have valves that prevent backflow
- Superior and inferior venae cavae collect venous blood for return to the heart

Key characteristics of capillaries
- Microscopic vessels
- Connect arterioles with venules
- Capillary walls serve as the exchange site for substances between blood and tissues

CIRCULATION

● **Key concepts**
  - The cardiovascular system includes the cardiac, pulmonary, systemic, and hepatic circulation
  - In pregnant women, it also includes fetal circulation

● **Cardiac circulation**
  - Blood enters the right atrium of the heart through the superior vena cava, inferior vena cava, and coronary sinus (see *Coronary circulation*, page 196)
    - As blood passes through the right AV (tricuspid) valve, it flows from the right atrium into the right ventricle
    - It exits through the pulmonary (semilunar) valve and enters the pulmonary circulation
  - Blood returns from pulmonary circulation to the left atrium
    - As it passes through the left AV (bicuspid or mitral) valve, it flows from the left atrium into the left ventricle
    - Blood exits the left ventricle through the aortic (semilunar) valve and enters the systemic circulation
  - The heart's functional blood supply comes from the right and left coronary arteries, which branch from the base of the aorta
    - Left coronary artery branches into the anterior interventricular artery and circumflex artery
    - Right coronary artery branches into the posterior interventricular artery and marginal artery
    - Extensive capillary beds join coronary arteries with cardiac veins, which empty into the coronary sinus

● **Pulmonary circulation**
  - Pulmonary circulation starts with blood flowing from the right ventricle into the pulmonary trunk (see *Pathways of oxygenated and deoxygenated blood,* page 197)
  - The pulmonary trunk bifurcates into right and left pulmonary arteries, which carry deoxygenated blood to lungs
  - In the lungs, pulmonary arteries divide into *lobar arteries*
    - Lobar arteries (three on right, two on left) branch profusely to form arterioles and pulmonary capillaries
    - Pulmonary capillaries drain into venules that join with pulmonary veins (two on right, two on left)
  - Pulmonary veins carry oxygenated blood to the heart's left atrium

Path of blood in cardiac circulation

- Right atrium
- Tricuspid valve
- Right ventricle
- Pulmonary valve
- Pulmonary circulation
- Left atrium
- Bicuspid valve
- Left ventricle
- Aortic valve
- Systemic circulation

Path of blood in pulmonary circulation

- Right ventricle
- Pulmonary trunk
- Right and left pulmonary arteries
- Lobar arteries
- Arterioles and pulmonary capillaries
- Venules
- Pulmonary veins
- Left atrium

Coronary circulation

These illustrations show the anterior and posterior views of the heart's blood vessels.

ANTERIOR VIEW

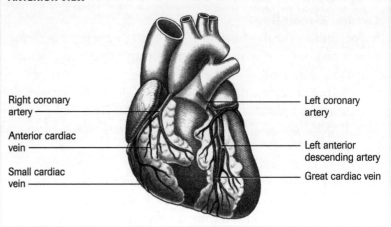

Right coronary artery

Anterior cardiac vein

Small cardiac vein

Left coronary artery

Left anterior descending artery

Great cardiac vein

POSTERIOR VIEW

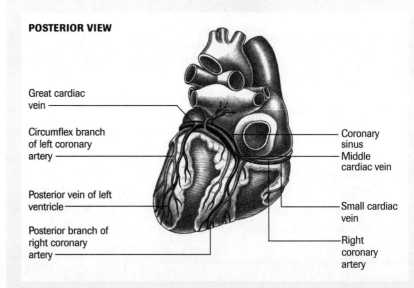

Great cardiac vein

Circumflex branch of left coronary artery

Posterior vein of left ventricle

Posterior branch of right coronary artery

Coronary sinus

Middle cardiac vein

Small cardiac vein

Right coronary artery

Key facts about systemic circulation

- Ascending aorta forms an arch with three branches
- Brachiocephalic artery branches to the heart's right side
- Left common carotid and left subclavian branch to the heart's left side
- The descending aorta becomes the thoracic aorta
- The thoracic aorta becomes the abdominal aorta

● **Systemic circulation**
  - Systemic circulation supplies blood to all body tissues (see *Arteries and veins of the systemic circulation,* page 198)
  - Starting at the heart, blood flow begins in the ascending aorta, which gives rise to the right and left coronary arteries
  - The ascending aorta forms an arch with three branches
    - The *brachiocephalic (innominate) artery* branches to the heart's right side

Pathways of oxygenated and deoxygenated blood

Oxygenated blood travels from the lungs to the left side of the heart, where it's pumped out to the body. Deoxygenated blood returns to the right side of the heart, where it's pumped back to the lungs.

OXYGENATED BLOOD PATH

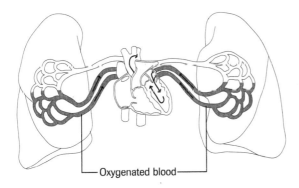

Oxygenated blood

DEOXYGENATED BLOOD PATH

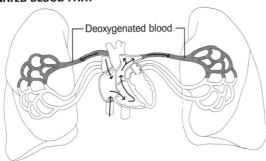

Deoxygenated blood

  - The *left common carotid artery* and *left subclavian artery* branch to the heart's left side
- The descending aorta becomes the *thoracic aorta,* which has four visceral and two parietal branches
- As the thoracic aorta continues through the body, it becomes the *abdominal aorta*
  - The abdominal aorta has several visceral and parietal branches
  - Ultimately, it bifurcates to form the right and left iliac arteries
- Small end-arteries (arteries that don't connect with other arteries) join arterioles and capillary beds, which in turn join venules and

Key systemic circulation arteries

- Temporal
- Common carotid
- Brachiocephalic
- Subclavian
- Pulmonary
- Renal
- Radial
- Common iliac
- Ulnar
- Exterior iliac
- Internal iliac
- Femoral
- Popliteal
- Posterior tibial
- Dorsalis pedis

Key systemic circulation veins

- Jugular
- Brachiocephalic
- Pulmonary
- Renal
- Iliac
- Femoral
- Popliteal

Arteries and veins of the systemic circulation

This illustration shows the major arteries and veins of the systemic circulation.

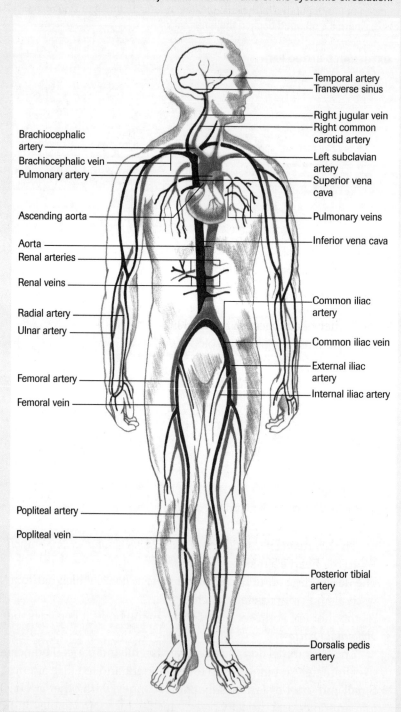

Brachiocephalic artery
Brachiocephalic vein
Pulmonary artery
Ascending aorta
Aorta
Renal arteries
Renal veins
Radial artery
Ulnar artery
Femoral artery
Femoral vein
Popliteal artery
Popliteal vein

Temporal artery
Transverse sinus
Right jugular vein
Right common carotid artery
Left subclavian artery
Superior vena cava
Pulmonary veins
Inferior vena cava
Common iliac artery
Common iliac vein
External iliac artery
Internal iliac artery
Posterior tibial artery
Dorsalis pedis artery

progressively larger veins that carry venous blood to the superior or inferior vena cava

● **Hepatic circulation**
- Hepatic circulation (also called *hepatic portal system*) circulates blood through the liver
- Veins from the digestive viscera empty blood into the hepatic portal vein
- This venous blood then passes through the liver before entering the systemic circulation via hepatic veins

● **Fetal circulation**
- Fetal circulation is a special circulatory system adaptation required for fetal development
- It includes umbilical vessels and three vascular shunts—ductus venosus, foramen ovale, and ductus arteriosus
- The umbilical vein carries oxygenated blood from the placenta to the fetus's liver
- Blood flows from the liver via the ductus venosus or hepatic veins to the inferior vena cava
    - The *ductus venosus* is a shunt that allows most blood to bypass the liver
    - It's necessary because the fetal liver doesn't process blood
- From the inferior vena cava, blood enters the heart's right atrium
    - Some blood entering the right atrium flows directly into the left atrium through the *foramen ovale,* a shunt in the interatrial septum
    - Blood entering the right ventricle is pumped out through the pulmonary artery
- Much of the blood in the pulmonary trunk passes through the ductus arteriosus
    - The *ductus arteriosus* is a vessel that connects the pulmonary artery directly to the descending aorta
    - It shunts blood away from the pulmonary circulation
- Blood flowing through the aorta passes through the internal iliac arteries into the umbilical arteries and back to the placenta
- At birth, the two umbilical arteries, the umbilical vein, and the three shunts are occluded (closed off)

BLOOD PRESSURE

● **Key concepts**
- In the pulmonary and systemic arteries, the pressure of blood varies with the phase of the cardiac cycle

---

Path of blood in hepatic circulation

- Veins from digestive viscera
- Hepatic portal vein
- Liver
- Hepatic veins
- Systemic circulation

Path of blood in fetal circulation

- Placenta
- Umbilical vein
- Fetus's liver
- Ductus venosus or hepatic veins
- Inferior vena cava
- Right atrium
- Some blood flows into left atrium through foramen ovale
- Right ventricle
- Pulmonary artery
- Ductus arteriosus
- Descending aorta

Key facts about blood pressure

- Refers to pressure of blood in the systemic circulation
- Pressure is highest during systole, lowest during diastole
- Systolic pressure depends on cardiac output
- Diastolic pressure depends on peripheral resistance

- It's highest when blood is ejected during systole (systolic pressure) and lowest during diastole immediately before the next cardiac contraction (diastolic pressure)
- The term *blood pressure* refers to the pressure of blood in systemic circulation; it's about six times higher than the pressure of blood in the pulmonary circulation
- A sphygmomanometer and stethoscope allow measurement of systolic and diastolic blood pressure
- Blood pressure varies rhythmically with the heartbeat
    – It's highest during ventricular systole, when blood is ejected from ventricles (systolic blood pressure)
    – It's lowest during ventricular diastole, when blood flows through arteries into capillaries (diastolic blood pressure)
- Systolic blood pressure depends primarily on *cardiac output* (force and volume of blood ejected from ventricles during systole); diastolic pressure depends on *peripheral resistance* (degree of impedance to blood flow; may be increased by vasoconstriction)
- Blood pressure is also influenced to a lesser degree by blood volume, blood viscosity, and arterial elasticity
- Systolic pressure is primarily a measure of the force of ventricular contraction; diastolic pressure is a measure of peripheral resistance caused by arteriolar vasoconstriction
- Blood pressure doesn't drop precipitously during diastole; it declines slowly as blood is released gradually into capillaries by arterioles, helping to maintain a fairly constant pressure
    – Relatively constant blood pressure is needed to maintain blood flow to tissues and prevent organ damage
    – Sustained high blood pressure (hypertension) can lead to heart failure and other disorders (see *Teaching a patient with hypertension*)

Cardiac output

- Cardiac output is the amount of blood ejected per minute from a ventricle
- Amount equals *stroke volume* (volume of blood ejected from a single ventricle at each contraction) multiplied by heart rate in beats per minute (bpm)
- Basal (resting) stroke volume is about 70 ml; basal heart rate, about 72 bpm
    – Cardiac output is about 5 L per minute (70 ml × 72 bpm = 5,040 ml)
    – Amount also equals total blood volume (approximately 5,000 ml)
- *End-diastolic volume* (EDV) (total blood volume in each ventricle before ventricular systole) is about 120 ml

Key facts about cardiac output

- Amount of blood ejected per minute from a ventricle
- EDV is the volume of blood in the ventricle before systole
- Ejection fraction is the amount of blood ejected during systole in relation to EDV

TIME-OUT FOR TEACHING

Teaching a patient with hypertension

Make sure you teach a patient with hypertension:
- factors that affect blood pressure
- the definition of hypertension and what type of hypertension he has
- what complications may occur
- what diagnostic tests to expect
- what exercise program and precautions to follow
- what dietary restrictions to follow, such as increasing potassium intake, decreasing salt intake, and decreasing calories (if necessary)
- how to use antihypertensives, diuretics, and other drugs
- how to monitor his blood pressure at home
- other measures he should take to prevent complications, such as stress reduction and smoking cessation (if necessary)
- the need for compliance with his regimen
- where to find sources of information and support.

- Ventricles don't completely empty of blood during systole; each ventricle ejects only about 70 ml of blood
  - *End-systolic volume* (unejected blood remaining in each ventricle) is about 50 ml (120 − 70 = 50 ml)
  - *Ejection fraction* is the amount of blood ejected during each ventricular contraction in relation to EDV
  - In this example, 70 ml (stroke volume) is divided by 120 ml (EDV), which equals an ejection fraction of 0.58, or 58%
- The heart can increase its rate and stroke volume as needed to raise cardiac output above the basal level (up to fourfold, if necessary)
  - Trained athletes can increase cardiac output even more
  - If cardiac output increases, blood pressure tends to rise because blood is delivered to arteries more rapidly than it leaves through arterioles

Peripheral resistance
- Degree of arteriolar vasoconstriction determines degree of peripheral resistance
- Arterioles restrict blood flow from arteries into capillaries
  - If arterioles constrict and peripheral resistance increases, blood can't flow readily from arteries into capillaries and arterial blood pressure increases
  - If arterioles relax and peripheral resistance decreases, blood flows more rapidly into capillaries and arterial blood pressure drops

● **Blood volume**
- Blood pressure tends to vary directly with total blood volume in the cardiovascular system
- Blood pressure tends to rise if blood volume increases (occurs in some diseases) and tends to drop if blood volume falls below normal (occurs in severe hemorrhage)

● **Blood viscosity**
- The greater the viscosity of a fluid, the slower the fluid flows through a narrow orifice; the less the viscosity, the more rapidly it flows
- In some diseases, blood viscosity rises because of increased proteins or number of erythrocytes in blood; this restricts blood flow through arterioles into capillaries, which tends to increase blood pressure

● **Arterial elasticity**
- Blood pressure changes if elasticity of large arteries changes
  - Normally, large artery distention absorbs some force of blood ejected during systole
  - Distention prevents excessive elevation of systolic pressure during each ventricular contraction
  - Arteries recoil during diastole and propel blood forward
- In some diseases, aorta and large arteries gradually lose elasticity and become more rigid
  - Rigid vessels can't distend and absorb impact of ejected blood
  - This can result in increase in systolic pressure

BLOOD PRESSURE REGULATION AND CARDIAC OUTPUT

● **Key concepts**
- For proper function of major body organs, the body must maintain adequate cardiac output and stable blood pressure
- Cardiac output normally varies in response to the body's requirements; blood pressure normally remains within a specific range
- Several mechanisms control cardiac output and blood pressure
  - The heart exerts control over its stroke volume, as described by Starling's law
  - The autonomic nervous system (ANS) controls nerve impulse discharge based on information that baroreceptors and chemoreceptors in major arteries relay to the brain
  - Kidneys secrete hormones that affect the heart

Starling's law

- According to Starling's law, the amount of stretching of cardiac muscle fibers helps regulate stroke volume and maintain equal output from both ventricles
- Muscle stretching typically occurs in two ways
  - If venous return to a ventricle increases, the ventricle overdistends and its muscles stretch
  - If diastolic pressure rises, the heart must eject blood against higher peripheral resistance; when this occurs, the ventricle tends to empty less completely and becomes overdistended, stretching cardiac muscles
- Stretching of fibers causes ventricle to contract more forcefully to expel additional blood
- More forceful ventricular contractions maintain normal cardiac output and supply adequate blood to tissues despite increased peripheral resistance

Regulation by baroreceptors

- ANS controls the heart and blood vessels
- Diffuse network of interconnecting neurons in the medulla regulates discharge of autonomic nerve impulses, mainly in response to impulses from *baroreceptors* (specialized pressure-sensitive receptors in carotid artery and walls of aortic arch)
- This medullary control center exerts opposing effects
  - *Cardioacceleratory* portion of medulla controls nerve impulse discharge from the sympathetic division of the ANS, which speeds the heart rate
  - *Cardioinhibitory* portion controls nerve impulse discharge from the parasympathetic division, which slows the heart rate
  - The net effect of the ANS on the heart and blood vessels reflects the combined response of both portions of the medullary control center
- In response to input from baroreceptors, the medullary center also sends regulatory impulses to the heart and blood vessels, which maintain a stable cardiac output and blood pressure
  - If intravascular pressure rises, baroreceptors send impulses to the medullary center
    - Impulses initiate discharge of parasympathetic impulses in the vagal nerve to slow heart rate and reduce the force of ventricular contraction (thereby reducing cardiac output) and to reduce arteriolar vasoconstriction (reducing intravascular pressure)
    - Impulses simultaneously inhibit sympathetic output from the cardioacceleratory portion of the medullary center

Key components of Starling's law

- Increased venous return or impaired ventricular emptying leads to increased ventricular volume
- Increased volume causes cardiac muscles to stretch
- Stretching results in a more forceful contraction

Key facts about regulation by baroreceptors

- Baroreceptors send impulses to the medulla
- Cardioacceleratory portion of the medulla sends impulses to speed heart rate
- Cardioinhibitory portion sends impulses to slow heart rate
- Medullary center also sends impulses to heart and blood vessels to maintain stable cardiac output and blood pressure

Key facts about regulation by chemoreceptors

- Chemical-sensitive receptors in the aortic arch and carotid sinus
- Respond to decreased blood oxygen, increased blood carbon dioxide, and decreased pH
- Respond to extreme changes by sending impulses to the medullary control center
- Medullary center sends impulses via the ANS to increase heart rate and blood pressure

Key facts about hormonal regulation

- Sustained drop in blood pressure triggers kidneys to release renin
- Renin is converted to angiotensin
- Angiotensin causes arteriolar constriction, raising blood pressure
- Angiotensin also stimulates the adrenal gland to release aldosterone
- Aldosterone causes sodium and water retention, also leading to increased blood pressure

– If intravascular pressure falls, baroreceptors relay fewer impulses to the medullary center
  · Medullary center responds by discharging sympathetic nerve impulses to increase heart rate and the force of ventricular contraction (thereby increasing cardiac output) and to constrict arterioles (increasing intravascular pressure)
  · Impulses simultaneously inhibit parasympathetic output from cardioinhibitory portion of medullary center

● **Regulation by chemoreceptors**
  • Chemoreceptors are chemical-sensitive receptors in the aortic arch and carotid sinus that respond to decreases in blood oxygen concentration and pH and to increases in blood carbon dioxide concentration
  • They don't play a major role in heart rate and blood pressure regulation under normal physiologic conditions; however, they respond to extreme partial pressure of oxygen and blood pH decreases and extreme partial pressure of carbon dioxide increases
  • They transmit impulses to the medullary control center using the same pathways that baroreceptors use; in response, the medullary center initiates impulses via the ANS to increase heart rate and blood pressure

● **Hormonal regulation**
  • In the kidneys, the hormones renin, angiotensin, and aldosterone help regulate blood pressure; the *renin-angiotensin-aldosterone mechanism* responds more slowly to blood pressure changes than reflex mechanisms do
  • A sustained drop in blood pressure causes kidneys to release renin, which is converted to angiotensin in the circulation
    – Angiotensin raises blood pressure by causing arteriolar constriction
    – It also stimulates the adrenal gland to release the steroid hormone aldosterone
      · Aldosterone causes kidneys to retain sodium and water, which increases blood volume and leads to a corresponding increase in blood pressure

FLUID MOVEMENT BETWEEN CAPILLARIES AND INTERSTITIUM

● **Key concepts**
  • Capillary blood and tissue cells exchange oxygen, nutrients, and cellular waste products

- These substances must pass in solution through the loose connective tissue (*interstitial space*) in which the cells are dispersed
- The interstitial space is filled with a semisolid matrix that contains connective tissue fibers and a little interstitial fluid that has filtered through the capillaries
- At the arterial end of the capillary, *hydrostatic pressure* (which pushes fluid out) is higher than *osmotic pressure* (which pulls fluid back), causing interstitial fluid to filter through the capillary's endothelium into the interstitial space
- At the venous end, hydrostatic pressure is lower than osmotic pressure, causing fluid to diffuse back into the capillary
- *Edema* (excess fluid in the interstitial space) may result from any disturbance in fluid transfer between the capillaries and interstitial tissue

● **Fluid movement**
- The cyclic flow of fluid from the interstitial space to the capillaries and back depends on capillary hydrostatic pressure, capillary permeability, osmotic pressure, and open lymphatic channels
- Blood in capillaries exerts capillary hydrostatic pressure
  - This tends to force fluid out from blood through the capillary endothelium and into interstitial fluid
  - It's much lower than pressure in larger arteries because arteriolar constriction restricts blood flow into the capillaries, functioning like a pressure reduction valve
  - This results in mean arterial pressure in larger arteries falling from about 85 mm Hg to about 35 mm Hg at the arterial end of the capillary and dropping to a low of 15 mm Hg at the venous end of the capillary
- Capillary permeability determines how easily fluid can pass through the capillary endothelium
- Osmotic pressure exerted by blood proteins (called *colloid osmotic pressure*) tends to attract interstitial fluid back into capillaries
- Open lymphatic channels collect some fluid forced out into interstitial tissues and return it to circulation; this occurs because pressure in lymphatic channels is lower than in interstitial tissues
- Edema may result from any disturbance in factors that regulate fluid transfer in the capillary–interstitial tissue–capillary cycle; may result from inflammation, decreased colloid osmotic pressure, increased capillary hydrostatic pressure, or lymphatic channel obstruction

Key facts about fluid movement between capillaries and interstitium

- Interstitial fluid filters through the capillary's endothelium into the interstitial space
- At the arterial end, hydrostatic pressure is higher than osmotic pressure, and fluid is pushed out
- At the venous end, hydrostatic pressure is lower than osmotic pressure, causing fluid to diffuse back into the capillary
- Edema results from a disturbance in fluid transfer between capillaries and interstitial fluid

TOP 10

Items to study for your next test on the cardiovascular system

1. Structures of the heart
2. Events of the cardiac cycle
3. Electrical conduction through the heart
4. Basic ECG waveforms
5. Types of blood vessels
6. Flow of blood through the cardiac, pulmonary, systemic, hepatic, and fetal circulatory systems
7. Factors affecting blood pressure
8. Mechanisms regulating blood pressure and cardiac output
9. Factors affecting fluid movement
10. Teaching tips for patients with an arrhythmia or hypertension

NCLEX CHECKS

It's never too soon to begin your NCLEX preparation. Now that you've reviewed this chapter, carefully read each of the following questions and choose the best answer. Then compare your responses with the correct answers.

1. While auscultating heart sounds, the nurse should keep in mind that the ventricles contract during systole, causing:
☐ **1.** all four heart valves to close.
☐ **2.** AV valves to close and semilunar valves to open.
☐ **3.** AV valves to open and semilunar valves to close.
☐ **4.** all four heart valves to open.

2. While teaching a client who will be receiving a permanent pacemaker, the nurse tells him that which structure is the heart's normal pacemaker?
☐ **1.** SA node
☐ **2.** AV node
☐ **3.** Bundle of His
☐ **4.** Purkinje fibers

3. The nurse is instructing a group of clients diagnosed with myocardial infarction about cardiac rehabilitation. The nurse tells the class that which vessels carry oxygenated blood from the lungs back to the heart?
☐ **1.** Capillaries
☐ **2.** Pulmonary veins
☐ **3.** Pulmonary arteries
☐ **4.** Superior and inferior venae cavae

4. The nurse is performing a cardiac assessment on a client with no known heart disease. Identify the area where the nurse expects the heart to be located.

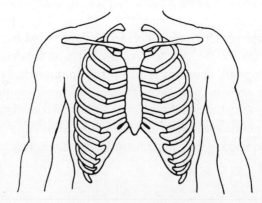

5. To evaluate the PR interval on a client's ECG, the nurse measures which distance?

☐ **1.** End of the P wave to the end of the QRS complex
☐ **2.** Beginning of the P wave to the beginning of the QRS complex
☐ **3.** End of the P wave to the beginning of the QRS complex
☐ **4.** Beginning of the P wave to the end of the QRS complex

6. While teaching about fetal circulation to a prenatal class, the nurse correctly identifies which structure that allows blood to flow from the right atrium to the left atrium in the fetus?

☐ **1.** Ductus venosus
☐ **2.** Foramen ovale
☐ **3.** Umbilical vein
☐ **4.** Ductus arteriosus

7. The nurse performing a blood pressure assessment should know that systolic blood pressure depends primarily on which factor?

☐ **1.** Blood volume
☐ **2.** Blood viscosity
☐ **3.** Cardiac output
☐ **4.** Arterial elasticity

8. Which formula would the nurse use to calculate a client's cardiac output?

☐ **1.** Stroke volume × heart rate
☐ **2.** Diastolic blood pressure × heart rate
☐ **3.** End-diastolic blood pressure × ejection fraction
☐ **4.** Stroke volume × heart rate

9. The nurse is caring for a client with severe, uncontrolled hemorrhage following a motor vehicle accident. Which trend in blood pressure would the nurse expect?

☐ **1.** Blood pressure will rise
☐ **2.** Blood pressure will remain the same
☐ **3.** Blood pressure will be variable
☐ **4.** Blood pressure will fall

10. The nurse explains to a client that stimulation of the vagal nerve through coughing or bearing down produces which response?

☐ **1.** Increased heart rate
☐ **2.** More forceful ventricular contraction
☐ **3.** Decreased heart rate
☐ **4.** Increased vasoconstriction

ANSWERS AND RATIONALES

1. CORRECT ANSWER: 2

During systole, the pressure is greater in the ventricles than in the atria, causing the AV valves (the tricuspid and mitral valves) to close. The pressure in the ventricles is also greater than the pressure in the aorta and pulmonary artery, forcing the semilunar valves (the pulmonic and aortic valves) to open.

2. CORRECT ANSWER: 1

The SA node normally sets the heart's pace. The AV node is the heart's secondary pacemaker. Electrical impulses from the SA node travel to the AV node. The impulses then pass to the bundle of His, bundle branches, and the Purkinje fibers.

3. CORRECT ANSWER: 2

Deoxygenated blood returns to the heart through the inferior and superior venae cavae. This blood then flows from the right atrium to the right ventricle and into the pulmonary arteries. These arteries branch into arterioles and pulmonary capillaries (where gas exchange takes place). Oxygenated blood then flows into venules that join with pulmonary veins and empty into the left atrium of the heart. The left ventricle then pumps this oxygenated blood out to the body.

4. CORRECT ANSWER:

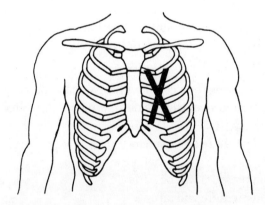

The heart of a person with no heart disease is typically situated slightly to the left of the body's midline, between the second rib and fifth intercostal space.

5. CORRECT ANSWER: 2

To determine the PR interval—the time needed for an impulse to travel from the atria to the ventricles through the bundle of His—measure from the beginning of the P wave to the beginning of the QRS complex.

6. CORRECT ANSWER: 2

In fetal circulation, most of the blood from the inferior vena cava enters the right atrium and flows through the foramen ovale (a shunt in the interatrial septum) into the left atrium. The ductus venosus is a shunt that allows most blood to bypass the fetal liver because the fetal liver doesn't process blood. The umbilical vein carries oxygenated blood from the placenta to the fetal liver. The ductus arteriosus connects the pulmonary artery directly to the descending aorta, shunting blood away from the pulmonary circulation.

7. CORRECT ANSWER: 3

Systolic blood pressure depends primarily on cardiac output—the force and volume of blood ejected from the ventricles during systole. Blood volume, blood viscosity, and arterial elasticity also influence blood pressure to a lesser degree.

8. CORRECT ANSWER: 4

Cardiac output equals the stroke volume (volume of blood ejected from a single ventricle at each contraction) multiplied by the heart rate in bpm.

9. CORRECT ANSWER: 4

Blood pressure tends to vary directly with the total blood volume. Consequently, blood pressure tends to drop if blood volume falls below normal, such as with severe hemorrhage, and tends to rise if blood volume increases.

10. CORRECT ANSWER: 3

When intravascular pressure rises, such as with coughing or bearing down, baroreceptors send impulses to the medullary center. These impulses initiate discharge of parasympathetic impulses in the vagal nerve to slow the heart rate, reduce the force of ventricular contraction, and reduce arteriolar vasoconstriction. Stimulation of the sympathetic nervous system increases heart rate and the force of ventricular contraction, and constricts the arterioles.

12

Respiratory system

CHAPTER OVERVIEW

Working closely with the cardiovascular system, the respiratory system provides tissues with oxygen and removes carbon dioxide. It must perform this function under widely varying external conditions and internal demands to ensure that body cells get the oxygen they need—or death would occur within minutes. To keep this system working efficiently, the nurse must understand its structures and functions. This chapter reviews airway structures, the lungs, ventilation, gas exchange, oxygen and carbon dioxide transport, and respiration control.

RESPIRATORY SYSTEM OVERVIEW

● **Key concepts**
  • The respiratory system consists of upper and lower airways and the lungs (see *Structures of the respiratory tract,* page 212)
    – *Upper airways* include the nose, pharynx, and larynx
    – *Lower airways* include the trachea and bronchi, which lead to the lungs
  • The respiratory system's main function is supplying body tissues with oxygen and eliminating carbon dioxide

● **Respiration**
  • Respiration consists of two processes
    – *Ventilation* refers to air movement through respiratory passages to and from the lungs
    – *Gas exchange* refers to oxygen and carbon dioxide transport between pulmonary alveoli and blood in pulmonary capillaries
  • Both processes must function properly for adequate tissue oxygenation and efficient carbon dioxide elimination

AIRWAY STRUCTURES

● **Nose**
  • The *nose* is formed superiorly by nasal and frontal bones, laterally by maxillary bones, and inferiorly by movable plates of hyaline cartilage (lateral and alar plates)
  • The usual site of inspiration (inhalation) and expiration (exhalation), the nose filters, warms, and moistens air inspired through the nostrils; it connects to the pharynx
  • Two *nasal cavities* open on the face through the anterior nasal apertures (nares); the *nasal septum* separates the cavities
    – The anterior portion of the nasal septum is composed of *hyaline cartilage*
    – The posterior portion consists of a flat bone called the *vomer* and the perpendicular plate of the *ethmoid* bone
  • Posteriorly, the nasal cavities join the pharynx through the *internal nares* (choanae)
  • Each cavity has three mucosa-covered passageways: superior, middle, and inferior conchae
  • Nasal cavities are lined with hairs that trap dust and foreign particles before they reach the lungs
    – Epithelial cells lining the nasal cavities secrete mucus, which collects foreign particles

Key respiratory tract structures

- Nasal cavity
- Pharynx
- Larynx
- Trachea
- Superior lobe
- Primary bronchus
- Right and left lung
- Horizontal fissure
- Secondary bronchus
- Middle lobe
- Tertiary bronchus
- Oblique fissure
- Inferior lobe
- Bronchiole
- Alveolus

Structures of the respiratory tract

This illustration shows the main structures of the respiratory tract.

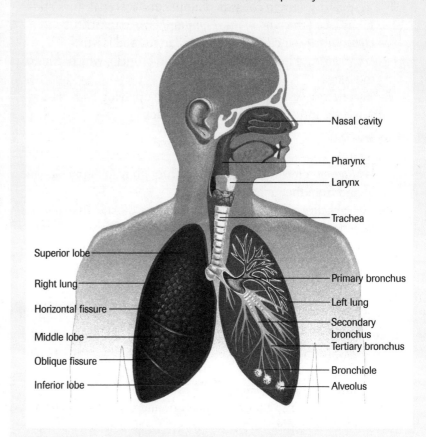

Key characteristics of the pharynx

- Cavity extending from base of skull to esophagus
- Passageway for air and food; also functions in speech
- Nasopharynx is superior division
- Oropharynx is middle division
- Laryngopharynx is inferior division

– Ciliated cells of the nasal mucosa move mucus toward the pharynx, where swallowing, sneezing, and spitting remove mucus
- *Paranasal sinuses,* which surround and drain into the nasal cavities, are in the frontal, sphenoid, and maxillary bones

● **Pharynx**
- The *pharynx* is a cavity that extends from the base of the skull to the esophagus (at the sixth cervical vertebra)
- It acts as a passageway for air entering the nose and for food entering the GI tract; also functions in speech, changing shape to allow phonation of vowel sounds
- It extends down from the juncture of the nasal and oral cavities and splits into the larynx and esophagus

- Entire pharynx is composed of striated muscle and lined with mucous membrane
- The pharynx has three divisions
  - The *nasopharynx* is the most superior division
    · Inferior to the sphenoid bone, it lies at the level of the soft palate
    · Walls have four openings
      - *Eustachian tubes* open out of the lateral walls to enter the middle ear (tympanic cavity)
      - Two openings lead to posterior nares
  - The *oropharynx* is the middle division
    · Continuous with the posterior oral cavity, it extends inferiorly from the soft palate to the hyoid bone
    · Anterolateral walls support the palatine tonsils
    · Lingual tonsils at the tongue's base protrude into it
  - The *laryngopharynx* is the most inferior division
    · It extends from the hyoid bone to the opening of the esophagus
    · It's lined with stratified squamous epithelium

● **Larynx**
- Also called the *voice box,* the *larynx* is a triangular organ in the neck's front, situated just below and in front of the most inferior part of the pharynx
  - It extends from the fourth to sixth cervical vertebrae, attaching to the hyoid bone
  - It connects the inferior part of the pharynx with the trachea
- The larynx is composed of muscle and numerous cartilages
  - Three single cartilages are the cricoid, epiglottic, and thyroid cartilages
  - Three paired cartilages are the arytenoid, corniculate, and cuneiform cartilages
  - Ligaments connect all the cartilages
- *True vocal cords,* a pair of horizontal folds that project into the laryngeal cavity, are separated by a space called the *glottis*
- The larynx functions mainly to provide a permanent airway to the lungs
  - The *epiglottis,* which overhangs the larynx, prevents food from entering the lungs
  - The glottis and vocal cords allow phonation; expired air vibrates vocal cords, causing sounds made in phonation

● **Trachea**
- Also called the *windpipe,* the *trachea* is a membranous tube that measures 4″ to 5″ (10 to 12.5 cm) long; it's located anterior to the esophagus and extends from the larynx at the level of the sixth cervical vertebra to the upper border of the fifth thoracic vertebra

Key characteristics of the larynx

● Also called the *voice box*
● True vocal cords project into the laryngeal cavity; separated by the glottis
● Provides a permanent airway to the lungs
● The epiglottis prevents food from entering the lungs

Key characteristics of the trachea

● Also called the *windpipe*
● Serves as a passageway for air to enter the lungs
● C-shaped cartilage rings strengthen the trachea

Bronchioles and alveoli

This illustration shows the bronchioles branching into progressively smaller tubes that eventually become alveolar ducts. These ducts terminate in clusters called *alveoli*. The alveoli are the basic functional units of the respiratory system and the site of gas exchange (exchange of oxygen and carbon dioxide) between the lungs and the bronchi.

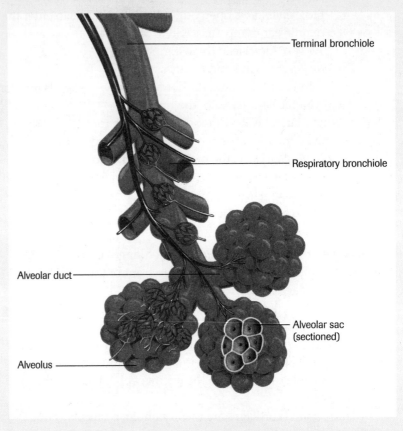

Terminal bronchiole

Respiratory bronchiole

Alveolar duct

Alveolar sac (sectioned)

Alveolus

- On entering the mediastinum, the trachea branches into right and left main bronchi at the fifth thoracic vertebrae
- Dorsally, it contacts the esophagus
• The trachea serves as an open passageway that lets air enter the lungs
• A series of C-shaped cartilage rings strengthens the trachea and prevents its collapse during inspiration
• The trachea is lined with ciliated pseudostratified columnar epithelium that contains mucus-secreting goblet cells, which trap and propel inhaled debris upward to the pharynx for removal through coughing

TIME-OUT FOR TEACHING

Teaching a patient with asthma

When teaching a patient with asthma, make sure you:

- explain how asthma causes bronchoconstriction, airway edema, and mucus production
- describe possible complications such as status asthmaticus
- prepare him as needed for diagnostic tests, such as arterial blood gas analysis and pulmonary function tests
- help him understand dietary changes, including increasing his fluid intake
- explain prevention methods for—and warning signs of—respiratory infections
- describe medications he may need such as theophylline (Bronkadyl)
- show him how to use a prescribed inhaler
- help him learn to identify and avoid asthma triggers
- show him methods to control an asthma attack
- provide sources of information and support.

Key teaching topics for a patient with asthma

- Explain diagnostic tests
- Discuss preventative measures and how to avoid triggers
- Review medications and dietary changes
- Demonstrate the use of an inhaler and how to control an attack

● Bronchi

- The lungs contain right and left *primary bronchi,* two larger air passages that branch from the trachea
- Primary bronchi branch into smaller *secondary bronchi*
  - Right primary bronchus divides into three secondary bronchi
  - Left primary bronchus divides into two secondary bronchi
- Secondary bronchi branch into *tertiary bronchi,* which, in turn, branch into increasingly smaller *bronchioles* (see *Bronchioles and alveoli*)
- Along with the trachea, bronchi and their branches constitute the *bronchial tree*
- The bronchis' main function is distributing air to the lungs
  - Some disorders, such as asthma, cause bronchoconstriction (partial or complete closure of bronchi and bronchioles), which typically produces dyspnea, wheezing, and coughing (see *Teaching a patient with asthma*)
  - Bronchitis (inflammation of bronchi) can result from a cold or other respiratory tract infection

Key characteristics of the bronchi

- Lungs contain right and left primary bronchi
- Primary bronchi branch into smaller secondary bronchi
- Secondary bronchi branch into tertiary bronchi
- Bronchi branch into bronchioles

LUNGS

● Key concepts

- The *lungs* are paired, cone-shaped organs that fill the pleural divisions of the thoracic cavity; they extend from the root of the neck to the diaphragm

Key facts about the lungs

- Primary bronchus enters the lung at the hilus
- Each lung is enclosed in the pleura
- The visceral pleura covers the lungs
- The parietal pleura lines the chest wall

- The main component of the respiratory system, lungs distribute air and exchange gases
- The right and left lungs are separated by the *mediastinum,* which contains the heart, blood vessels, and other midline structures; fissures divide each lung into lobes
- Each primary bronchus enters its respective lung at the *hilus,* an indentation on the mediastinal surface; connective tissue binds together bronchi and pulmonary blood vessels to form the root of the lung
  - The *base,* the lung's inferior surface, rests on the diaphragm
  - The *apex,* the lung's most superior portion, projects above the clavicle
- Each lung is enclosed in a *pleura,* a protective, double-layered serous membrane
  - The *visceral pleura* covers the lungs and dips into fissures
  - At the hilus, the visceral pleura folds back to form the *parietal pleura,* which lines the chest wall and covers the diaphragm
  - The space between the lungs and chest wall is the *pleural cavity*
    - This space usually contains a little fluid, which lubricates the lungs as they expand and contract
    - Pleurisy (inflammation of the parietal and visceral pleura) may result from pneumonia or another disorder and may lead to respiratory failure
    - When fully expanded, the lungs completely fill the pleural cavity and the parietal and visceral pleurae come in contact

● **Lobes**
- *Fissures* divide the lungs into lobes
  - The right lung is separated into three lobes (superior, middle, and inferior) by horizontal and oblique fissures
  - The smaller left lung is separated into two lobes (upper and lower) by an oblique fissure, which contains a concavity (cardiac notch) molded to accommodate the heart
- Functionally, each lobe is divided into *bronchopulmonary segments*
  - Right lung has 10 bronchopulmonary segments
  - Left lung has eight bronchopulmonary segments

● **Bronchioles**
- Flexible tubes that extend from bronchi, bronchioles allow air to travel to gas exchange sites in the lungs
  - Like bronchi, they branch repeatedly, becoming progressively smaller; unlike bronchi, they contain no cartilage in their walls

Key characteristics of the lobes of the lungs

- Fissures divide the lungs into lobes
- The larger right lung has three lobes
- The smaller left lung has two lobes

Key characteristics of the bronchioles

- Allow air to travel to gas exchange sites in the lungs
- Branch repeatedly, becoming progressively smaller
- Eventually branch into alveolar ducts, which terminate in alveoli

- They progress to form terminal bronchioles (smallest bronchioles that conduct air only)
- They also form respiratory bronchioles (tubes distal to terminal bronchioles that conduct air and participate in gas exchange)
  – Diameter of bronchioles varies with the respiratory phase—increasing slightly during inspiration and decreasing slightly during expiration
- Eventually, bronchioles branch into alveolar ducts, which terminate in clusters called *alveoli*

Alveoli

- Tiny grapclike clusters of air sacs at the ends of bronchioles, alveoli are surrounded by an extensive network of capillaries; alveoli exchange oxygen and carbon dioxide with this network by diffusion
- Alveoli are separated by thin vascular partitions called *alveolar septa*, which are lined by flat squamous cells and a small number of secretory cells that produce surfactant
  – The lipoprotein surfactant reduces surface tension, allowing fluid that lines alveoli to spread as a thin film rather than coalescing into droplets
  – Surfactant reduces the cohesive surface tension of water molecules in alveoli, allowing alveoli to expand uniformly during inspiration
    - Without surfactant, surface tension could restrict alveolar expansion or cause alveolar collapse during expiration
    - This condition commonly occurs in neonates born before 28 weeks' gestation, producing infant respiratory distress syndrome; decreased surfactant in adults also causes alveolar collapse and acute respiratory distress syndrome

Blood supply

- Blood circulates through the lungs via pulmonary and systemic circulatory systems (see *Tracing pulmonary circulation,* page 218)
- In pulmonary circulation, pulmonary arteries branch profusely into pulmonary capillaries, which surround alveoli
  – Pulmonary arteries carry deoxygenated blood to the lungs
  – Pulmonary veins return oxygenated blood from the lungs to the heart
- Systemic circulation supplies blood directly to lung tissues
  – This blood travels through bronchial arteries (one artery on the right and two on the left)
  – Venous blood returns through bronchial veins

Key characteristics of the alveoli

- Clusters of air sacs at the ends of bronchioles
- Exchange oxygen and carbon dioxide with surrounding network of capillaries
- Surfactant around alveoli reduces surface tension and keeps alveoli from collapsing

Key facts about blood supply to the lungs

- The lungs receive blood from the pulmonary and systemic circulation
- In pulmonary circulation, pulmonary capillaries surround alveoli
- Systemic circulation supplies blood directly to lung tissue

Tracing pulmonary circulation

The right and left pulmonary arteries carry deoxygenated blood from the right side of the heart to the lungs. These arteries divide into distal branches, called *arterioles,* which eventually terminate as a concentrated capillary network in the alveoli and alveolar sac, where gas exchange occurs.

Pulmonary venules—the end branches of the pulmonary veins—collect oxygenated blood from capillaries and transport it to larger vessels that, in turn, lead to the pulmonary veins. The pulmonary veins enter the left side of the heart and distribute oxygenated blood throughout the body.

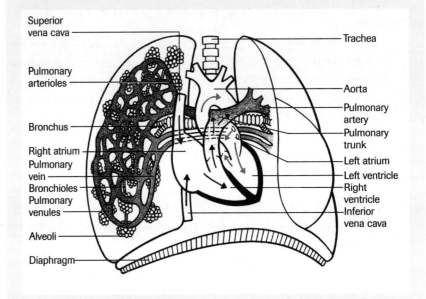

● **Lung pressures**
- The lungs remain expanded in the pleural cavity because *intrapleural pressure* (pressure in the pleural cavity) is less than *intrapulmonary pressure* (air pressure in the lungs)
- These pressure differences develop at birth when the thoracic cavity enlarges and respiration begins
- As the lungs expand and fill with air at atmospheric pressure, the elastic tissue of the lungs stretches
- Stretched lungs tend to pull away from the chest wall and return to their original state; this creates a slight vacuum in the pleural cavity and makes intrapleural pressure slightly less than atmospheric pressure
- Because intrapleural pressure is slightly less than atmospheric pressure, it's commonly called *negative* or *subatmospheric pressure;* without this pressure to keep the lungs expanded, the elastic tissue would contract and the lungs would collapse

VENTILATION

● **Key concepts**
  • The diaphragm and intercostal muscles produce the normal inspiratory and expiratory movement of the lungs and ribs, which allows ventilation (see *The mechanics of breathing,* page 220)
  • During respiration, intrapulmonary and intrapleural pressures change from resting levels (760 and 756 mm Hg, respectively); atmospheric pressure remains constant at about 760 mm Hg
  • The volume of air in the lungs varies during the two phases of respiration—*inspiration* (air movement into the lungs) and *expiration* (air movement out of the lungs)
  • Pulmonary volume (amount of air in lungs) varies greatly between normal inspiration and expiration; it varies even more with forced inspiration and expiration

● **Inspiration**
  • Stimulated by the central nervous system (CNS), the diaphragm contracts and descends, pulling down the lung's lower surfaces
  • At the same time, external intercostal muscles contract and raise the rib cage; this expands lungs by lifting the sternum up and forward
  • Thoracic expansion lowers intrapleural pressure to 754 mm Hg and lungs expand to fill the enlarged thoracic cavity
  • Intrapulmonary pressure decreases to 758 mm Hg; intrapulmonary-atmospheric pressure gradient pulls air into the lungs

● **Expiration**
  • Normally, expiration is passive
  • As CNS impulses stop after inspiration, the diaphragm slowly relaxes and moves up
  • External intercostal muscles relax and the rib cage descends
  • These actions let the lungs and thorax return to their resting size and position
  • Lung and thorax relaxation causes intrapulmonary pressure to rise above atmospheric pressure to 763 mm Hg; intrapleural pressure rises to 756 mm Hg
  • Intrapulmonary-atmospheric pressure gradient forces air out of the lungs until the two pressures equalize
  • During vigorous exertion, the lungs can expel air more actively
    – Contraction of internal intercostal muscles actively forces down the ribs
    – Abdominal muscle contraction pushes abdominal contents up against the bottom of the diaphragm, expelling air more rapidly than can happen with normal diaphragm and intercostal muscle relaxation

Key steps in inspiration
● CNS stimulates the diaphragm to contract and descend
● Intercostal muscles contract and raise the rib cage
● Intrapleural pressure drops to 754 mm Hg and lungs expand
● Intrapulmonary pressure decreases to 758 mm Hg
● Intrapulmonary-atmospheric pressure gradient pulls air into the lungs

Key steps in expiration
● CNS impulses stop after inspiration
● Diaphragm relaxes; external intercostal muscles relax
● Lungs return to resting size
● Intrapulmonary pressure rises above atmospheric pressure to 763 mm Hg
● Intrapleural pressure rises to 756 mm Hg
● Pressure gradient forces air out of the lungs until pressures equalize

The mechanics of breathing

These illustrations show how mechanical forces, such as the movement of the diaphragm and intercostal muscles, produce a breath. A plus sign (+) indicates positive pressure, and a minus sign (−) indicates negative pressure.

AT REST
- Inspiratory muscles relax.
- Atmospheric pressure is maintained in the tracheobronchial tree.
- No air movement occurs.

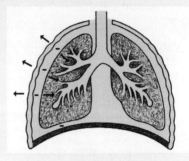

INHALATION
- Inspiratory muscles contract.
- The diaphragm descends.
- Negative alveolar pressure is maintained.
- Air moves into the lungs.

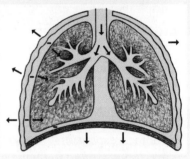

EXHALATION
- Inspiratory muscles relax, causing lungs to recoil to their resting size and position.
- The diaphragm ascends.
- Positive alveolar pressure is maintained.
- Air moves out of the lungs.

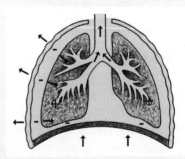

Key facts about pulmonary volumes and capacities

- Tidal volume: amount of air inspired and expired during normal breathing
- Residual volume: amount of air lungs still hold after forceful expiration
- Vital capacity: maximum amount of air that can be moved out of the lungs after a maximum inspiration and expiration

● **Pulmonary volumes and capacities**
- Pulmonary volumes and capacities vary with a person's size, which influences the size of the lungs and thorax
- *Tidal volume* is the amount an average adult inspires and expires during normal quiet breathing (about 500 ml of air with each breath)
- *Inspiratory reserve volume* is the amount an adult can forcefully inhale at the end of normal tidal inspiration (another 3,000 ml of air)
- *Expiratory reserve volume* is the amount an adult can forcefully exhale at the end of normal tidal expiration (about 1,300 ml of air)
- *Residual volume* is the amount lungs still hold even after expelling expiratory reserve volume (about 1,200 ml of air)

- *Vital capacity* is the maximum amount of air that can be moved out of the lungs after a maximum inspiration and expiration (about 4,800 ml); vital capacity = tidal volume + inspiratory reserve volume + expiratory reserve volume, or 500 ml + 3,000 ml + 1,300 ml
- *Total lung capacity* is approximately 6,000 ml
- Although tidal volume is 500 ml of air, about 150 ml never reaches the alveoli; instead, it fills upper respiratory passages until it's exhaled with the next breath
    - The portion of the upper airway containing air that doesn't enter the alveoli is called the *dead space;* the volume of air it contains is called the *dead space volume*
    - Because of this dead space, only about 350 ml of air actually enters the alveoli with each breath and mixes with the 2,500 ml of air already in the lungs (expiratory reserve volume + residual volume)
    - Consequently, with each breath, new atmospheric air replaces less than 15% of alveolar air
    - This slow replacement offers several advantages
        - Slow admixture of atmospheric air with alveolar air prevents wide fluctuations in oxygen and carbon dioxide concentration in alveolar air, which could produce adverse effects
        - Concentration of oxygen and carbon dioxide in blood remain in balance with concentrations in alveolar air, promoting stable concentrations of oxygen and carbon dioxide in arterial blood

GAS EXCHANGE

- **Key concepts**
    - Oxygen and carbon dioxide diffusion (exchange) between alveoli, blood, and tissues depends on concentrations and pressures of these gases
    - In a mixture of gases, the pressure each gas exerts (*partial pressure*) is independent of the pressure that other gases exert; pressure directly corresponds to the percentage of that gas in the total mixture (*concentration*)
        - For example, air exerts a total pressure of 760 mm Hg (atmospheric pressure) at sea level
        - Air contains about 21% oxygen, so partial pressure of oxygen (Po_2) is 21% of atmospheric pressure: $0.21 \times 760 = 159.6$ mm Hg
    - Oxygen and carbon dioxide exist in three physiologically important areas: in the atmosphere and pulmonary alveoli as gases and in the blood in solution

Key facts about gas exchange

- Gas exchange depends on concentrations and pressures of the gases
- The partial pressure of a gas is the pressure that the gas exerts in a mixture of gases
- The pressure corresponds to the concentration of that gas in the mixture

● **Gas concentrations in inspired air**
- Inspired air contains nearly 79% nitrogen (an inert gas) and about 21% oxygen
- The remainder is a mixture of water vapor (about 0.5%) and carbon dioxide (about 0.04%)

● **Gas concentrations in alveolar air**
- Alveolar air contains more water vapor (about 6.2%) than inspired air because of the moist secretions in respiratory passages
- It has a lower oxygen content (about 13.6%) than inspired air because red blood cells (RBCs) take up oxygen as they pass through pulmonary capillaries
- It has a higher carbon dioxide concentration (about 5.3%) than inspired air because the gas diffuses continually from pulmonary capillaries into alveolar air
- Nitrogen accounts for about 74.9% of alveolar air

● **Gas concentrations in expired air**
- Expired air contains about the same amount of water vapor as alveolar air (about 6.2%)
- It contains more oxygen (about 15.7%) and less carbon dioxide (about 3.6%) than alveolar air because it's a mixture of alveolar air and atmospheric air from dead space
- Nitrogen accounts for about 74.5% of expired air

● **Gas diffusion**
- *Diffusion* refers to the exchange of gases—particularly oxygen and carbon dioxide—between alveoli and capillaries and between body cells and RBCs
- In diffusion, substances move from an area of higher concentration to one of lower concentration; a gas diffuses from an area with a high partial pressure of the gas to one with a low partial pressure
- Inspired air has a P_{O_2} of 158 mm Hg and a partial pressure of carbon dioxide (P_{CO_2}) of 0.3 mm Hg
- When blood returns to the heart, the right ventricle pumps it to the lungs, where it passes through the pulmonary capillaries
- P_{O_2} in venous blood, which is returned to the heart through the vena cavae, is 40 mm Hg; P_{CO_2} is 47 mm Hg
- Because alveolar air has a higher P_{O_2} (100 mm Hg) and a lower P_{CO_2} (40 mm Hg) than blood in pulmonary capillaries, oxygen diffuses from alveolar air into pulmonary capillaries, and carbon dioxide diffuses in the opposite direction
- As a result, arterial blood has a P_{O_2} of 97 mm Hg, which is almost the same as alveolar P_{O_2}; it also has a P_{CO_2} of 40 mm Hg, the same as alveolar P_{CO_2}
- Tissues have a lower P_{O_2} (40 mm Hg) and a higher P_{CO_2} (about 60 mm Hg) than arterial blood

TIME-OUT FOR TEACHING

Teaching a patient with pneumonia

When teaching a patient with pneumonia, make sure you:
- explain respiratory defense mechanisms and how pneumonia develops
- describe the classifications, risk factors, and signs and symptoms of pneumonia
- prepare him as needed for diagnostic tests, such as chest X-rays and sputum analysis

- explain treatments, including activity restrictions, drug therapy, breathing and coughing exercises, chest physiotherapy, hydration, and oxygen therapy
- describe methods for preventing pneumonia, such as influenza vaccinations, and for preventing its spread, such as proper hand washing and tissue disposal
- provide sources of information and support.

- As a result, oxygen diffuses into tissues from arterial blood, and carbon dioxide diffuses in the opposite direction, from tissues into blood
- In pneumonia, inflammatory exudate accumulates in the alveoli and causes consolidation, filling one or more lobes with mucus, pus, and other substances (see *Teaching a patient with pneumonia*)

OXYGEN AND CARBON DIOXIDE TRANSPORT

● Key concepts
- When diffusion occurs, arterial blood transports oxygen to tissues in two ways: physically dissolved in plasma and chemically bound to hemoglobin
- Tissues release carbon dioxide into the bloodstream, where it travels to the lungs in three forms: dissolved in plasma, combined with hemoglobin, and combined with water as carbonic acid and its component ions
- In the lungs, oxygen and carbon dioxide transport is the reverse of that in the tissues

● Oxygen transport in blood
- Only about 3% of oxygen is dissolved in blood plasma
- The remaining 97% is chemically bound with hemoglobin in a ratio of 1 g of hemoglobin to approximately 1.34 cc of oxygen

– 100 ml of blood contains about 15 g of hemoglobin, so 100 ml of blood should combine with about 20 cc of oxygen ($15 \times 1.34 = 20.1$)

– In reality, oxygenated blood normally carries slightly less than the predicted 20 cc of oxygen because it's only about 97% oxygen saturated (the hemoglobin doesn't carry its full complement of oxygen)

- Tissues remove about 5 cc of oxygen from each 100 ml of blood; blood returning to the heart contains about 15 cc of oxygen per 100 ml of blood (75% oxygen saturation)
- During vigorous exercise, muscles remove more oxygen from the blood, and the rate of blood flow to tissues increases greatly, increasing the amount of oxygen available to tissues
- Oxygen uptake by hemoglobin works most efficiently in the lungs, which have a high oxygen concentration; oxygen release occurs most readily in tissues, which have a low oxygen concentration
- Lower acidity (pH) and higher temperature of actively metabolizing tissue (such as during vigorous exercise) also enhances oxygen release from hemoglobin

● Carbon dioxide transport in blood

- Blood transports carbon dioxide in several forms
    - A small amount is dissolved in plasma
    - Some loosely combines with amino groups in the hemoglobin molecule
    - Most is converted in RBCs to bicarbonate by the enzyme carbonic anhydrase
        · Conversion occurs when hemoglobin liberates oxygen
        · Bicarbonate combines with sodium, and plasma transports it as sodium bicarbonate
- RBC uptake of carbon dioxide begins in capillaries
    - In RBCs, hemoglobin liberates oxygen to supply tissues
    - Simultaneously, carbon dioxide diffuses from tissues into RBCs, where carbonic anhydrase rapidly catalyzes carbonic acid formation by combining with carbon dioxide and water
    - Then carbonic acid dissociates into hydrogen ions (H^+) and bicarbonate ions (HCO_3^-)
    - During oxygen release to tissues, hemoglobin molecules take up H^+; after releasing oxygen, the molecule is reduced and has an increased capacity to combine with H^+
    - The remaining HCO_3^- accumulates until their concentration in RBCs exceeds their concentration in plasma; then HCO_3^- diffuses from RBCs into plasma

- Simultaneously, chloride ions diffuse into RBCs to replace HCO_3^-; this exchange is called the *chloride shift*
- Then HCO_3^- combines with plasma sodium ions to form sodium bicarbonate

● **Gas transport in the lungs**
- In the lungs, carbon dioxide–oxygen exchanges are the reverse of those in tissues
- Reduced hemoglobin takes up oxygen, decreasing hemoglobin's capacity to combine with H^+
  - Then hemoglobin releases H^+
  - Simultaneously, HCO_3^- diffuses into RBCs and chloride ions diffuse out
  - As HCO_3^- moves into RBCs, the ions combine with H^+ liberated from hemoglobin to form carbonic acid
  - Carbonic acid rapidly decomposes, liberating carbon dioxide
  - Carbon dioxide diffuses from RBCs into plasma
  - Some carbon dioxide travels to alveoli, where the lungs excrete it
  - Most remains in plasma as part of HCO_3^-, which plays an essential role in maintaining blood's acid-base balance

CONTROL OF RESPIRATION

● **Key concepts**
- The *respiratory center,* a control center in the brain stem, regulates respiratory rate and depth
- This center discharges impulses to neurons that innervate the diaphragm and intercostal muscles
- The chemical composition of arterial blood and nerve impulses sent to the respiratory center influence the center's impulse discharge rate

● **Arterial blood concentration**
- Arterial concentrations of carbon dioxide and H^+ directly stimulate neurons in the respiratory center
- Normally, arterial P_{CO_2} serves as the primary regulator of the respiratory center; variations in P_{CO_2} levels cause the center to automatically adjust respirations
- During exercise, the body produces more carbon dioxide and arterial P_{CO_2} rises
  - This stimulates the respiratory center to increase respiratory rate and depth
  - This increase causes the lungs to eliminate carbon dioxide more rapidly, allowing arterial P_{CO_2} to decrease to normal

Key facts about gas transport in the lungs

- In the lungs, carbon dioxide–oxygen exchanges are the reverse of those in tissues
- Reduced hemoglobin takes up oxygen and releases H^+
- HCO_3^- combines with H^+ to form carbonic acid
- Carbonic acid releases carbon dioxide

Key facts about the control of respiration

- The respiratory center in the brain regulates respiratory rate and depth
- Chemical composition of blood and nerve impulses influence center's discharge rate

Key facts about arterial blood concentration as a control of respirations

- Arterial concentrations of carbon dioxide and H^+ stimulate neurons in the respiratory center
- Variations in P_{CO_2} levels cause the center to adjust respirations

– Chemoreceptors in the aortic arch and carotid sinus also convey impulses to the respiratory center
– These chemoreceptors respond to arterial blood changes in P_{CO_2}, H^+ concentration (acidity), and P_{O_2}; they signal the respiratory center to adjust respiratory rate and depth as needed

● Nervous system control

- Cranial nerves control functions related to breathing; the pulmonary plexus, a network of nerves made up of tributaries from the vagus nerve (cranial nerve X), innervates the lungs
- Phrenic and intercostal nerves regulate muscles of respiration
  – Innervated by the phrenic nerve, the *diaphragm* is the chief muscle of respiration; this dome-shaped muscle separates the thoracic and abdominopelvic cavities
  – Innervated by the intercostal nerves, the *intercostal muscles* connect the ribs
    · When these muscles contract, they pull the rib cage upward and outward, expanding the lungs and pulling air into them
    · They work in concert (synergistically) with the diaphragm
  – In forced expiration, the scalene and sternocleidomastoid muscles lift the ribs and the quadratus and lumborum muscles of the abdominal wall to aid expiration
- The respiratory center controls respiratory rate and depth and regulates smooth transitions from inspiration to expiration
- Nerve impulses from the lungs, cerebral cortex, and sensory nerve endings affect the rate of impulse discharge from the respiratory center
  – Receptors in the lungs respond to stretching as the lungs inflate, sending impulses to the respiratory center to inhibit further inspiration
    · When the lungs deflate (expiration), the stretch receptors are no longer stimulated
    · Inhibitory impulses no longer travel to the respiratory center
    · Inspiration follows automatically
    · This pulmonary reflex mechanism prevents lung overinflation and helps maintain normal respiratory rhythm
  – The cerebral cortex sends impulses to the respiratory center in response to strong emotions, such as anxiety, fear, and anger; these impulses increase the respiratory rate
  – Some sensory stimuli, such as irritating vapors in the upper respiratory passages, may cause reflex inhibition of respiration

NCLEX CHECKS

It's never too soon to begin your NCLEX preparation. Now that you've reviewed this chapter, carefully read each of the following questions and choose the best answer. Then compare your responses with the correct answers.

1. When assessing a client's lungs, the nurse needs to keep in mind that the right lung has how many lobes?
- ☐ **1.** One
- ☐ **2.** Two
- ☐ **3.** Three
- ☐ **4.** Four

2. Which of the following would the nurse discuss when teaching a client with asthma?
- ☐ **1.** Decrease of fluid intake
- ☐ **2.** Use of an inhaler
- ☐ **3.** Methods to prevent bronchodilation
- ☐ **4.** Methods to promote mucus production

3. The nurse is caring for a neonate with respiratory distress syndrome born at 26 weeks' gestation. The nurse explains to the parents that this disorder results from:
- ☐ **1.** reduced surfactant production.
- ☐ **2.** decreased number of alveoli.
- ☐ **3.** small size of fetal lung structures.
- ☐ **4.** incompletely formed fetal lungs.

4. A client is undergoing pulmonary function tests. The nurse explains to the client that he'll be asked to forcefully exhale after a normal exhalation. Which volume is the nurse testing?
- ☐ **1.** Tidal
- ☐ **2.** Inspiratory reserve
- ☐ **3.** Residual
- ☐ **4.** Expiratory reserve

5. When teaching a client about the respiratory system, the nurse correctly explains that which is the basic unit of gas exchange?
- ☐ **1.** Alveolus
- ☐ **2.** Larynx
- ☐ **3.** Bronchiole
- ☐ **4.** Surfactant

TOP 7

Items to study for your next test on the respiratory system

1. Structures and functions of the respiratory tract
2. Mechanics of inspiration and expiration
3. Pulmonary volumes and capacities
4. Gas exchange in the alveoli
5. Oxygen and carbon dioxide transport
6. Respiratory control mechanisms
7. Teaching tips for patients with asthma or pneumonia

6. For arterial blood gas assessment, which result would the nurse consider normal?

- [ ] **1.** Po_2 97 mm Hg, Pco_2 40 mm Hg
- [ ] **2.** Po_2 40 mm Hg, Pco_2 47 mm Hg
- [ ] **3.** Po_2 97 mm Hg, Pco_2 47 mm Hg
- [ ] **4.** Po_2 40 mm Hg, Pco_2 60 mm Hg

7. A client tells the nurse that he has been following a vigorous exercise program. Which statement would be appropriate for the nurse to make?

- [ ] **1.** "During exercise, increased body temperature inhibits release of oxygen from hemoglobin."
- [ ] **2.** "During exercise, muscles remove more oxygen from the blood."
- [ ] **3.** "During exercise, the rate of blood flow to the tissues drops."
- [ ] **4.** "During exercise, the higher acidity of exercising muscle improves oxygen release from hemoglobin."

8. In the adult without lung disease, the nurse understands that the respiratory center of the brain is regulated primarily by:

- [ ] **1.** venous Pco_2.
- [ ] **2.** venous Po_2.
- [ ] **3.** arterial Pco_2.
- [ ] **4.** arterial Po_2.

9. During a routine respiratory assessment, the nurse keeps in mind that which is the chief respiratory muscle?

- [ ] **1.** Intercostal
- [ ] **2.** Scalene
- [ ] **3.** Sternocleidomastoid
- [ ] **4.** Diaphragm

10. The nurse is caring for a client undergoing pulmonary function tests. The client has a tidal volume of 600 ml of air, an inspiratory reserve volume of 2,900 ml of air, and an expiratory reserve volume of 1,200 ml of air. How many milliliters of air is this client's vital capacity?

_____

ANSWERS AND RATIONALES

1. CORRECT ANSWER: 3
The right lung has three lobes; the left lung has two.

2. CORRECT ANSWER: 2
The nurse would teach the client how to use an inhaler properly to prevent or treat asthma attacks. The nurse should also advise the client to

increase fluid intake and teach him methods to prevent bronchoconstriction and decrease mucus production.

3. CORRECT ANSWER: 1
Neonates born before 28 weeks' gestation have decreased surfactant production. Without sufficient surfactant, surface tension restricts alveolar expansion and may cause alveolar collapse during expiration. Decreased number of alveoli, small lung size, and incompletely formed lungs don't cause respiratory distress syndrome in neonates.

4. CORRECT ANSWER: 4
Forceful expiration at the end of a normal tidal expiration is called expiratory reserve volume—about 1,300 ml of air in a typical adult. Tidal volume is the amount of air an adult inspires and expires with each breath during normal quiet breathing (about 500 ml). Forceful inhalation at the end of a normal tidal inspiration is called inspiratory reserve volume (about 3,000 ml in an adult). Residual volume is the amount of air left after the lungs expel the expiratory reserve volume (about 1,200 ml).

5. CORRECT ANSWER: 1
The alveolus is the basic unit of gas exchange in the lungs. The larynx contains the vocal cords that produce sounds and initiate the cough reflex. Bronchioles are flexible tubes that extend from the bronchi, branching repeatedly and becoming progressively smaller until they branch into the alveolar ducts. Surfactant reduces surface tension to keep alveoli from collapsing.

6. CORRECT ANSWER: 1
Arterial blood has a Po_2 of 97 mm Hg and a Pco_2 of 40 mm Hg. Venous blood has a Po_2 of 40 mm Hg and a Pco_2 of 47 mm Hg. In the tissues, Po_2 is 40 mm Hg and the Pco_2 is about 60 mm Hg.

7. CORRECT ANSWER: 2
During exercise, muscles remove more oxygen from the blood and the rate of blood flow to the tissues increases greatly, increasing the amount of oxygen available to the tissues. The lower acidity and higher temperature of actively metabolizing tissue, which may occur during vigorous exercise, also enhances oxygen release from hemoglobin.

8. CORRECT ANSWER: 3
Normally, the respiratory center (located in the brain stem) is regulated primarily by arterial Pco_2. It adjusts respirations automatically to variations in Pco_2 levels.

9. CORRECT ANSWER: 4
The diaphragm is the chief muscle of respiration; this dome-shaped muscle separates the thoracic and abdominopelvic cavities. The intercostal muscles connect the ribs; when these muscles contract, they pull

the rib cage upward and outward, expanding the lungs and pulling air into them. The scalene and sternocleidomastoid muscles lift the ribs and the quadratus and lumborum muscles of the abdominal wall to aid expiration.

10. CORRECT ANSWER: 4700

The maximum amount of air that can be moved out of the lungs after a maximum inspiration and expiration is called the *vital capacity*. It's calculated by adding together the tidal volume, inspiratory reserve volume, and expiratory reserve volume. In this case: 600 + 2,900 + 1,200 = 4,700.

13

Hematologic system

LEARNING OBJECTIVES

After studying this chapter, you should be able to:

- List the functions of blood.
- Explain the development of formed elements in the blood.
- Discuss the structure and function of the formed elements of the blood.
- Understand the process of the clotting cascade, hemostasis, and fibrinolysis.
- Describe the role of genetics, antigens, and antibodies in blood groups.

CHAPTER OVERVIEW

The hematologic system performs most of its functions through the cardiovascular system. In this system, the blood acts as the body's major transport mechanism, bringing oxygen, nutrients, and hormones to the cells and carrying away cellular wastes. These and other functions make the hematologic system a key factor in maintaining homeostasis. Because blood can provide clues to many hematologic and other disorders, the nurse should be familiar with its structures and normal functions. This chapter reviews blood composition and functions, red and white blood cells, platelets, hemostasis, and blood groups.

Key functions of blood

- Delivers oxygen and nutrients to body cells
- Transports wastes for elimination
- Transports hormones to target tissues
- Maintains body temperature
- Maintains acid-base balance
- Maintains fluid volume
- Helps prevent blood loss through hemostasis
- Helps prevent infection

Key facts about plasma

- Accounts for 55% of total blood volume
- Contains the proteins albumin, globulin, fibrinogen

BLOOD COMPOSITION AND FUNCTIONS

● **Key concepts**
- Blood is a specialized type of connective tissue; it consists of formed elements suspended in a viscous fluid called blood *plasma*
  - Formed elements include red blood cells (RBCs, or erythrocytes), white blood cells (WBCs, or leukocytes), and platelets (thrombocytes)
  - Plasma is a liquid containing dissolved substances
- Slightly alkaline (pH 7.35 to 7.45), blood is red due to its rich oxygen content
- Blood accounts for about 8% of total body weight; the body of an average adult contains about 1.3 gallons (5 liters) of blood
- Blood chiefly functions to:
  - Deliver oxygen to body cells from the lungs and deliver nutrients to body cells from the GI tract
  - Transport carbon dioxide to the lungs and nitrogenous wastes to the kidneys for elimination
  - Transport hormones from endocrine glands to their target tissues
  - Maintain body temperature by absorbing and distributing body heat
  - Maintain acid-base balance
    - Blood proteins and other solutes act as buffers to prevent sudden changes in blood pH
    - Blood also stores bicarbonate atoms (an important component of the blood-buffer system needed to maintain normal blood pH)
  - Maintain adequate fluid volume; salts (such as sodium chloride) and proteins (such as albumin) in blood prevent excessive fluid loss
  - Help prevent blood loss through *hemostasis,* a mechanism that involves a vascular spasm, platelet plug formation, and coagulation
  - Help prevent infection through the action of the antibodies, complement proteins, and WBCs

● **Plasma**
- Plasma accounts for about 55% of total blood volume; contains about 7% proteins and about 93% water with dissolved minerals, nutrients (such as glucose and amino acids), and cellular wastes
- It contains the proteins albumin, globulin, and fibrinogen
  - *Albumin* makes up about one-half of total plasma proteins
    - It's essential in maintaining the blood's colloid osmotic pressure

- This pressure plays a major role in regulating fluid flow between capillaries and interstitial tissues
  – *Globulins* are divided into alpha, beta, and gamma globulins based on physical and chemical characteristics; each type has a specific function
    - Some alpha and beta globulins play a role in blood coagulation; others transport enzymes, hormones, vitamins, and other substances
    - Gamma globulins act as antibodies, defending the body against infection
  – *Fibrinogen* plays a major role in blood coagulation; it's converted to fibrin when blood coagulates

Serum

- Serum is the fluid expressed from clots
- Like plasma, it contains no formed elements
- Unlike plasma, it lacks fibrinogen and other proteins that are depleted by blood coagulation

Formed elements

- Formed elements of blood consist of RBCs, WBCs (granulocytes and agranulocytes), and platelets
- Each type of cell has a characteristic structure and staining reaction when examined microscopically
- All formed elements develop from a common precursor cell — the stem cell — found in red bone marrow of certain bones
  – Stem cells transform into immature versions of each formed element, which then mature
  – This process, called *hematopoiesis*, produces the various types of blood cells (see *Tracing blood cell formation*, pages 234 and 235)
- The quantity of each type of blood cell in circulation stays within narrow limits (varying with a person's age and physical demands)
  – 4.5 to 5.5 $\times$ 10^6 RBCs/mm^3
  – 5,000 to 10,000 WBCs/mm^3
  – 150,000 to 350,000 platelets/mm^3

RED BLOOD CELLS

Key concepts

- RBCs are the most numerous formed element in blood, accounting for about 45% of total blood volume; the measurement of their percentage in blood is called the *hematocrit*
  – These flexible, biconcave disks measure about 7 microns in diameter (1 mm = 1,000 microns)
  – They lack nuclei; nuclei disappear as cells mature
- Maturation of RBCs requires hemoglobin formation

(Text continues on page 236.)

Tracing blood cell formation

Blood cells form and develop in bone marrow by a process called *hematopoiesis*. This chart traces the process, starting with the "birth" of five unipotential stem cells from a multipotential stem cell and ending when they each reach "adulthood" as fully formed cells—erythrocytes, granulocytes, agranulocytes, or platelets.

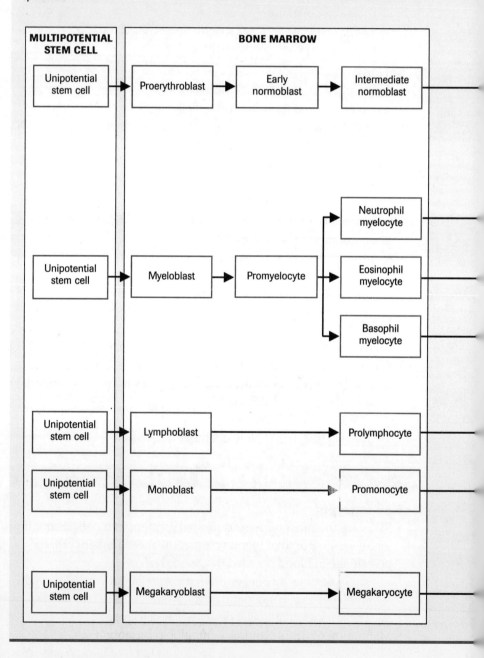

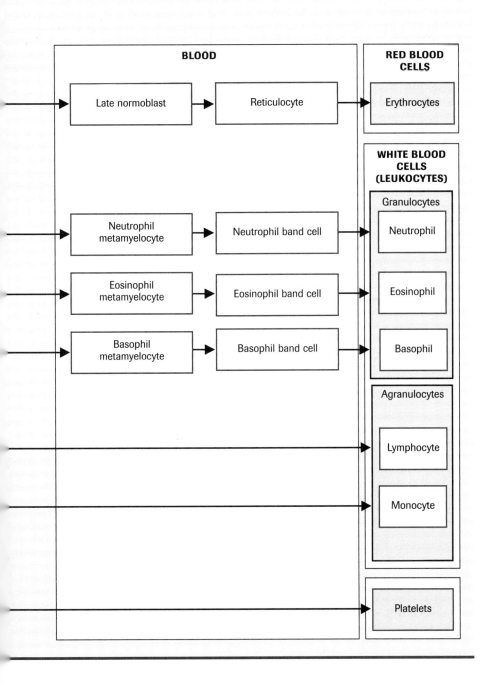

- Hemoglobin is a protein composed of *heme* and *globin*
  - Heme is an ironcontaining porphyrin compound
  - Globin is a protein composed of amino acids
- Mature RBCs consist of a hemoglobin solution enclosed in a protein framework surrounded by a lipoprotein cell membrane
  - Mature RBCs circulate through the cardiovascular system, carrying oxygen to tissues and removing carbon dioxide
  - They contain enzymes that let them perform essential metabolic functions
- RBCs lack mitochondria and can't obtain energy from mitochondrial enzyme systems the way other cells do; instead, they derive energy from glucose breakdown via other enzyme pathways
- Mature RBCs can't synthesize proteins because they don't have nuclei and so can't make new enzymes to replace those that wear out
- RBC aging results, in part, from progressive deterioration of enzyme systems
  - After about 4 months, cells can no longer function
  - In the spleen, the *mononuclear phagocyte (reticuloendothelial) system* removes aged RBCs from circulation and breaks them down into components that the body recycles or discards
    - Globin chains break down and their component amino acids are used to make other proteins
    - Iron is extracted and recycled to make new hemoglobin
    - In the heme molecule, the porphyrin ring can't be salvaged; instead, it's broken down and transported to the liver, which excretes it as bile pigment (bilirubin)

● Functions of RBCs

- RBCs transport oxygen to body tissues
  - Hemoglobin in RBCs combines with oxygen from the lungs, forming oxyhemoglobin
  - When RBCs reach body tissues, hemoglobin releases oxygen, which then diffuses into tissue cells
  - The shape and flexibility of an RBC makes this process easier
    - Biconcave shape gives an RBC a relatively large surface area for oxygen diffusion
    - Flexibility lets it squeeze through narrow capillaries
    - In sickle cell anemia, RBCs assume a sickle shape, making them more rigid; as a result, they can wedge in small capillaries, leading to painful sickle cell crises, chronic fatigue, dyspnea, joint swelling, and frequent infection
- RBCs transport carbon dioxide to the lungs
  - In capillaries, hemoglobin in RBCs combines with carbon dioxide to form carbaminohemoglobin

Key functions of RBCs

- Transport oxygen to body tissues
- Transport carbon dioxide to the lungs
- Contribute to blood viscosity

– When RBCs reach the lungs, hemoglobin releases carbon dioxide, which the lungs exhale
- RBCs also contribute to blood viscosity, with an increase in number leading to more viscous blood, and a decrease leading to less viscous blood

● RBC production and maturation

- *Erythropoiesis* (production of RBCs) occurs in the marrow of certain bones; it's regulated by the oxygen content of arterial blood
  - If the number of circulating RBCs falls below normal, blood delivers less oxygen to tissues; the marrow responds to this oxygen decrease by increasing RBC output
  - The kidneys mediate this marrow response
    · Specialized kidney cells respond to low oxygen tension by liberating the enzyme *renal erythropoietic factor,* which acts on blood protein to form erythropoietin
    · Erythropoietin stimulates stem cells in bone marrow to produce erythroblasts
- *Erythroblasts* (precursors to RBCs) develop over several stages
- As each erythroblast matures, hemoglobin accumulates in the cytoplasm and the nuclear chromatin condenses; normal RBC maturation (*normoblastic erythropoiesis*) differs from abnormal maturation (*megaloblastic erythropoiesis*)
  - When the cell has synthesized most of its hemoglobin, it extrudes its nucleus and becomes a *reticulocyte*
  - The reticulocyte then enters one of the sinusoids in bone marrow and is carried into the circulatory system
    · In a microscopic examination of stained blood, the reticulocyte appears slightly larger than a mature RBC and has a faint blue color because it contains less red-staining hemoglobin
    · Special stains highlight reticulocytes by precipitating and clumping the mitochondria and other organelles within the cytoplasm, causing them to appear as a meshwork (reticulum) of irregular, blue-staining strands and granules in the cytoplasm; the name *reticulocyte* comes from this meshwork
- Final cell maturation occurs in circulation
  - After losing its nucleus, the cell retains its organelles and continues to synthesize hemoglobin
  - The reticulocyte matures into an RBC over the next 24 to 48 hours; the cell gradually decreases in size and loses its blue tinge as it synthesizes more hemoglobin
- The proportion of reticulocytes serves as a useful index of RBC production

Key facts about RBC production and maturation

- Erythropoiesis occurs in marrow of certain bones
- Erythroblasts develop over several stages
- Reticulocyte develops before RBC
- Final cell maturation occurs in circulation
- Proportion of reticulocytes serves as index of RBC production

– Because RBCs survive in circulation for about 100 days (actually 120 days, but considered as 100 days to simplify calculations), the body must produce about 1% of its total RBCs each day to replace those that wear out and are eliminated from the circulation
– This means that the percentage of reticulocytes in normal circulation should be about 1%
– RBC production increases to compensate for increased blood loss (such as after blood donation) or reduced RBC survival (as in some types of anemia); the percentage of circulating reticulocytes increases correspondingly

● **Iron structure and formation**
• Iron constitutes an essential part of hemoglobin and appears in *myoglobin,* a similar compound in muscle
• The body contains about 4 grams of iron; hemoglobin contains about 75% of this amount
• The bone marrow, liver, and spleen store extra iron, where it combines with the protein *apoferritin* to form two different iron-protein complexes
    – *Ferritin* contains about 20% iron
    – *Hemosiderin* contains about 25% iron
• Small amounts of iron circulate in plasma with the iron-binding transport protein *transferrin;* this protein transports iron from the intestinal tract (where iron is absorbed) and mononuclear phagocytes (where iron is recovered from RBC breakdown) to the bone marrow, liver, and spleen (where extra iron is stored)
• The body absorbs and excretes only small amounts of iron; intestinal mucosal cells closely control iron absorption to ensure an adequate — but not excessive — iron supply
    – Dietary iron absorption occurs principally in the duodenum; it's regulated by the iron content of intestinal mucosal cells
    – When iron stores are high, mucosal cells contain ferritin, which inhibits their uptake of additional iron
    – When iron stores are low, mucosal cells absorb more iron, which enters plasma; transferrin then carries iron to bone marrow and storage sites until the body needs it for hemoglobin synthesis
• The usual diet provides about 10 to 20 mg of iron daily
    – Men absorb about 1 mg per day
    – Women and children absorb slightly more
        · Women require more iron to compensate for blood loss during menstruation and for fetal needs during pregnancy

Key facts about iron structure and formation

● Iron is an essential part of hemoglobin
● Bone marrow, liver, and spleen store extra iron
● Small amounts of iron circulate with transferrin
● The body absorbs and secretes small amounts of iron

- Children require extra iron to synthesize hemoglobin during periods of growth when blood volume increases
- Pregnancy, childhood growth, or chronic or excessive blood loss may deplete iron stores; if dietary iron intake doesn't compensate for this depletion, iron deficiency anemia may result
- Normally, iron from RBC breakdown is recycled to make new hemoglobin
- One milliliter of blood contains approximately 0.5 mg of iron

● Hemoglobin structure and formation

- Hemoglobin is the oxygen-carrying protein formed in the cytoplasm of developing RBCs
- It consists of four monomers fitted together to form a tetramer, like the sections of an apple cut into quarters
- Each monomer is a complex composed of the iron-containing compound heme and the protein globin
- Heme is constructed from four nitrogen-containing ring compounds called *pyrrole rings,* which join to form a more complex ring structure called a *porphyrin ring*
  - An atom of iron with six binding sites occupies the central position of the porphyrin ring
    - Nitrogen atoms bind to four of these sites
    - The amino acid histidine binds the globin chain to the iron at the fifth site
    - The sixth binding site remains available for reversible combination with oxygen
- Globin forms the largest part of the hemoglobin monomer
  - It's composed of an amino acid chain joined together to form a coiled polypeptide chain
  - Heme is tucked into one of the bends in the globin coil and held there by the bond between the iron atom and histidine in the globin chain
- Heme and globin are synthesized in different locations in the cell
  - Transferrin brings iron to the erythroblast
  - When inside the mitochondria, iron is incorporated into the porphyrin ring to form heme (nearby reticuloendothelial cells remove excess iron not used in heme synthesis)
  - At the same time, ribosomes in the cytoplasm produce globin chains
  - Globin chains and heme join to form a hemoglobin monomer
  - The four monomers aggregate to form the complete hemoglobin tetramer

Key facts about hemoglobin structure and formation

- Hemoglobin forms in cytoplasm of developing RBCs
- Consists of four monomers fitted together as a tetramer
- Each monomer is composed of iron-containing compound heme and protein globin
- Globin forms the largest part of the monomer

● Globin chains

- The five types of globin chains—alpha, beta, gamma, delta, and epsilon—have different amino acid compositions
- The body produces globin chains at different times and in different proportions, beginning when an embryo and extending into adulthood
- In most hemoglobin tetramers, two subunits contain one type of globin chain; the other two subunits have a different type
- Adults produce two types of hemoglobin
  - About 98% of hemoglobin consists of tetramers with two subunits containing alpha chains and two containing beta chains; this is *hemoglobin A* (adult hemoglobin)
  - The other 2% consists of tetramers containing alpha and delta chains; this is *hemoglobin A$_2$*
- The embryo and fetus produce different hemoglobins
  - An embryo initially produces hemoglobin containing only epsilon chains
  - The fetus soon replaces this tetramer with a tetramer containing alpha and gamma chains—*hemoglobin F* (fetal hemoglobin), the predominant hemoglobin in the fetus
  - Late in the fetal period, the fetus produces beta chains of adult hemoglobin in small quantities
- Fetal hemoglobin can take up and release oxygen at lower oxygen tensions than hemoglobin A—an advantage because fetal blood has a relatively low oxygen tension
- After birth, gamma-chain synthesis declines and beta-chain synthesis increases in hemoglobin production
  - Hemoglobin F in RBCs gradually declines
  - Hemoglobin A rises correspondingly
- Genes control globin chain structure by directing the order of amino acid incorporation into the chains
  - Mutation of these genes can alter the amino acid sequence, causing hemoglobin abnormalities such as sickle cell anemia

WHITE BLOOD CELLS

● Key concepts

- WBCs (leukocytes) are nucleated blood cells that play an important role in the body's defenses (inflammation) and immune responses
  - WBCs defend the body against viruses, bacteria, and other foreign particles
  - Counts above 11,000/mm^3 usually signal viral or bacterial infection

Comparing granulocytes and agranulocytes

White blood cells protect the body from invading organisms. Each type works differently.

PRIMARY RESPONSE
Granulocytes, including basophils, neutrophils, and eosinophils, are the first forces marshaled against invading organisms.

Basophils fire histamine at inflammatory and immune stimuli.

Neutrophils eat foreign bodies.

Eosinophils eat antigens and antibodies.

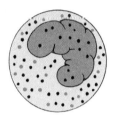 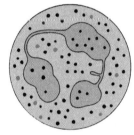 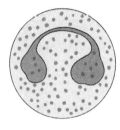

SECONDARY RESPONSE
Agranulocytes—lymphocytes and monocytes—may patrol when inflammation occurs, but they mainly defend against invaders at structures that filter large amounts of fluid such as the liver.

Lymphocytes eat the invading organism or produce antibodies.

Monocytes eat bacteria, cellular debris, and necrotic tissue.

 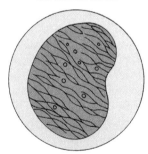

Key characteristics of granulocytes

- Act as a primary response to invading organisms
- Subdivided into neutrophils, eosinophils, and basophils

Key characteristics of agranulocytes

- Defend against invading organisms at structures that filter large amounts of fluid
- Subdivided into lymphocytes and monocytes

- They're generally classified according to their structure, each having a specific function
  - *Granulocytes* contain cytoplasmic granules; they're subdivided into *neutrophils, eosinophils,* and *basophils*
  - Agranulocytes lack cytoplasmic granules; they're subdivided into lymphocytes and monocytes (see *Comparing granulocytes and agranulocytes*)

• Normally, the WBC differential count (a percentage count of
WBCs) is 40% to 60% neutrophils, 0% to 1% basophils, 1% to 3%
eosinophils, 20% to 40% lymphocytes, and 4% to 8% monocytes
• WBCs mature in bone marrow
 – Maturation is characterized by condensation of nuclear
chromatins and an increase in cytoplasm
 – Several types of WBCs develop different kinds of cytoplasmic
granules and multilobed nuclei
• Fewer WBCs than RBCs circulate in the body, and most have a
short life span
 – WBCs circulate about 4 to 8 hours after release from bone marrow; then they leave the circulation and enter various body tissues, where they live another 4 to 5 days (they may have a total
life span of just a few hours in a person with a severe infection)
 – They use an amoeboid motion to move in and out of blood
vessels and through tissue spaces

● **Neutrophils**
• Also called *polymorphonuclear WBCs, neutrophils* have a segmented
nucleus and cytoplasm containing fine granules
• Relatively large cells (twice the size of RBCs), neutrophils are the
largest group of circulating WBCs (constituting about 65% of all
WBCs); their numbers increase in response to infection
• Neutrophils are phagocytic, destroying bacteria, viruses, and other
foreign substances by engulfing, ingesting, and digesting them
• Worn-out neutrophils form the main component of pus

● **Eosinophils**
• *Eosinophils,* which account for about 2% of all WBCs, contain large,
bright red-staining (eosinophilic) granules
• Their main function is the phagocytosis of antigen-antibody complexes, which form as an allergic reaction when antibodies combine with the antigens that trigger their release
• The number of eosinophils increases in many allergic conditions
and in response to some parasitic infections

● **Basophils**
• The least abundant of all WBCs (constituting less than 1%), *basophils* are slightly larger than RBCs and contain dark purple (basophilic) granules
• They play an essential role in some allergic reactions
• In a sensitized individual, basophils rupture in response to specific
antigens, such as penicillin and bee venom
 – Rupture releases large quantities of histamine, bradykinin, heparin, and some lysosomal enzymes

— These substances produce the tissue and vascular reactions that cause allergy signs and symptoms

● **Lymphocytes**
- Small, mononuclear, nonphagocytic WBCs, *lymphocytes* have a deep-staining nucleus that contains dense chromatin and a pale blue–staining cytoplasm
- The second most abundant type of WBC (constituting about 30% of all WBCs), lymphocytes are more common in lymphoid tissues than in blood; they increase in number in response to some infections
- Lymphocytes play a major role in the body's immune response
  - *T lymphocytes* (thymus-dependent lymphocytes) act directly against infected cells and tumors
  - *B lymphocytes* (bursa-dependent lymphocytes) give rise to plasma cells, which produce humoral antibodies called immunoglobulins
- Lymphocytes can be divided into two groups based on their life span
  - One group has a relatively short life span compared with other WBCs
  - The other group survives for several years; cells in this group are known as *memory cells*

● **Monocytes**
- The largest of all WBCs, *monocytes* are phagocytic cells that form part of the mononuclear phagocyte system
- Constituting about 3% of all WBCs, they have a single, U-shaped nucleus
- Monocytes differentiate into *macrophages,* phagocytic cells that serve as the first-line defense against viruses, certain bacteria, some chronic infections (such as tuberculosis), and some systemic fungal infections
  - They leave the circulation and function as scavenger cells, cleaning up debris after acute inflammation
  - They also participate (along with lymphocytes) in the body's immune response

PLATELETS

● **Key concepts**
- Named for their resemblance to small plates, *platelets* are also called *thrombocytes*
- Small and anucleated (containing no nucleus), these cells are about one-third the size of RBCs

● **Functions**
- Platelets play an essential role in blood clotting and in plugging blood vessel breaks
- Insufficient quantity or dysfunction of platelets can cause serious bleeding problems

● **Platelet life cycle**
- Platelets form from large, multinucleated cells called *megakaryocytes* in bone marrow
  - Megakaryocytes are extremely large cells that develop from stem cells
  - On the surface of megakaryocytes, platelets form as buds that pinch off to enter the circulation
  - Blood normally contains 150,000 to 350,000 platelets/mm^3
- Platelets are motile and can store and release biochemicals and change shape
- They have a life span of about 10 to 14 days

HEMOSTASIS

● **Key concepts**
- Hemostasis is the process by which bleeding stops; the body arrests all bleeding as quickly as possible to prevent life-threatening hemorrhage
- Blood vessels, platelets, and coagulation factors help blood to clot, which stops bleeding
- After a blood vessel has healed and no longer needs a clot, the clot must be lysed (dissolved)
- The body normally maintains a balance between clotting and clot fibrinolysis, which is controlled largely by substances that inhibit and activate clotting and lysis

● **Role of blood vessels and platelets**
- Blood vessels and platelets function together to prevent bleeding
- Injury to a blood vessel causes it to constrict, narrowing its diameter, which makes it easier for a blood clot to close it off
- Vessel injury also disrupts the endothelium and exposes the underlying connective tissue, stimulating platelets and coagulation factors to react
- Platelets aggregate and adhere to the injury site
  - They release vasoconstrictors, causing vessels to constrict further
  - These platelets also release phospholipids that initiate *coagulation* (clotting of blood)
- Platelets also play an important role in preventing capillary bleeding

---

Key facts about platelets

- Play an essential role in blood clotting and in plugging blood vessel breaks
- Form from megakaryocytes in bone marrow
- Can store and release chemicals and change shape

Key role of blood vessels and platelets in hemostasis

- Injury to a vessel causes it to constrict
- Vessel injury also stimulates platelets and coagulation factors to react
- Platelets aggregate and adhere to the injury site

TIME-OUT FOR TEACHING

Teaching a patient with thrombocytopenia

When teaching a patient with thrombocytopenia, make sure you:
- describe platelets and explain their role in clotting
- discuss possible causes of thrombocytopenia
- describe the severity of thrombocytopenia
- tell him what signs and symptoms of bleeding and complications to report
- describe platelet counts and other diagnostic tests
- discuss treatments he may undergo, such as platelet infusion, administration of immunosuppressive agents, and splenectomy
- explain bleeding precautions and activity restrictions
- provide sources of information and support

- Small breaks in capillaries occur frequently, but formation of a platelet plug (rather than a blood clot) promptly seals the break
- If there aren't enough platelets (thrombocytopenia) or if they don't function properly, pinpoint areas of bleeding (petechiae) develop in the skin and internal organs and more serious bleeding may follow (see *Teaching a patient with thrombocytopenia*)

● **Coagulation factors**
- Coagulation factors are precursor compounds that are activated and circulated during coagulation; they're designated by name and Roman numeral (see *Coagulation factors,* page 246)
- Coagulation occurs as a chain reaction in which each coagulation factor sequentially activates the next coagulation factor in the chain
- The liver manufactures several coagulation factors and requires vitamin K for their synthesis
  - Vitamin K deficiency can inhibit their synthesis and disrupt normal coagulation
- All phases of coagulation require calcium ions; however, coagulation disturbances don't result from abnormally low blood calcium levels because a calcium level low enough to interfere with coagulation would cause death

● **Coagulation factor activation**
- Although a continuous sequence, the coagulation cascade can be thought of as three phases (see *How blood clots,* pages 248 and 249)
- In phase 1, prothrombin activator forms

Key teaching topics for a patient with thrombocytopenia
- Describe signs and symptoms
- Explain diagnostic tests
- Review treatments and bleeding precautions

Key facts about coagulation factors
- Designated by name and Roman numeral
- Each coagulation factor sequentially activates the next factor
- Because synthesis requires vitamin K, vitamin K deficiency can disrupt normal coagulation

Key facts about phases of coagulation factor activation
- Phase 1: Prothrombin activator forms
- Phase 2: Prothrombin activator converts prothrombin to thrombin
- Phase 3: Thrombin converts fibrinogen to fibrin

Key coagulation factors

- Fibrogen
- Prothrombin
- Tissue thromboplastin
- Calcium ions
- Proaccelerin
- Serum prothrombin conversion accelerator
- Antihemophilic factor
- Plasma thromboplastin component
- Stuart factor
- Plasma thromboplastin antecedent
- Hageman factor
- Fibrin stabilizing factor

Coagulation factors

Various factors perform vital functions in the coagulation process, as described in this chart.

FACTOR NUMBER AND NAME	DESCRIPTION AND FUNCTION
I (fibrinogen)	High-molecular-weight protein synthesized in liver; converted to fibrin in phase 3 (a common phase)
II (prothrombin)	Protein synthesized in liver (requires vitamin K); converted to thrombin in phase 2 (a common phase)
III (tissue thromboplastin)	Factor released from damaged tissue; required in phase 1 of the extrinsic system
IV (calcium ions)	Factor required throughout the entire clotting sequence
V (proaccelerin, or labile factor)	Protein synthesized in liver; functions in phases 1 and 2 of the intrinsic and extrinsic systems
VII (serum prothrombin conversion accelerator, stable factor, or proconvertin)	Protein synthesized in liver (requires vitamin K); functions in phase 1 of the extrinsic system
VIII (antihemophilic factor, or antihemophilic globulin)	Protein synthesized in liver; required in phase 1 of the intrinsic system
IX (plasma thromboplastin component)	Protein synthesized in liver (requires vitamin K); required in phase 1 of the intrinsic system
X (Stuart factor or Stuart-Prower factor)	Protein synthesized in liver (requires vitamin K); required in phase 1 of the intrinsic and extrinsic systems
XI (plasma thromboplastin antecedent)	Protein synthesized in liver; required in phase 1 of the intrinsic system
XII (Hageman factor)	Protein required in phase 1 of the intrinsic system
XIII (fibrin stabilizing factor)	Protein required to stabilize the fibrin strands in phase 3

- Two different mechanisms produce prothrombin activator—the intrinsic system and the extrinsic system
- The *intrinsic system* is so named because all of its components come from the blood
  - Platelets accumulate at the injury site and release phospholipids, which interact with coagulation factors
  - Factors are activated in sequence to yield prothrombin activator

– In the *extrinsic system,* tissue injury liberates thromboplastin (factor III), which interacts with coagulation factors to produce factor X_a
  · The extrinsic system is so named because prothrombin activator derives primarily from injured tissue rather than blood
  · This system requires about one-half the number of coagulation factors as the intrinsic system; it requires no platelets
• Phase 2 involves conversion of prothrombin (factor II) to thrombin by prothrombin activator, which was formed in phase 1
  – *Prothrombin* is a protein made in the liver
  – Prothrombin activator splits prothrombin into fragments
  – Fragmentation produces thrombin, a protein-digesting enzyme
• Phase 3 involves conversion of fibrinogen (factor 1) to fibrin by thrombin
  – *Fibrinogen* is a high-molecular-weight protein produced by the liver
  – Thrombin cleaves part of the fibrinogen molecule to form a smaller molecule, called a *fibrin monomer*
  – Then fibrin monomers join end-to-end and cross-link from side-to-side to form a meshwork of fibrin threads containing plasma, RBCs, WBCs, and platelets; this meshwork is a *clot*
  – Another plasma factor (XIII) strengthens the bonds between the fibrin molecules and increases the strength of the clot

● **Coagulation inhibition**
• Certain inhibitors and anticoagulants retard clotting to counterbalance coagulation factors, preventing excessive intravascular coagulation
• Antithrombin in plasma inhibits thrombin formation
• Heparin, which is found in basophils and mast cells, has anticoagulant properties
• Prostaglandin derivatives inhibit the platelet aggregation and phospholipid release that initiate coagulation

● **Fibrinolytic system**
• This clot-dissolving system is activated simultaneously with the coagulation mechanism; it restricts clotting to a limited area, preventing excessive intravascular coagulation
• The precursor compound *plasminogen* (profibrinolysin) is converted to *plasmin* (fibrinolysin) by various substances
  – Factor XII_a, which forms during phase 1 of coagulation by the intrinsic system, activates plasminogen conversion
  – Components from injured tissues activate the extrinsic system as well as plasminogen conversion
  – *Thrombin,* which converts fibrinogen to fibrin, also converts plasminogen to plasmin

Key coagulation inhibitors
• Antithrombin: Inhibits thrombin formation
• Heparin: Has anticoagulant properties
• Prostaglandin derivatives: inhibit platelet aggregation and phospholipid release

Key facts about the fibrinolytic system
• Restricts clotting to a limited area
• Activated along with coagulation mechanism
• Plasminogen is converted to plasmin
• Plasmin breaks down fibrin strands in a clot

GO WITH THE FLOW

How blood clots

When a blood vessel is severed or injured, three interrelated processes take place.

CONSTRICTION AND AGGREGATION

Immediately, the vessels affected by the injury contract (*constriction*), reducing blood flow. Also, platelets, stimulated by the exposed collagen of the damaged cells, begin to clump together (*aggregation*). Aggregation provides a temporary seal and a site for clotting to take place. The platelets release a number of substances that enhance constriction and aggregation.

CLOTTING PATHWAYS

Clotting, or *coagulation*—the transformation of blood from a liquid to a solid—may be initiated through two different pathways: the intrinsic pathway or the extrinsic pathway. The *intrinsic pathway* is activated when plasma comes in contact with damaged vessel surfaces. The *extrinsic pathway* is activated when tissue factor (a substance released by damaged endothelial cells) comes in contact with one of the clotting factors.

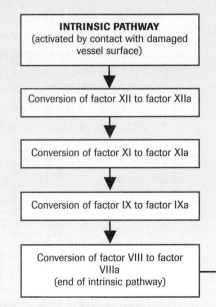

INTRINSIC PATHWAY
(activated by contact with damaged vessel surface)

↓

Conversion of factor XII to factor XIIa

↓

Conversion of factor XI to factor XIa

↓

Conversion of factor IX to factor IXa

↓

Conversion of factor VIII to factor VIIIa
(end of intrinsic pathway)

- Plasmin is a proteolytic (protein-digesting) enzyme that breaks down the fibrin strands in the clot
- Circulating inhibitors (alpha globulins) inactivate plasmin
  - Alpha globulins combine with plasmin to form inactive complexes; this prevents unwanted clot breakdown by inactivating plasmin trapped in the fibrin clot
  - These inhibitors also inactivate plasmin that diffuses from the coagulation sites; this prevents plasmin from attacking and degrading other clotting factors

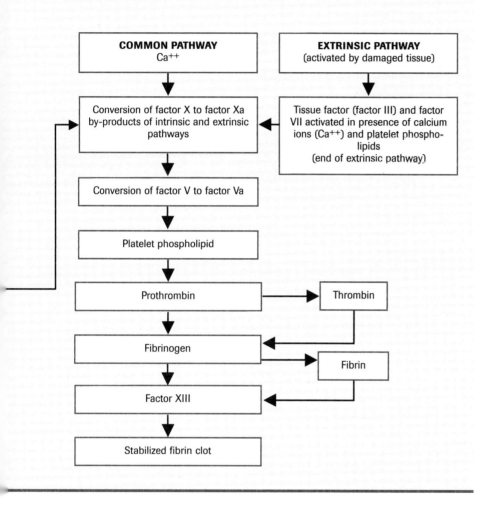

COMMON PATHWAY	EXTRINSIC PATHWAY
Ca^{++}	(activated by damaged tissue)

Conversion of factor X to factor Xa by-products of intrinsic and extrinsic pathways ← Tissue factor (factor III) and factor VII activated in presence of calcium ions (Ca^{++}) and platelet phospholipids (end of extrinsic pathway)

Conversion of factor V to factor Va

Platelet phospholipid

Prothrombin → Thrombin

Fibrinogen ← (Thrombin)

Fibrin

Factor XIII ← (Fibrin)

Stabilized fibrin clot

BLOOD GROUPS

- **Key concepts**
  - The surface of RBCs contains antigens or agglutinogens (glycoproteins) that are inherited through Mendelian patterns; an *antigen* is a substance that stimulates formation of antibodies that can combine with the antigen
  - When exposed to certain antibodies, these antigens cause reactions that are the basis for classifying blood groups (blood typing)
  - Many different blood group systems have been described; the ABO and Rh systems are the most important

Key facts about blood groups

- The surface of RBCs contains antigens or agglutinogens
- Antigens cause reactions when exposed to certain antibodies
- Blood is classified according to the reactions that occur

Key facts about ABO blood group system

- Identifies blood type by testing for A and B antigens on surface of RBCs and for anti-A and anti-B antibodies in serum
- Blood belongs to one of four groups: A, B, O, or AB
- Genetics determine ABO antigens

● ABO blood group system

- ABO group identifies a person's blood type by testing for A and B antigens on the surface of RBCs and for anti-A and anti-B antibodies in serum
- Each person's blood belongs to one of four groups—A, B, O, or AB (see *Blood type compatibility*)
- Individuals normally have antibodies directed against antigens their RBCs lack
    - Group A individuals (41% of the population) have A antigen on RBCs and anti-B antibody in serum
    - Group B individuals (10% of the population) have B antigen on RBCs and anti-A antibody in serum
    - Group O individuals (45% of the population) have no A or B antigens on RBCs; they have anti-A and anti-B antibodies in serum
        - Type O is the most common blood type among white Americans
        - People with type O blood are called *universal donors* because their blood may be given to people with any other ABO type
    - Group AB individuals (4% of the population) have both A and B antigens on the RBCs and no anti-A or anti-B antibodies in serum
        - AB is the rarest blood type
        - People with type AB blood are called *universal recipients* because they may receive blood of any other ABO type
- Antigens are identified by mixing a sample of RBCs with anti-A typing serum and another sample with anti-B typing serum; this ABO antigen typing is known as *direct typing*
    - RBC clumping (*agglutination*) in the typing serum determines the antigens
    - For example, if cells agglutinate with anti-A typing serum but not anti-B typing serum, then a person's RBCs contain A antigen
- Serum antibodies are determined by mixing one serum sample with a suspension of known group A test cells and another sample with a suspension of known group B test cells; this antibody typing, known as *reverse typing,* confirms direct typing
    - Test cell agglutination indicates the corresponding antibody in the serum
    - For example, if the serum sample agglutinates group B test cells but not group A test cells, the serum contains only anti-B antibody
- Genetics determine ABO antigens

Blood type compatibility

Precise blood typing and crossmatching can prevent the transfusion of incompatible blood, which can be fatal. Usually, typing the recipient's blood and crossmatching it with available donor blood takes less than 1 hour.

MAKING A MATCH

Agglutinogen (an antigen in red blood cells) and agglutinin (an antibody in plasma) distinguish the four ABO blood groups. This chart shows ABO compatibility from the perspectives of the recipient and the donor.

BLOOD GROUP	ANTIBODIES PRESENT IN PLASMA	COMPATIBLE RBCS	COMPATIBLE PLASMA
Recipient			
O	Anti-A and anti-B	O	O, A, B, AB
A	Anti-B	A, O	A, AB
B	Anti-A	B, O	B, AB
AB	Neither anti-A nor anti-B	AB, A, B, O	AB
Donor			
O	Anti-A and anti-B	O, A, B, AB	O
A	Anti-B	A, AB	A, O
B	Anti-A	B, AB	B, O
AB	Neither anti-A nor anti-B	AB	AB, A, B, O

- The gene locus on each chromosome may be occupied by an A, B, or O gene; Mendelian inheritance patterns determine which genes the offspring inherits
  - A person is homozygous for ABO genes if the alleles are the same on both chromosomes (AA, BB, or OO)
  - A person is heterozygous if the genes are different (AO, BO, AB)
- The gene combination on the chromosomes determines the ABO *genotype*
- The blood type obtained by testing RBCs with anti-A and anti-B typing serum determines the ABO *phenotype*
  - A phenotype may include more than one genotype
  - For example, the phenotype B may represent genotype BB (homozygous) or BO (heterozygous)
- Because parents may transmit either allele to their offspring, an infant may not have the same ABO genotype or phenotype as either parent

Key facts about genetic blood type

- The gene combination on the chromosomes determines the ABO genotype
- The blood type obtained by testing RBCs with anti-A and anti-B typing serum determines the ABO phenotype
- A phenotype may include more than one genotype

Key facts about the Rh blood group system

- Classifies RBCs according to group of inherited antigens on their surface
- If an Rh-negative individual is exposed to Rh-positive blood, she may form anti-Rh antibodies
- If she becomes exposed to Rh-positive blood at some time in the future, the anti-Rh antibodies will destroy the Rh-positive RBCs

- For example, two heterozygous type A (AO) parents may produce type O (OO) infant; the same pattern is true for two heterozygous type B (BO) parents
- Two type AB parents may produce a homozygous type A (AA), homozygous type B (BB), or type AB infant
- A heterozygous type A (AO) parent and a type AB parent can produce a homozygous type A (AA), heterozygous type A (AO), heterozygous type B (BO), or type AB infant

● **Rh blood group system**
- Rh system classifies RBCs according to a group of inherited antigens on their surface
- Scientists performed the original Rh studies by immunizing rabbits and guinea pigs with blood from rhesus monkeys
  - The immunized animals formed anti-rhesus antibodies that reacted not only with the rhesus monkey RBCs but with the RBCs of about 85% of white individuals and 95% of black individuals
  - Those whose RBCs were agglutinated by the anti-rhesus antibodies were called rhesus-positive (Rh-positive); those whose RBCs didn't react with the anti-rhesus antibodies were called rhesus-negative (Rh-negative)
- When exposed to Rh-positive blood by blood transfusion or pregnancy with an Rh-positive fetus, an Rh-negative individual may form anti-Rh antibodies
  - Subsequent transfusion of Rh-positive blood to such a person leads to rapid destruction of the transfused cells (transfusion reaction)
  - If a woman whose blood contains anti-Rh antibodies becomes pregnant with an Rh-positive fetus, the anti-Rh antibodies cross the placenta and destroy fetal RBCs, causing hemolytic disease of the newborn
- Although many genes and RBC antigens are involved in the Rh system, the Rh antigen described first is the most important clinically; it's called the D antigen or the Rh_o antigen (the subscript "o" stands for *original*)
  - Of the eight types of Rh antigens, only C, D, and E are common
  - Normally, blood contains the Rh antigen (in other words, it's Rh-positive and lacks anti-Rh antibodies)
- The gene D and its allele determine the presence of D antigen on RBCs
- People whose RBCs contain the D antigen (genotype DD or Dd) are considered Rh-positive (regardless of other Rh antigens on the

RBCs); those who lack the D antigen (genotype dd) are considered Rh-negative

- An Rh-positive person may be homozygous (DD) or heterozygous (Dd); the latter is more common
- Because each parent transmits one of two alleles to offspring, an infant may not have the same Rh genotype or phenotype as either parent
    - Two heterozygous Rh-positive (Dd) parents may produce a homozygous Rh-positive (DD), heterozygous Rh-positive (Dd), or Rh-negative (dd) infant
    - A homozygous Rh-positive (DD) parent and a heterozygous Rh-positive (Dd) parent may produce a homozygous Rh-positive (DD) or heterozygous Rh-positive (Dd) infant
    - A heterozygous Rh-positive (Dd) parent and an Rh-negative (dd) parent may produce an Rh-positive (Dd) or Rh-negative (dd) infant

NCLEX CHECKS

It's never too soon to begin your NCLEX preparation. Now that you've reviewed this chapter, carefully read each of the following questions and choose the best answer. Then compare your responses with the correct answers.

1. A client who's being seen for a possible infection asks the nurse to describe the different blood components that will be analyzed in his blood test. The nurse correctly explains that infections are primarily prevented by the presence of which component?
- ☐ **1.** RBC
- ☐ **2.** WBC
- ☐ **3.** Platelet
- ☐ **4.** Fibrin

2. The nurse is infusing platelets into a child with a low platelet count. The nurse explains to the mother that platelets have a life span of how long?
- ☐ **1.** 4 to 8 hours
- ☐ **2.** 4 to 5 days
- ☐ **3.** 10 to 14 days
- ☐ **4.** 120 days

3. The nurse should notify the physician if a client's laboratory results indicate which value?
- ☐ **1.** 100,000 platelets/mm^3
- ☐ **2.** 5×10^6 RBCs/mm^3
- ☐ **3.** 6,000 WBCs/mm^3
- ☐ **4.** 45% hematocrit

TOP 9

Items to study for your next test on the hematologic system

1. General functions of the blood
2. Process of hematopoiesis
3. Structure and function of RBCs
4. Structure and function of iron and hemoglobin
5. Types of WBCs and their functions
6. Structure and function of platelets
7. Coagulation factors and the clotting cascade
8. ABO and Rh blood grouping systems
9. Teaching tips for patients with thrombocytopenia

4. Which information should the nurse include when teaching a client with sickle cell anemia? Select all that apply.

☐ **1.** The sickle shape makes RBCs more flexible.

☐ **2.** The sickle shape makes blood flow more easily in the arteries.

☐ **3.** The sickle shape causes RBCs to occlude small capillaries.

☐ **4.** Sickle cell disease can lead to painful crises.

☐ **5.** Sickle cell disease can cause chronic fatigue.

☐ **6.** Sickle cell disease can cause joint swelling.

5. The nurse is providing nutritional counseling to a female client who has two children under age 5. Which statement is the nurse most likely to make about iron requirements?

☐ **1.** "A woman needs more iron during pregnancy."

☐ **2.** "Increased iron intake during pregnancy is unhealthy for the developing fetus."

☐ **3.** "Children require less iron than adults."

☐ **4.** "Menstruation reduces iron needs."

6. The nurse is reviewing a client's WBC differential count. In the absence of illness, which type of WBCs would the nurse expect to be most abundant?

☐ **1.** Basophils

☐ **2.** Lymphocytes

☐ **3.** Neutrophils

☐ **4.** Eosinophils

7. Which intervention would the nurse most likely include in the care plan for a client with thrombocytopenia?

☐ **1.** Encourage the client to resume all activities after discharge.

☐ **2.** Advise the client to take aspirin for headaches.

☐ **3.** Teach the client which signs and symptoms of bleeding to report.

☐ **4.** Discuss ways the client can reduce the risk of infection.

8. The nurse is drawing blood to send to the laboratory to type and crossmatch for a potential blood transfusion. The client asks the nurse many questions about which blood types are universal donors and recipients. How does the nurse respond to the client's questions?

☐ **1.** People with type O blood are universal donors.

☐ **2.** People with type O blood are universal recipients.

☐ **3.** People with type AB blood are universal donors.

☐ **4.** People with type AB blood may receive blood only from type A or type B donors.

9. After a client receives genetic counseling, the nurse clarifies for the client that it's possible for two heterozygous blood type A parents to produce offspring with which blood type?

☐ **1.** AO
☐ **2.** BB
☐ **3.** AB
☐ **4.** BO

10. The nurse teaches a client that, for normal blood clotting to occur, it's important to have a sufficient amount of which vitamin?

☐ **1.** Vitamin A
☐ **2.** Vitamin C
☐ **3.** Vitamin D
☐ **4.** Vitamin K

ANSWERS AND RATIONALES

1. CORRECT ANSWER: 2

WBCs participate in the inflammatory and immune responses and defend the body against viruses, bacteria, and other foreign particles. RBCs transport oxygen to body tissues. Platelets play an essential role in blood clotting and in plugging vessel breaks. Fibrin joins together to form a meshwork of fibrin threads that contains plasma, RBCs, WBCs, and platelets to form a clot.

2. CORRECT ANSWER: 3

Platelets have a life span of about 10 to 14 days. WBCs circulate about 4 to 8 hours after they're released from the bone marrow; they live another 4 to 5 days in tissues. RBCs have a life span of 120 days.

3. CORRECT ANSWER: 1

Blood normally contains 150,000 to 350,000 platelets/mm^3; 4.5 to 5.5 $\times$ 10^6 RBCs/mm^3; and 5,000 to 10,000 WBCs/mm^3 in adults. The average hematocrit (percentage of RBCs in blood) is 45%.

4. CORRECT ANSWER: 3, 4, 5, 6

In sickle cell anemia, the RBCs develop a sickle shape, making them more rigid and prone to getting stuck in small capillaries. This blood vessel occlusion leads to painful sickle cell crisis, chronic fatigue, joint swelling, and frequent infection.

5. CORRECT ANSWER: 1

Women require more iron to meet fetal needs during pregnancy and to compensate for blood loss during menstruation. Children require extra iron to synthesize hemoglobin during periods of growth when blood volume increases.

6. CORRECT ANSWER: 3
Neutrophils make up about 65% of all WBCs. Basophils account for less than 1% of all WBCs. Lymphocytes are the second-most common type, accounting for about 30% of WBCs. Eosinophils constitute only 2% of all types of WBCs.

7. CORRECT ANSWER: 3
The nursing care plan should include an intervention for teaching the client the signs and symptoms of bleeding to report because thrombocytopenia indicates a reduced platelet count, which increases the risk of bleeding and serious hemorrhage. The care plan should also include interventions for teaching the client to avoid activities that could promote bleeding (such as contact sports) and to avoid aspirin use. Because thrombocytopenia doesn't affect WBCs, the client isn't at increased risk for infection.

8. CORRECT ANSWER: 1
People with type O blood are universal donors because their blood may be given to people with any other ABO type; they aren't universal recipients and may only receive type O blood. People with type AB blood are universal recipients and may receive blood from any ABO blood type.

9. CORRECT ANSWER: 1
A person is heterozygous for ABO genes if the genes are different. Two heterozygous type A (AO) parents may produce a homozygous type A (AA), heterozygous type A (AO), or type O (OO) offspring.

10. CORRECT ANSWER: 4
Several coagulation factors are manufactured in the liver that require vitamin K for their synthesis. A vitamin K deficiency can inhibit synthesis of these coagulation factors and disrupt normal coagulation.

14

Lymphatic system

LEARNING OBJECTIVES

After studying this chapter, you should be able to:

- Identify the structure and function of lymph tissues.
- Describe the function, formation, and flow of lymph.
- Discuss the formation and function of T and B lymphocytes.
- Explain the mechanisms of nonspecific resistance to disease.
- Compare and contrast cell-mediated immunity and humoral immunity.

CHAPTER OVERVIEW

The lymphatic system parallels the circulatory system, returning excess fluid and protein from interstitial fluid to the circulatory system. Perhaps more important, the lymphatic system provides several lines of defense against disease. Without a properly functioning lymphatic system, an injury as mild as a paper cut could be life-threatening. Because this system is so vital to homeostasis and immunity, the nurse should be aware of its basic structures and functions. This chapter reviews lymph tissue, lymphatic fluid and vessels, lymphocytes, nonspecific resistance to disease, and acquired immunity (cell-mediated and humoral).

Key facts about the lymphatic system

- Serves as the second circulatory system
- Acts as the body's primary defense against invading pathogens

Key characteristics of the lymph nodes

- Composed of reticular connective tissue, lymphocytes, and sinuses
- Hundreds exist throughout the body
- Lymph flows through lymph nodes

LYMPH TISSUE

● Key concepts

- The *lymphatic system* serves as the second circulatory system and one of the body's primary defenses against invasion by harmful organisms and chemical toxins; it's composed of lymphocyte-containing (lymphoid) tissues, lymph, and a network of lymphatic vessels
- Lymph tissue is the cornerstone of the immune system
  - It consists of reticular connective tissue and free cells (lymphocytes and macrophages)
  - Mainly concentrated in the lymph nodes, spleen, and thymus, it's also found in mucous membranes of the respiratory and GI tracts
- *Lymph*—a clear fluid containing white blood cells (WBCs) and antigens—bathes body tissues and helps filter and transport substances; it's collected from body tissues and seeps into lymphatic vessels

● Lymph nodes

- Small, bean-shaped structures, *lymph nodes* are composed of reticular connective tissue, lymphocytes, and sinuses (see *Lymphatic vessels and lymph nodes*)
- Hundreds exist throughout the body
  - They are located along lymphatic vessels, where they act as filters
  - Many appear along the surface of the GI tract; large clusters are also found in the inguinal, axillary, and cervical regions
- Each node consists of a mass of lymphocytes supported by a meshwork of reticular fibers; it's enclosed by a fibrous capsule and divided into an outer cortex and inner medulla
  - Outer cortex divides into superficial and deep cortex
    - Superficial cortex contains follicles composed predominantly of B cells (the follicles expand and develop clusters of proliferating cells, called *germinal centers,* in an immune response)
    - Deep cortex and interfollicular areas contain mostly T cells
  - Inner medulla contains loosely arranged lymphocytes and scattered groups of mononuclear phagocytes derived from monocytes
- Lymph nodes receive lymph via afferent lymphatic vessels; lymph empties into the subcapsular sinus at the periphery of the node
- Lymph nodes drain lymph through efferent lymphatic channels, which exit the node at an indentation on the concave side (hilus)
  - As lymph filters slowly through the node, mononuclear phagocytes filter out and destroy foreign substances

Lymphatic vessels and lymph nodes

Lymphatic tissues are connected by a network of thin-walled drainage channels called lymphatic vessels. Resembling veins, the afferent lymphatic vessels carry lymph into lymph nodes; lymph slowly filters through the node and is collected into efferent lymphatic vessels. Lymphatic capillaries are located throughout most of the body. Wider than blood capillaries, they permit interstitial fluid to flow into them but not out.

LYMPHATIC VESSELS AND CAPILLARIES

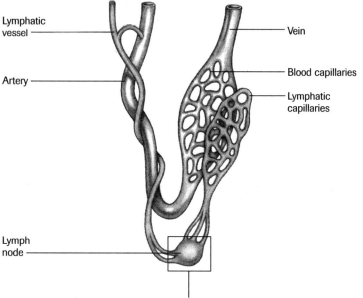

Lymphatic vessel
Artery
Vein
Blood capillaries
Lymphatic capillaries
Lymph node

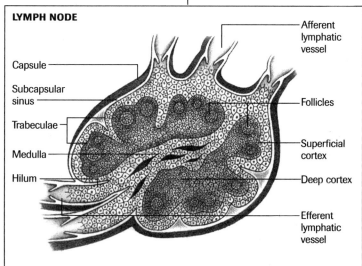

LYMPH NODE

Capsule
Subcapsular sinus
Trabeculae
Medulla
Hilum
Afferent lymphatic vessel
Follicles
Superficial cortex
Deep cortex
Efferent lymphatic vessel

Key lymph node structures

- Afferent lymphatic vessel
- Capsule
- Subcapsular sinus
- Follicles
- Trabeculae
- Superficial cortex
- Deep cortex
- Medulla
- Hilum
- Efferent lymphatic vessel

– These phagocytes also interact with lymphocytes to generate an immune response

● Spleen

- A dark red, ovoid, fist-sized structure in the left upper abdominal quadrant (posterior and inferior to the stomach), the *spleen* filters antigens and other particles from the blood
- The spleen is surrounded by a dense fibrous capsule and contains bands of connective tissue that extend from the capsule into the spleen's interior (called the *splenic pulp*)
- Splenic pulp is made up of both white and red matter
    - White pulp consists of compact masses of lymphocytes that surround branches of the splenic artery
    - Red pulp contains a network of blood-filled sinusoids supported by a framework of reticular fibers and star-shaped mononuclear phagocytes (lymphocytes, plasma cells, and monocytes also appear in the framework)
        - Pulp cords surround and separate the sinusoids
        - Long, narrow endothelial cells line the splenic sinusoids; they lie parallel to the long axis of the sinusoids and are supported by a fenestrated basement membrane
- Blood is transported to the spleen through branches of the splenic arteries
    - Some flows directly into the splenic sinusoids; most discharges into the pulp cords
    - Blood passes from the area between the pulp cords (which consists of a meshwork of cells and fibers) into the sinusoid lumens
        - As it does so, blood cells must squeeze through long, slitlike openings between adjacent endothelial cells
        - This forces the blood to flow through the framework of reticular fibers, macrophages, and other cells before entering the sinusoids
- The spleen filters blood and promotes immunity through phagocytic mechanisms
    - Splenic phagocytes engulf and break down worn-out red blood cells (RBCs); this releases hemoglobin (Hb), which is broken down into its components
    - Phagocytes selectively retain and destroy damaged or abnormal RBCs and cells with a large amount of abnormal Hb
    - Phagocytes remove bacteria and other foreign substances that the spleen has filtered out of the bloodstream
    - Phagocytes also interact with lymphocytes to initiate an immune response

- Removal of the spleen may be necessary after injury or disease
  - Injury or disease dampens efficiency of bacteria elimination and antibody production
  - In turn, this increases susceptibility to serious blood infections from various pathogenic organisms

● **Thymus**
  - The *thymus* is a double-lobed mass of lymphoid tissue located over the base of the heart in the mediastinum, below the sternum
  - It helps develop T lymphocytes in the fetus and in the infant for a few months after birth; it has no function in the body's immune defenses after this time
  - A large structure during infancy, it gradually atrophies when no longer required; only a remnant persists in adulthood

● **Other lymph tissues**
  - Structures include the tonsils, adenoids, appendix, and Peyer's patches
  - They're distributed in mucous membranes where they can intercept invading organisms or toxins before they can spread widely
    - Tissues in the throat and pharynx (tonsils and adenoids) intercept antigens that enter by the upper respiratory tract
    - Tissues in the GI tract (appendix and Peyer's patches) intercept antigens that attempt to enter via the gut

LYMPH

● **Key concepts**
  - Lymph (also called *lymphatic fluid*) is a transparent, colorless, alkaline fluid containing lymphocytes, interstitial fluid, and plasma proteins
  - It travels through lymphatic vessels to large ducts, where it empties into the subclavian vein
  - The osmotic pressure of lymph slightly exceeds that of plasma; consequently, fluid moves from blood into the interstitial space and, ultimately, into the lymphatic system

● **Functions of lymph**
  - Lymph helps maintain homeostasis by conveying invading foreign substances (such as viruses and bacteria) to the lymph nodes, where lymphocytes attack them
  - It maintains osmotic pressure of interstitial fluid by transporting protein that leaks from the arteriolar ends of capillaries back to the bloodstream and plasma

**Key facts about
the formation and
flow of lymph**

- Forms from excess fluid seepage from capillaries
- Skeletal muscle contractions, one-way valves in vessels, and respiratory movements ensure proper flow

**Key facts about
lymphatic vessels**

- Form a complex network that connects lymph tissue
- Drain excess fluid from interstitial spaces and return it to the circulation
- Small lymphatic channels converge to form larger vessels
- Carry lymph toward the heart and eventually empty into the subclavian vein

**Key facts about
lymphatic capillaries**

- Found throughout most of the body
- Allow interstitial fluid to flow in but not out
- Anchoring filaments attach lymphatic endothelium to surrounding tissue

- It transports nutrients, such as fats, that have been absorbed from the digestive tract

● **Formation and flow**
  - More fluid seeps out of capillaries into interstitial fluid than is absorbed by them; excess fluid (about 3 L daily) forms lymph
  - Fluid flows from lymphatic capillaries to lymphatic vessels to the thoracic duct or right lymphatic duct to the subclavian veins
  - Several mechanisms cause proper flow
    – Skeletal muscle contractions (compress lymphatic vessels to propel lymph forward)
    – One-way valves in lymphatic vessels (prevent backward flow)
    – Respiratory movements (create a pressure gradient in the lymphatic system, forcing lymph to flow from abdominal area to thoracic area)

LYMPHATIC VESSELS

● **Key concepts**
  - Thin-walled drainage channels similar to veins, *lymphatic vessels* form a complex network that connects lymph tissue
  - Vessels drain excess fluid from interstitial spaces and return it to the circulation; they also absorb fats from the GI tract and transport them into the bloodstream
  - Small lymphatic channels converge to form larger vessels with valves that prevent reflux

● **Functions of lymphatic vessels**
  - Lymphatic vessels carry lymph toward the heart, eventually emptying into the right or left subclavian vein
  - Beginning with tiny lymphatic capillaries, lymph flows through progressively larger vessels
    – From the left side of the body, lymph passes to the thoracic duct; this duct joins the venous circulation at the junction of the internal jugular vein and subclavian vein on the left side
    – From the right side of the body, lymph passes to the right lymphatic duct; this duct joins the venous circulation at the junction of the internal jugular vein and subclavian vein on the right side

● **Lymphatic capillaries**
  - *Lymphatic capillaries* are found throughout most of the body, except in avascular tissue, bone marrow, central nervous system structures, or splenic pulp
  - Wider than blood capillaries, they allow interstitial fluid to flow in but not out

- When interstitial fluid pressure exceeds pressure in the lymphatic capillaries, capillary cells separate slightly to let fluid enter
- When lymphatic capillary fluid pressure exceeds interstitial fluid pressure, cells cling together to prevent fluid from leaving the lymphatic capillaries
• Anchoring filaments attach the lymphatic endothelium to surrounding tissues
• In edema, excess interstitial fluid causes tissues to swell, which pulls on the anchoring filaments; this separates the lymphatic capillary cells further, allowing more fluid to enter the capillaries

LYMPHOCYTES

● **Key concepts**
  • *Lymphocytes* are a type of leukocyte (or WBC) that develops from stem cells in the bone marrow and differentiates into lymphocyte precursor cells
  • Precursor cells develop into two types of lymphocytes—T lymphocytes and B lymphocytes; both types perform specific immune functions

● **Types of lymphocytes**
  • *T (thymus-dependent) lymphocytes* arise from precursor cells that migrate from the bone marrow to the thymus, where they undergo further differentiation
  • *B (bone marrow–dependent)* lymphocytes arise from precursor cells that continue to differentiate in the bone marrow
  • T and B lymphocytes migrate into the lymph nodes, spleen, and other lymph tissues, where they proliferate to form the mature lymphocytes that populate these lymph tissues
    - These lymphocytes don't remain permanently in a specific lymphatic organ; they continually recirculate between blood and various lymphatic tissues and organs
    - About 70% of these circulating cells are T lymphocytes; most of the remainder are B lymphocytes
  • A small proportion of lymphocytes called *null cells* can't be classified as T or B lymphocytes
    - They're hematopoietic stem cells and may include T- and B-lymphocyte precursors and precursor, myeloid, and platelet cells
    - They can destroy tumor cells spontaneously or through an antibody-dependent cellular cytotoxic mechanism

Types of lymphocytes
● T lymphocytes: thymus dependent
● B lymphocytes: bone marrow dependent
● Null cells: neither T nor B lymphocytes

Key functions of lymphocytes

- T lymphocytes provide cell-mediated immunity
- Mature B lymphocytes differentiate into plasma cells and memory cells, providing humoral immunity

Key protective mechanisms against disease

- Nonspecific resistance: general protective mechanisms that function without prior exposure
- Acquired immunity: depends on the lymphatic system

Key roles of the skin and mucous membranes in disease resistance

- Mechanical: block, trap, and wash away organisms
- Chemical: kill organisms and discourage bacterial growth

● **Functions of lymphocytes**
- T lymphocytes also have initial and ultimate functions
  - Initially, they seek, recognize, and attach to antigens that fit their surface receptors
  - Later, they produce *cell-mediated immunity*
- B lymphocytes have distinct initial and ultimate functions
  - Initially, they synthesize and insert antibodies on their surface
  - Mature B lymphocytes differentiate into plasma cells and memory cells, providing humoral immunity
    · Plasma cells secrete antibodies in response to antigens
    · Memory cells (longer-lived than plasma cells) produce antibodies during subsequent exposure to an antigen

NONSPECIFIC RESISTANCE TO DISEASE

● **Key concepts**
- The body has two mechanisms to protect against microorganisms and other potentially harmful substances
- The first is a group of general protective mechanisms that function without prior exposure to harmful agents; these mechanisms provide *nonspecific resistance*
  - *Resistance* is the body's ability to fend off disease (*susceptibility* refers to lack of resistance)
  - Nonspecific resistance wards off a wide range of pathogens, using a variety of physiologic responses
  - This type of resistance incorporates factors in the skin and mucous membranes, antimicrobial substances, phagocytosis, inflammation, and fever
- The second mechanism depends on the lymphatic system and provides acquired immunity

● **Skin and mucous membranes**
- These structures provide mechanical and chemical protection
- Mechanical protection occurs in several ways
  - Intact skin prevents the attachment of invading organisms
  - Skin desquamation and low pH impede bacterial colonization
  - Mucus in the respiratory and other tracts traps bacteria and other foreign substances
  - Body fluids (such as tears, saliva, urine, and vaginal secretions) help wash away or dilute microorganisms
- Chemical protection typically results from body secretions
  - Gastric acid secretions and digestive enzymes destroy organisms swallowed into the stomach
  - Chemical compounds in the blood attach to and destroy foreign substances or toxins

- The enzyme lysozyme (present in tears, nasal secretions, perspiration, and saliva) acts as an antibacterial agent
- Basic polypeptides inactivate certain gram-positive bacteria
- The serum protein properdin destroys gram-negative bacteria
  – Sebaceous gland secretions, which are slightly acidic, discourage bacterial growth

Antimicrobial substances

- Antimicrobials provide a second line of defense when organisms penetrate the skin and mucous membranes
- Lymphocytes, macrophages, and fibroblasts produce proteins called *interferons* in response to viral infection
  – Interferons bind to surface receptors on uninfected neighboring cells
  – This causes uninfected cells to synthesize antiviral proteins, which inhibit viral replication
- The *complement system* is a group of about 20 proteins in blood plasma and on cell membranes
  – Normally, these proteins are inactive
  – When activated, they enhance certain immune, allergic, and inflammatory reactions

Phagocytosis

- *Phagocytosis* refers to the ingestion of organisms or foreign substances by cells called *phagocytes*
- Phagocytes include granulocytes (neutrophils, eosinophils, and basophils) and macrophages
- Three phases of phagocytosis include chemotaxis, adherence, and ingestion
  – During *chemotaxis* (movement toward a chemical stimulus), phagocytes are attracted to the invasion site by chemicals, such as microbial products and activated complement proteins
  – During *adherence,* the phagocyte's cell membrane attaches to the organism's surface
  – During *ingestion,* the phagocyte's cell membrane extends projections (pseudopods) that engulf the organism; pseudopods fuse together and surround the organism in a phagocytic vesicle
- After ingestion, the phagocyte releases chemicals that kill the organism

Inflammation

- The *inflammatory response* mobilizes WBCs to engulf and destroy bacteria and other foreign substances (see *The inflammatory response,* page 266)

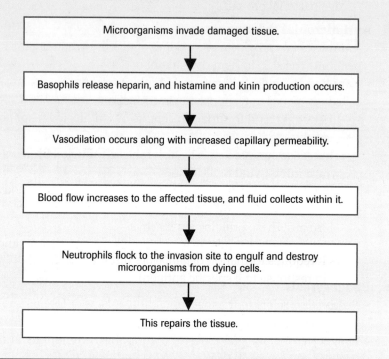

GO WITH THE FLOW

The inflammatory response

This flowchart outlines the sequence of events in the inflammatory process.

> Microorganisms invade damaged tissue.
>
> ↓
>
> Basophils release heparin, and histamine and kinin production occurs.
>
> ↓
>
> Vasodilation occurs along with increased capillary permeability.
>
> ↓
>
> Blood flow increases to the affected tissue, and fluid collects within it.
>
> ↓
>
> Neutrophils flock to the invasion site to engulf and destroy microorganisms from dying cells.
>
> ↓
>
> This repairs the tissue.

Key facts about inflammation

- Mobilizes WBCs to engulf and destroy bacteria
- Helps remove organisms, toxins, and foreign substances from an affected site

Key facts about fever

- Intensifies the effects of interferons
- Prepares the site for tissue repair

- – After organisms invade, tissue injury leads to release of histamine, kinins, and prostaglandins, which cause vasodilation and increased capillary permeability
- – This increases blood flow to the affected tissues, where fluid collects
- – Neutrophils and other WBCs are attracted to the invasion site
- – These cells engulf and destroy the organisms, foreign substances, and debris
- Inflammation usually causes redness, pain, heat, and swelling and may produce loss of function in the affected area, depending on the site and degree of the damage
- Inflammation helps remove organisms, toxins, and foreign substances from the affected site, inhibiting their spread and preparing the site for tissue repair

● **Fever**
  - Increased body temperature intensifies the effects of interferons
  - It prevents the growth of some organisms and hastens tissue repair

ACQUIRED IMMUNITY

- ● **Key concepts**
  - *Acquired immunity*—the body's second (specific) mechanism for warding off microorganisms and disease—involves a specific immune response directed against a specific invading agent (virus, bacterium, toxin, or other foreign substance)
  - Usually, previous exposure to an invading agent is necessary to cause antibody formation or lymphatic activation
  - There are two types of acquired immunity: cell-mediated immunity and humoral immunity
    - *Cell-mediated immunity* is carried out by T lymphocytes
      - It requires formation of large numbers of sensitized lymphocytes
      - In this process, phagocytic cells (macrophages) present processed antigens to the lymphocytes, thereby sensitizing the T lymphocytes to that antigen; sensitization allows T lymphocytes to destroy the antigen on subsequent exposure
    - *Humoral immunity* is carried out by B lymphocytes
      - It requires formation of *antibodies* (immunoglobulins formed in response to a specific antigen)
      - In this process, macrophages present processed antigens to the lymphocytes; B lymphocytes then differentiate into plasma cells that produce antibodies
    - Both types of immunity interact to protect the body against invading antigens
      - Some B and T lymphocytes retain a memory of the sensitizing antigen, which they pass on to succeeding generations of lymphocytes
      - Later contact with this antigen leads to rapid proliferation of sensitized lymphocytes or antibody-forming plasma cells

- ● **The immune response**
  - Acquired immunity develops after the first invasion by a foreign organism or first contact with a toxin
    - Each toxin or type of organism contains specific chemical compounds that make it different from all other substances
    - These compounds, called *antigens*, cause acquired immunity; they usually are high-molecular-weight proteins, polysaccharides, or lipids
  - Initial phase of the immune response involves macrophage and lymphocyte interaction; both types of cells are distributed widely throughout the body and can respond to a foreign substance wherever they encounter it (see *The immune response*, page 268)

Key facts about acquired immunity

- ● Involves a specific immune response against a specific invading agent
- ● Requires previous exposure for antibody formation

Types of acquired immunity

- ● Cell-mediated: involves sensitization of T lymphocytes
- ● Humoral: carried out by B lymphocytes and involves the formation of antibodies

Key facts about antigens and antibodies

- ● Antigens: chemical compounds specific to each organism that cause acquired immunity
- ● Antibodies: immunoglobulins formed in response to a specific antigen

Phases of the immune response

- In the initial phase, macrophages and lymphocytes are distributed throughout the body
- Macrophages ingest and process the antigen
- Lymphocytes produce antibodies to the antigen over a several week period
- Memory cells retain the ability to respond promptly to the same antigens on subsequent exposure

GO WITH THE FLOW

The immune response

When foreign substances invade the body, humoral and cell-mediated immunity can come to the body's defense. Both types of immunity involve lymphocytes that share a common origin in stem cells of the bone marrow. These lymphocytes undergo differential development to become B cells and T cells. This chart shows how these cells evolve to perform their immune functions.

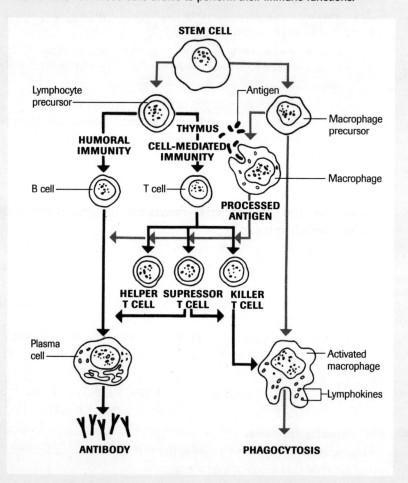

– Macrophages ingest the foreign material, process its antigens, and present the processed material to the lymphocytes
– Lymphocytes respond and transform into antibody-forming plasma cells and sensitized lymphocytes, respectively, which proliferate rapidly to perform immune functions

- Following initial contact with an antigen, several weeks are needed for macrophages to process the antigen and for lymphocytes to respond
- After reaction to the antigen, some lymphocytes (called *memory cells*) retain the ability to respond promptly to the same antigen on subsequent exposure
  - Successive generations of lymphocytes derived from these memory cells also retain this ability
  - Subsequent contact with the sensitizing antigen provokes a renewed immune response
  - This response is rapid because earlier exposure to the antigen has primed the immune system
- Ability to generate an immune response is controlled genetically; immune-response genes regulate T- and B-lymphocyte proliferation

CELL-MEDIATED IMMUNITY

● **Key concepts**
- Cell-mediated immunity—the body's main defense against viruses, parasites, and some bacteria—results from the function of sensitized T lymphocytes
- Cell-mediated immunity also eliminates abnormal cells that may arise during cell division; these cells can develop into tumors if not destroyed
- This mechanism also causes organ transplant rejection
- Hypersensitivity to bacterial antigens or other foreign substances is common with this type of immunity; reaction is characterized by an intense inflammatory reaction at the site of contact with the foreign substance

● **Cell-mediated immune response**
- Response involves specific functions performed by three types of sensitized T lymphocytes: cytotoxic T cells, helper T cells, and suppressor T cells
  - *Cytotoxic T cells* (also called *killer cells*) directly kill organisms or other invading cells
    · These cells bind tightly to the invading cell, swell, and release cytotoxic substances directly into the attacked cell
    · They can attack and kill many organisms in succession, without being harmed
  - *Helper T cells* interact with other T and B lymphocytes to enhance the immune response

- When activated, helper T cells secrete lymphokines, which increase activation of B cells, cytotoxic T cells, and suppressor T cells by antigens
- They attract macrophages and promote more efficient phagocytosis
  - *Suppressor T cells* inhibit the immune response
    - They suppress the actions of cytotoxic and helper T cells
    - This regulates the other T cells, preventing them from causing excessive immune reactions and severe tissue damage
- Sensitized T lymphocytes are classified into two major groups according to specific antigens on their membranes
  - One group, the CD4 lymphocytes, are helper T cells; they account for about 70% of all T cells
  - The other group, the CD8 lymphocytes, consists of suppressor and cytotoxic T cells; they account for about 30% of all T cells
  - A normal ratio of CD4 to CD8 lymphocytes (which reflects the normal proportions of helper to suppressor and cytotoxic T cells) is essential for proper immune function
    - Loss or destruction of helper T cells (as in acquired immunodeficiency syndrome [AIDS]) leads to a relative excess of suppressor T cells, inhibiting the immune response and increasing susceptibility to infection (see *Teaching a patient with AIDS*)

Key teaching topics for a patient with AIDS

- Explain diagnostic criteria and tests
- Stress the importance of nutrition, rest, and moderate exercise
- Describe how to prevent infection and practice safer sex
- Review medications

TIME-OUT FOR TEACHING

Teaching a patient with AIDS

Make sure you teach a patient with acquired immunodeficiency syndrome (AIDS):
- the effects of human immunodeficiency virus on the immune response
- the affects of opportunistic infections, cancer, and other disorders associated with AIDS
- diagnostic criteria for AIDS
- diagnostic tests to anticipate, such as Western blot and helper T-cell count

- activity modifications, including the need for adequate rest and moderate exercise
- the importance of adequate nutrition to prevent opportunistic infections
- techniques for preventing infection
- drug therapy, such as zidovudine (Retrovir), co-trimoxazole (Bactrim, Septra), and pentamidine (NebuPent, Pentam 300)
- safer sex practices, including condom use
- resources for finding additional information and support.

• A relative lack of suppressor T cells allows the immune system to respond unchecked, increasing the likelihood of autoimmune disease in which the immune defenses attack the body's own cells and tissues

HUMORAL IMMUNITY

● **Key concepts**
  • Humoral immunity—the major defense against many bacteria and bacterial toxins—results from B-lymphocyte function
  • In response to antigen stimulation, B lymphocytes differentiate into plasma cells; these plasma cells produce antibodies (immunoglobulins) that can combine with and eliminate the foreign substance

● **Antibody mechanisms of action**
  • Antibodies directly attack the invader or activate the complement system, which destroys the invader
  • Antibodies can directly inactivate an invader in one of four ways
    – Through *agglutination,* antibodies can cause clumping of multiple large structures with antigens on their surfaces, such as RBCs or bacteria
    – Through *precipitation,* antibodies produce an antigen-antibody complex so large that it's insoluble and precipitates; tetanus toxin is a soluble antigen that's susceptible to precipitation
    – Through *neutralization,* antibodies cover the toxic sites on an antigen
    – Through *lysis,* potent antibodies attack the cell membrane of an antigen, causing it to rupture; this process requires complement activation
  • The complement system augments the effects of the direct actions of antibodies
    – Exposure to an antigen activates the complement system, triggering a complex cascade of sequential reactions
    – The cascade ultimately produces many end products, some of which help prevent antigen-induced damage
      • Some end products increase phagocytosis through opsonization, which can increase bacteria destruction by many hundredfold
      • One end product (lytic complex) directly causes cell lysis by rupturing the membrane of bacteria and other organisms
      • Some end products cause invading organisms to adhere to each other by altering their surfaces, producing agglutination

- Enzymes and other end products can neutralize viruses by attacking their structures
- One end product attracts many neutrophils and macrophages to the area affected by the antigen through chemotaxis

Immunoglobulins

- *Immunoglobulins* are proteins produced by the plasma cells derived from B lymphocytes
- Although they differ in chemical composition, molecular weight, and size, they all have the same basic structure: two matched pairs of polypeptide (protein) chains bound together by chemical bonds
- Chains are arranged to resemble a fork with four tines
  - The two central chains (heavy chains) form the handle and inner tines of the fork
  - The two outer chains (light chains) form the outer tines of the fork
  - The open end of each tine is different for each immunoglobulin; this variable part gives the immunoglobulin its specificity (ability to respond to a particular antigen)
  - The handle end is the constant part of the immunoglobulin; it's the same in every immunoglobulin
  - The constant part doesn't combine with an antigen; however, it determines other properties of the immunoglobulin, such as its ability to activate complement and attach to the surface of an antigen's cell membrane
- All consist of the same basic four-chain units, but some aggregate to form clusters of two, three, or five units
- Five types of antibodies exist: immunoglobulin M (IgM), immunoglobulin G (IgG), immunoglobulin A (IgA), immunoglobulin D (IgD), and immunoglobulin E (IgE)
  - IgM—an aggregate of five basic immunoglobulin units—is the first immunoglobulin produced during an immune response
    - It's the largest immunoglobulin; commonly called a *macroglobulin* because of its large size and high molecular weight
    - IgM is particularly efficient in combining with large particulate antigens
  - IgG—composed of a single basic immunoglobulin unit—is the principal immunoglobulin molecule formed in response to most infectious agents
    - It combines with antigens and activates complement
    - It's the major antibacterial and antiviral antibody

- IgA—an aggregate of two basic immunoglobulin units—is produced by antibody-forming cells in the respiratory system, GI tract, and other mucous membranes
    - It appears in secretions and combines with potentially harmful ingested or inhaled antigens, preventing their absorption
    - It defends against pathogens on body surfaces
- IgD—composed of one basic immunoglobulin unit—coats the surface of B lymphocytes
    - Its prongs (antigen-binding sites) can attach antigens to the surface of B lymphocytes, stimulating them to produce antibodies
    - It's mainly an antigen receptor
- IgE—composed of a single immunoglobulin unit—is involved in immediate hypersensitivity reactions or allergic reactions
    - It's usually present in small amounts in the blood of most people
    - In allergic individuals, it appears in much larger amounts

● Allergic reaction

- Some individuals form specific IgE antibodies (become allergic) to ragweed, plant pollens, and other substances that don't affect most people (see *Allergic response,* page 274)
    - The allergy-prone individual is called *atopic*
    - The sensitizing antigen is called an *allergen*
- Primary response begins with initial exposure to an antigen; it ends with sensitization of mast cells
    - The handle end of IgE attaches to the membrane of mast cells and basophils
    - The tine ends project from the cell membrane
- Secondary response begins with reexposure to the sensitizing antigen
    - Reexposure causes the antigen to fix to the antigen-combining sites on the projecting ends of IgE molecules
    - This event triggers basophil and mast cell granules to release histamine and other chemicals; because these chemicals incite an inflammatory reaction, they're called *mediators of inflammation*
- Histamine and other chemicals typically produce allergic manifestations, such as sneezing, stuffy nose, and itchy eyes
- A more severe allergic reaction, called *anaphylaxis,* can be life-threatening, causing acute respiratory failure and vascular collapse (see *Teaching a patient with anaphylaxis,* page 275)

Key facts about allergic reactions

- Primary response begins with initial exposure to antigen
- Ends with sensitization of mast cells
- Reexposure to antigen triggers secondary response
- Histamine and other chemicals produce allergy symptoms

GO WITH THE FLOW

Allergic response

An allergen is an antigen that triggers an allergic response. The first exposure to an allergen causes lymphocytes and plasma cells to produce specific immunoglobulin E antibodies, which bind to mast cells and basophils. Subsequent exposure to this allergen leads to antigen-antibody interaction, causing mast cells and basophils to release histamine and other mediators. These mediators produce allergic manifestations.

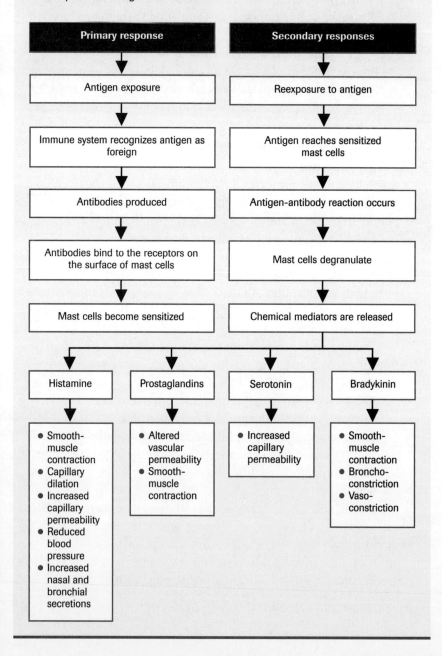

Primary response	Secondary responses
Antigen exposure	Reexposure to antigen
Immune system recognizes antigen as foreign	Antigen reaches sensitized mast cells
Antibodies produced	Antigen-antibody reaction occurs
Antibodies bind to the receptors on the surface of mast cells	Mast cells degranulate
Mast cells become sensitized	Chemical mediators are released

Histamine	Prostaglandins	Serotonin	Bradykinin
• Smooth-muscle contraction • Capillary dilation • Increased capillary permeability • Reduced blood pressure • Increased nasal and bronchial secretions	• Altered vascular permeability • Smooth-muscle contraction	• Increased capillary permeability	• Smooth-muscle contraction • Broncho-constriction • Vaso-constriction

TIME-OUT FOR TEACHING

Teaching a patient with anaphylaxis

Make sure you teach a patient with anaphylaxis:
- the causes, signs, and symptoms of anaphylaxis
- which complications, including respiratory failure and cardio-vascular collapse, are possible
- the need for skin testing and an elimination diet to identify allergens
- the importance of immediate treat-ment after reexposure to an allergen
- how to use an anaphylaxis kit
- how to apply a tourniquet
- the importance of avoiding known allergens
- the need to wear medical identifi-cation such as a bracelet
- how to find additional information and support.

NCLEX CHECKS

It's never too soon to begin your NCLEX preparation. Now that you've reviewed this chapter, carefully read each of the following questions and choose the best answer. Then compare your responses with the correct answers.

1. The nurse is assessing the lymphatic system of a client with Hodgkin's lymphoma. Which tissues and organs should the nurse assess? Select all that apply.
- ☐ **1.** Spleen
- ☐ **2.** Thyroid
- ☐ **3.** Thymus
- ☐ **4.** Lymph nodes
- ☐ **5.** Liver
- ☐ **6.** Kidneys

2. The nurse is assessing a client's spleen. In which abdominal quadrant will the nurse palpate the spleen?
- ☐ **1.** Left lower
- ☐ **2.** Right lower
- ☐ **3.** Left upper
- ☐ **4.** Right upper

3. The nurse is teaching a client who's scheduled for a splenectomy. Which information about spleen removal should be part of the discussion?
- ☐ **1.** Without a spleen, he'll be more likely to develop an infection.
- ☐ **2.** Without a spleen, he'll be more prone to bleeding.
- ☐ **3.** Without a spleen, he'll be more likely to form blood clots.
- ☐ **4.** Without a spleen, he'll be more resistant to foreign organisms.

Key teaching topics for a patient with anaphylaxis
- Review causes, signs and symp-toms, and complications
- Stress the importance of imme-diate treatment, avoiding known allergens, and wearing medical identification
- Explain how to use an anaphy-laxis kit

TOP 8

Items to study for your next test on the lymphatic system
1. Structure and function of lymphatic tissues
2. Structure and function of lymphatic fluid and vessels
3. Types of lymphocytes
4. Comparison of nonspecific resistance and acquired immunity
5. Comparison of cell-mediated and humoral immunity
6. Types of immunoglobulins
7. Processes that occur in an allergic response
8. Teaching tips for patients with AIDS or anaphylaxis

4. A client is having several lymph nodes removed for biopsy. In answer to the client's questions, the nurse explains that lymph flows through the body in which order?

☐ **1.** Subclavian veins, right lymphatic duct, lymphatic vessels, lymphatic capillaries
☐ **2.** Lymphatic capillaries, thoracic duct, lymphatic vessels, subclavian veins
☐ **3.** Lymphatic vessels, thoracic duct, lymphatic capillaries, subclavian veins
☐ **4.** Lymphatic capillaries, lymphatic vessels, right lymphatic duct, subclavian veins

5. The nurse explains to a client that the skin offers mechanical protection from invading organisms by which mechanism?

☐ **1.** Skin prevents invasion and attachment of organisms.
☐ **2.** Lysozyme, present in perspiration, acts as an antibacterial agent.
☐ **3.** Properdin, a serum protein, destroys bacteria.
☐ **4.** Sebaceous gland secretions discourage bacterial growth.

6. While caring for a client with an infection, the nurse keeps in mind that macrophages are attracted to the invasion site by chemicals during which phase of phagocytosis?

☐ **1.** Chemotaxis
☐ **2.** Adherence
☐ **3.** Ingestion
☐ **4.** Inflammation

7. A client has inflammation around the site of an insect bite. Which signs and symptoms is the nurse most likely to assess?

☐ **1.** Paleness, swelling, numbness
☐ **2.** Coolness, pain, swelling
☐ **3.** Pain, heat, swelling
☐ **4.** Redness, coolness, pain

8. Which immunoglobulin would the nurse expect to be responsible for a client's allergic reaction?

☐ **1.** IgA
☐ **2.** IgM
☐ **3.** IgG
☐ **4.** IgE

9. Which information is most important to include in a teaching plan for a client with anaphylaxis?

☐ **1.** The need to report signs and symptoms within 24 hours of reexposure to the allergen

☐ **2.** The need to reduce contact with known allergens

☐ **3.** Use of an anaphylaxis kit

☐ **4.** Complications of anaphylaxis, such as renal and hepatic failure

10. When assessing a client's thymus gland, the nurse would expect to palpate the gland in which location?

☐ **1.** Around the thyroid gland

☐ **2.** Just to the left of the sternum

☐ **3.** At the apex of the heart

☐ **4.** At the base of the heart

ANSWERS AND RATIONALES

1. CORRECT ANSWER: 1, 3, 4
Lymph tissues are concentrated in the spleen, thymus, and lymph nodes, but are also found in the mucous membranes of the respiratory and GI tracts.

2. CORRECT ANSWER: 3
The spleen is located in the upper left abdominal quadrant, posterior and inferior to the stomach.

3. CORRECT ANSWER: 1
The spleen filters out bacteria and other foreign substances that enter the bloodstream. After spleen removal, bacteria elimination and antibody production are less efficient, making the client more susceptible to infection from foreign organisms. Removal of the spleen doesn't increase the risk of bleeding or blood clot formation.

4. CORRECT ANSWER: 4
Lymph flows from the lymphatic capillaries to the lymphatic vessels, then to the thoracic duct or right lymphatic duct, and finally to the subclavian veins.

5. CORRECT ANSWER: 1
The skin provides both mechanical and chemical protection from invading organisms. Skin offers mechanical protection by preventing organisms from attaching to skin surfaces and through skin desquamation. Chemical protection occurs from body secretions, such as lysozyme, properdin, and sebaceous gland secretions.

6. CORRECT ANSWER: 1

Phagocytosis occurs in three phases: chemotaxis, adherence, and ingestion. During chemotaxis, macrophages are attracted to the invasion site by chemicals. During adherence, the macrophage's cell membrane attaches to the organism's surface. During ingestion, the macrophage's cell membrane extends projections, called *pseudopods,* that engulf the organism; these pseudopods then fuse and surround the organism in a phagocytic vesicle. After ingestion, the macrophage releases chemicals that kill the organism. Inflammation isn't a phase of phagocytosis.

7. CORRECT ANSWER: 3

Inflammation causes redness, pain, heat, and swelling. It may also produce loss of function in the affected area.

8. CORRECT ANSWER: 4

IgE is involved in immediate hypersensitivity and allergic reactions. IgA defends against pathogens on body surfaces. IgM is the first immunoglobulin produced during an immune response. IgG is formed in response to infectious agents.

9. CORRECT ANSWER: 3

It's imperative to teach a client with anaphylaxis how to use an anaphylaxis kit. Other important areas to cover include the need to seek immediate treatment after reexposure to known allergens, to avoid known allergens, and to watch for complications, such as respiratory failure and cardiovascular collapse. The client should also be taught the causes and signs and symptoms of anaphylaxis, the need for skin testing and an elimination diet to identify allergens, and the importance of wearing medical identification such as a bracelet.

10. CORRECT ANSWER: 4

The thymus gland is located over the base of the heart, below the sternum.

15

Gastrointestinal system

After studying this chapter, you should be able to:

- Identify the structures and functions of the GI tract.
- Describe the structures and functions of the accessory organs of the GI tract.
- Explain the process of digestion and absorption.
- Discuss the phases of glucose metabolism.
- Explain protein and lipid metabolism.
- Discuss hormone regulation of metabolism.

CHAPTER OVERVIEW

Through the GI system, the body obtains and processes almost all of the nutrients it needs. These nutrients supply all of the energy and building materials required by the body for daily activities, growth, and repair. For these reasons, the nurse should recognize GI structures and understand the processes of digestion, absorption, and metabolism. This chapter reviews the GI tract, accessory organs, nutrient digestion and absorption, carbohydrate metabolism, protein metabolism, lipid metabolism, and hormonal regulation of metabolism.

Key facts about the GI tract

- Includes organs of the GI tract and accessory GI organs
- Extends as a continuous tube from the mouth to the anus
- Purpose is to modify and prepare food for use by body cells

GI TRACT

● **Key concepts**
- The *GI system,* also called the *digestive system,* consists of structures that ingest, digest, and absorb food
- It includes organs of the GI tract and accessory GI organs (see *Structures of the GI system*)
- The GI tract (or *alimentary canal*) is a continuous tube open at both ends; it extends through the ventral cavities from the mouth to the anus
- Consisting of the oral cavity, pharynx, esophagus, stomach, and small and large intestines, the GI tract is surrounded by the peritoneum

Structures of the GI system

This illustration shows the major organs of the GI tract (mouth, pharynx, esophagus, stomach, small intestine, and large intestine) as well as several accessory GI organs (liver, gallbladder, and pancreas).

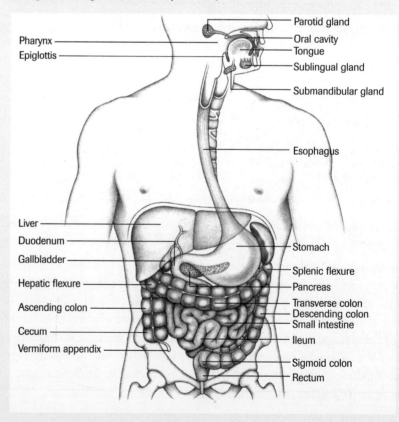

● **Functions of the GI system**
  • Overall purpose of the GI system is to modify and prepare food chemically and physically for use by body cells
  • It accomplishes this through five main functions
    – It ingests food (via the oral cavity)
    – It propels food through the pharynx and esophagus into the stomach
    – It digests food mechanically and chemically
    – It absorbs food molecules
    – It eliminates indigestible materials from the body (via defecation)

GI STRUCTURES

● **Oral cavity**
  • Bounded by the lips, cheeks, palate, and tongue, the *oral cavity* also includes the salivary glands and 32 permanent teeth (see *The oral cavity,* page 282)
  • It joins the pharynx at a junction called the *fauces*
  • The oral cavity prepares food for swallowing and begins digestion
    – Teeth cut and grind food into small particles
    – Salivary glands pour saliva into the mouth
    – Food mixes with saliva to form a pliable mass (bolus) for swallowing
    – Saliva contains amylase, an enzyme that begins starch digestion

● **Pharynx**
  • The *pharynx* is a cavity that extends from the base of the skull to the esophagus (about the level of the sixth vertebra); it's lined with mucous membrane
  • It aids swallowing by grasping food and moving it toward the esophagus
    – Food leaving the mouth is propelled into the oropharynx and laryngopharynx (the middle and inferior portions of the pharynx, respectively)
    – Normally, food doesn't pass through the nasopharynx (the superior portion of the pharynx), which connects the oral cavity to the nasal cavities

● **Esophagus**
  • The *esophagus* is a collapsible, muscular tube that extends from the laryngopharynx through the mediastinum to the stomach
  • It conducts food from the pharynx to the stomach
    – Swallowing triggers food passage from the laryngopharynx into the esophagus

Key characteristics of the oral cavity
  • Prepares food for swallowing and begins digestion
  • Includes salivary glands and 32 teeth

Key characteristics of the pharynx
  • Cavity extending from the base of the skull to the esophagus
  • Aids swallowing

Key characteristics of the esophagus
  • Conducts food from the pharynx to the stomach
  • Lower esophageal sphincter closes after food enters the stomach to prevent reflux

The oral cavity

The mouth, or oral cavity, is bounded by the lips (labia), cheeks, palate (roof of the mouth), and tongue. The mouth initiates the mechanical breakdown of food.

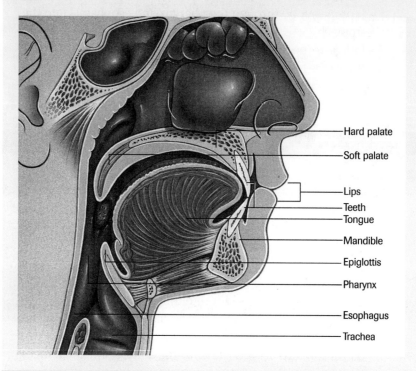

- Hard palate
- Soft palate
- Lips
- Teeth
- Tongue
- Mandible
- Epiglottis
- Pharynx
- Esophagus
- Trachea

– Peristalsis—rhythmic contraction of smooth muscle—propels liquids and solids through the esophagus into the stomach
– Normally, the lower esophageal sphincter closes after food enters the stomach
  • If it fails to close or remains closed, gastric juices can flow backward into the esophagus, causing gastroesophageal reflux

● Stomach

- The *stomach* is a collapsible, pouchlike structure that attaches to the lower end of the esophagus; it's immediately inferior to the diaphragm
- It serves as a temporary storage area for food, which remains there until it's partially digested
- The stomach churns ingested food and mixes it with gastric juices (composed of digestive enzymes and hydrochloric acid); this results in a thick, acidic fluid called *chyme*
  – GI hormones, such as gastrin, gastric inhibitory peptides, secretin, and cholecystokinin, regulate gastric secretion and motility

Key characteristics of the stomach

- Pouchlike structure attached to lower end of the esophagus
- Serves as temporary storage area for food
- Mixes food with gastric juices to form chyme

– Stimulation of gastric acid secretion occurs during two phases
  · In the cephalic phase, secretion is stimulated by the sight, smell, or anticipation of food
  · In the gastric phase, secretion is stimulated by *gastrin,* the GI hormone released in response to food in the stomach and duodenum
– Gastric acid activates the gastric enzyme precursor pepsinogen to form pepsin, which digests proteins by breaking peptide bonds
– Intrinsic factor (IF) in gastric acid combines with vitamin B_{12}; the vitamin B_{12}–IF complex is absorbed later in the small intestine
– Stomach walls are protected by mucus secreted by mucous cells of the gastric glands

● **Small intestine**
  • The *small intestine,* the longest organ of the GI tract, joins to the pylorus of the stomach at the pyloric sphincter
  • It has three major divisions—the duodenum, jejunum, and ileum
  • Its main function is to complete food digestion
    – The stomach expels chyme through the pylorus into the upper part of the small intestine (duodenum)
    – Segmenting contractions (alternating contractions and relaxations of adjacent segments of the small intestine) mix the contents of the small intestine
      · The small intestine's contents are propelled by peristalsis
      · Abnormal peristalsis can lead to constipation, diarrhea, or both—as in irritable bowel syndrome (see *Teaching a patient with irritable bowel syndrome*)

> **Key characteristics of the small intestine**
> - Longest organ of the GI tract
> - Three divisions: duodenum, jejunum, ileum
> - Main function is to complete food digestion
> - Absorbs most of the nutrients, water, and electrolytes in food

---

 TIME-OUT FOR TEACHING

Teaching a patient with irritable bowel syndrome

Make sure you teach a patient with irritable bowel syndrome:
- the nature of the disorder (including excessive peristalsis and spasms) and factors that promote exacerbations
- how to prepare for tests, such as a barium enema, that may be necessary to rule out other disorders
- dietary changes to minimize pain, bloating, constipation, and diarrhea
- the proper use of prescribed drugs, such as antispasmodics, laxatives, antidiarrheals, and tranquilizers
- self-care measures, such as stress-reduction techniques and smoking cessation.

> **Key teaching topics for a patient with irritable bowel syndrome**
> - Explain diagnostic tests and how to prepare for them
> - Review dietary changes and medications
> - Discuss stress reduction and smoking cessation

Small intestine: Digestion and absorption

Nearly all digestion and absorption takes place in the 20′ (6.1 m) of small intestine. The structure of the small intestine, as shown here, is key to digestion and absorption.

SPECIALIZED MUCOSA

Multiple projections of the intestinal mucosa increase the surface area for absorption several hundredfold.

Circular projections (Kerckring's folds) are covered by villi. Each villus contains a lymphatic vessel (lacteal), a venule, capillaries, an arteriole, nerve fibers, and smooth muscle.

Each villus is densely fringed with about 2,000 microvilli, making it resem- ble a fine brush. The villi are lined with columnar epithelial cells, which dip into the lamina propria between the villi to form intestinal glands (crypts of Lieberkühn).

TYPES OF EPITHELIAL CELLS

The type of epithelial cell dictates its function. Mucus-secreting goblet cells are found on and between the villi on the crypt mucosa. In the proximal duo-

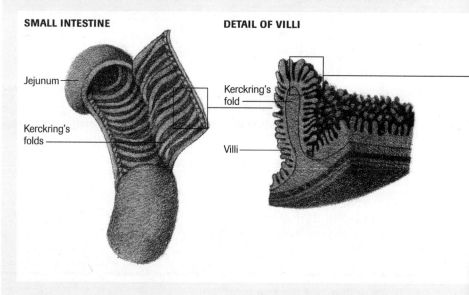

SMALL INTESTINE

Jejunum

Kerckring's folds

DETAIL OF VILLI

Kerckring's fold

Villi

- Most of the nutrients, water, and electrolytes in foods are digested and absorbed during the 6- to 8-hour passage through the small intestine (see *Small intestine: Digestion and absorption*)
- Intestinal glands secrete enzymes that further digest various nutrients
- The intestinal hormones cholecystokinin and secretin also regulate gallbladder function and pancreatic fluid and bile secretion
- Bile and pancreatic fluid mix with intestinal contents to continue digestion

denum, specialized Brunner's glands also secrete large amounts of mucus to lubricate and protect the duodenum from potentially corrosive acidic chyme and gastric juices.

Duodenal argentaffin cells produce the hormones secretin and cholecystokinin. Undifferentiated cells deep within the intestinal glands replace the epithelium. Absorptive cells consist of large numbers of tightly packed microvilli over a plasma membrane that contains transport mechanisms for absorption and produces enzymes for the final step in digestion.

INTESTINAL GLANDS

The intestinal glands primarily secrete a watery fluid that bathes the villi with chyme particles. Fluid production results from local irritation of nerve cells and, possibly, from hormonal stimulation by secretin and cholecystokinin. The microvillous brush border secretes various hormones and digestive enzymes that catalyze final nutrient breakdown.

DETAIL OF INTESTINAL MUCOSA

TRANSVERSE SECTION OF VILLUS

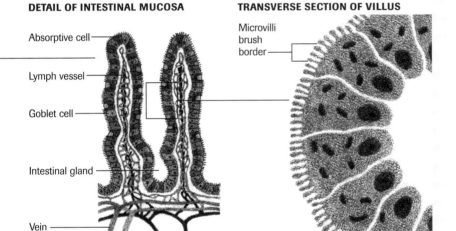

Absorptive cell

Lymph vessel

Goblet cell

Intestinal gland

Vein
Artery

Microvilli brush border

- After digestion, food molecules are absorbed through the wall of the small intestine into the circulatory system for delivery to body cells

● **Large intestine**
  - The *large intestine* extends from the ileocecal valve of the small intestine to the anus
  - Consists of segments—the cecum, vermiform appendix, ascending colon, transverse colon, descending colon, and sigmoid colon

- The rectum—the last several inches of the large intestine—extends to the anus, which allows passage of feces
- The large intestine mainly functions to absorb water and eliminate digestive waste products
    - Peristalsis and segmenting contractions move intestinal contents slowly; water and minerals are absorbed from the contents, leaving a residue of fecal material
        · Intestinal bacteria act on the residue, releasing decomposition products and intestinal gases
        · These bacteria also synthesize vitamin K and some B vitamins, which are absorbed in the colon
    - Peristalsis propels fecal material into the rectum; this causes reflex contraction of rectal smooth muscle and relaxation of the internal anal sphincter (defecation reflex)
    - Voluntary relaxation of the external anal sphincter combined with bearing-down efforts results in evacuation of rectal contents

● **Peritoneum**
- A strong, colorless membrane that completely lines the walls of the abdominal cavity, the *peritoneum* includes the parietal peritoneum and visceral peritoneum
    - *Parietal peritoneum* lines the abdominal and pelvic walls and the underside of the diaphragm
    - *Visceral peritoneum,* a continuation of the parietal peritoneum, covers the external surfaces of most abdominal organs, including the stomach, spleen, and liver
- Folds of peritoneum called *mesenteries* hold the intestines and other GI organs in place; they contain blood vessels, lymphatic vessels, and nerves
- Other peritoneal folds, called *omenta,* attach to the stomach
- Additional peritoneal folds form the *ligaments* of the liver, spleen, and stomach

ACCESSORY ORGANS

● **Key concepts**
- Accessory organs include the salivary glands, intestinal glands, liver, gallbladder, and pancreas
- Most produce or store secretions needed for digestion
- The liver, gallbladder, and pancreas lie outside the GI tract

● **Gastric glands and intestinal glands**
- *Gastric glands* are located in the mucosal lining of the stomach; they produce the hormone gastrin when stimulated by partially digested proteins

- They secrete gastrin directly into capillaries in the stomach
- Circulating gastrin stimulates secretion of gastric juice, which has a high content of pepsin and hydrochloric acid
- Gastrin triggers histamine release, causing increased gastric secretion; it also stimulates mucosal cell growth
- *Intestinal glands* include intestinal crypts and Brunner's glands
  - Intestinal crypts, found in the intestinal mucosa, secrete intestinal juice (a mixture of digestive enzymes, mucus, and hormones)
  - Brunner's glands, found in the duodenal submucosa, secrete an alkaline mucus that helps neutralize the acidic chyme entering the duodenum from the stomach

Liver
- The largest gland in the body, the *liver* is located immediately inferior to the diaphragm and partially anterior to the stomach
- It consists of a right lobe, left lobe, caudate lobe (behind the right lobe), and quadrate lobe (below the left lobe)
- It contains lobules, the liver's functional unit (see *The liver lobule*)
- The liver is covered almost entirely by a fold of peritoneum called the *lesser omentum;* the hepatic artery and hepatic portal vein (which enter the liver) and the common bile duct and hepatic veins (which leave the liver) all pass through the lesser omentum

Key characteristics of the liver
- Largest gland in the body
- Contains lobules, the liver's functional unit
- Chief digestive function is production of bile
- Detoxifies or excretes many wastes and toxins

The liver lobule

The liver's functional unit is called a *lobule.* It consists of a plate of hepatic cells, or hepatocytes, that encircle a central vein and radiate outward. Separating the hepatocyte plates from each other are sinusoids, which serve as the liver's capillary system. Sinusoids carry oxygenated blood from the hepatic artery and nutrient-rich blood from the portal vein.

Key liver lobule structures
- Hepatic cells plate
- Bile canaliculi
- Sinusoids
- Portal vein branch
- Hepatic artery branch
- Central vein
- Lymph vessel
- Venule
- Arteriole
- Bile duct

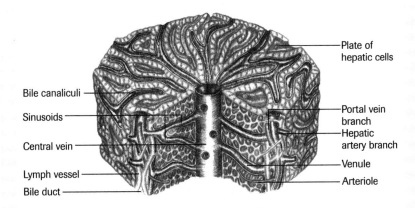

Plate of hepatic cells
Bile canaliculi
Sinusoids
Central vein
Lymph vessel
Bile duct
Portal vein branch
Hepatic artery branch
Venule
Arteriole

- A specialized accessory organ, the liver has digestive, metabolic, storage, and regulatory functions; its chief digestive function is production of bile, which acts as a fat emulsifier in the small intestine
- The liver receives digestive products through the portal vein
  - It can convert the absorbed hexoses, amino acids, and lipid digestion products into whatever nutrient mixture the body needs for metabolic processes
  - It also forms ketone bodies from products of lipid metabolism
  - It produces blood proteins (such as albumin and globulin), lipoproteins, and proteins involved with blood coagulation; it stores a small reserve of fat and glycogen, iron, and vitamins A, B_{12}, D, E, and K
- The liver secretes 500 to 1,000 ml of bile daily to promote fat digestion (see *Functions of digestive secretions*)
  - Bile is a complex secretion composed of cholesterol, lecithin (a phospholipid), bile salts (composed of cholesterol and amino acid derivatives), minerals, bile pigments (derived from hemoglobin breakdown), and water
  - Bile emulsifies fats into small globules for more efficient digestion; bile salts promote the absorption of fats and fat-soluble vitamins
- The liver detoxifies or excretes many wastes and toxins
  - It converts potentially toxic compounds, such as ammonia, to nontoxic compounds
  - It inactivates such substances as drugs, antibiotics, and steroid hormones
  - It excretes bilirubin derived from red blood cell breakdown; in the colon, intestinal bacteria break down bilirubin into various compounds that produce the normal color of feces
  - It also excretes cholesterol and other inactivated or detoxified products

Gallbladder

- The *gallbladder* is a muscular sac located on the ventral surface of the liver, between the right and quadrate lobes; it's covered by visceral peritoneum and joined to the common bile duct by the cystic duct (see *The gallbladder and pancreas*, page 290)
- The gallbladder stores and concentrates bile secreted by the liver
  - Bile travels through the cystic duct and enters the gallbladder, where it's stored and concentrated tenfold through water absorption
  - Bile can enter the duodenum only when the ampullary Oddi's sphincter is open, during digestion

Key characteristics of the gallbladder

- Muscular sac located on ventral surface of the liver
- Stores and concentrates bile
- A fatty meal induces cholecystokinin release
- Cholesterol may precipitate from bile and form gallstones

Functions of digestive secretions

Most digestive secretions contain enzymes that have specific digestive functions, as shown below. Only one secretion (bile) performs its functions without enzymes.

DIGESTIVE SECRETION	ENZYME	FUNCTION
Saliva	• Amylase	• Digests starch
Gastric acid	• Pepsin	• Digests protein
	• Intrinsic factor	• Promotes vitamin B_{12} absorption
Small intestine secretions	• Disaccharidases (such as maltase, sucrase, and lactase)	• Digest carbohydrates
	• Peptidases	• Digest proteins
	• Amylase	• Digests starch further
	• Enterokinase	• Activates pancreatic trypsinogen to form trypsin, which continues protein digestion
Bile	• None	• Emulsifies fats and other lipids
Pancreatic secretions	• Trypsin, chymotrypsin, and carboxypeptidase	• Digest protein
	• Ribonuclease and deoxyribonuclease	• Digest nucleic acids
	• Amylase	• Digests starch further
	• Lipase	• Digests fats and other lipids
	• Cholesterol esterase	• Splits cholesterol esters to cholesterol and fatty acids

Key digestive secretions

- Saliva
- Gastric acid
- Small intestine secretions
- Bile
- Pacreatic secretions

- A fatty meal induces cholecystokinin release
  - This stimulates gallbladder contraction
  - Simultaneously, the ampullary sphincter relaxes, permitting bile to enter the small intestine
- Various factors regulate cholesterol solubility in bile
  - Micelles formed from bile salts have a lipid-soluble center and a water-soluble periphery
  - Cholesterol remains in solution in bile by dissolving in the lipid-soluble centers of the micelles

The gallbladder and pancreas

Together, the gallbladder and pancreas constitute the biliary tract. This illustration shows the structures of the biliary tract.

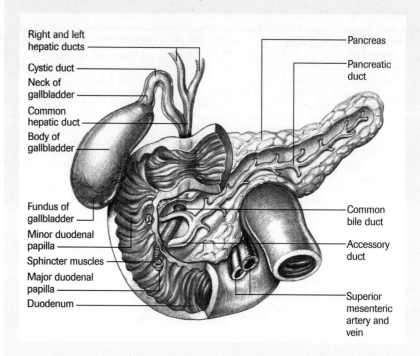

Key characteristics of the pancreas

- Exocrine pancreas secretes digestive enzymes into the duodenum through the pancreatic duct
- Endocrine pancreas contains cells that secrete hormones directly into the bloodstream
- Chronic pancreatitis can cause enzymes to back up into the pancreas and destroy pancreatic tissue

· Cholesterol may precipitate from bile and form gallstones if the cholesterol concentration in bile exceeds the capacity of the micelles to hold cholesterol in solution

● Pancreas

- The *pancreas* is an elongated, triangular gland located transversely behind the stomach, between the spleen and duodenum
- It consists of the exocrine pancreas and the endocrine pancreas
- The *exocrine pancreas* contains cells that secrete digestive enzymes into the duodenum through the pancreatic duct (secretes about 1,500 ml of alkaline pancreatic fluid into the duodenum daily)
  – Pancreatic fluid contains potent digestive enzymes
    · Amylase digests starch and glycogen
    · Trypsin, chymotrypsin, and carboxypeptidase digest proteins
    · Lipase digests certain lipids
    · Cholesterol esterase digests cholesterol esters
    · Ribonuclease and deoxyribonuclease digest nucleic acids
  – The pancreas secretes proteolytic (protein-digesting) enzymes as inactive precursors

- · The intestinal enzyme enterokinase activates trypsinogen to trypsin
  - · In turn, trypsin activates chymotrypsinogen and procarboxy-peptidase to form chymotrypsin and carboxypeptidase
  - – The small intestine releases the hormone secretin when acidic chyme is expelled into the duodenum; this hormone stimulates the pancreas to secrete a large volume of pancreatic fluid that's low in enzymes
  - – The small intestine also releases cholecystokinin when lipids and proteins enter the duodenum; this stimulates secretion of pancreatic fluid, which is rich in digestive enzymes, and stimulates gallbladder contraction
  - – In chronic pancreatitis, the duct through which enzymes leave the pancreas becomes blocked; this can cause enzymes to back up into the pancreas and destroy pancreatic tissue
- • The *endocrine pancreas* contains about 1 million small clusters of endocrine cells (islets of Langerhans) that secrete hormones directly into the bloodstream; each cluster is composed of three major cell types
  - – Alpha cells secrete glucagon to increase blood glucose in response to decreased blood glucose levels
  - – Beta cells secrete insulin to lower blood glucose in response to increased blood glucose levels
    - · These cells are absent or defective in people with diabetes mellitus, resulting in elevated blood glucose
  - – Delta cells secrete somatostatin (growth hormone inhibitory hormone), which inhibits glucagon and insulin secretion

NUTRIENT DIGESTION AND ABSORPTION

- ● **Key concepts**
  - • The body needs a continual supply of water and various nutrients to maintain its functions; virtually all nutrients come from digested food
  - • Three major types of nutrients the body needs are *carbohydrates*, *proteins*, and *lipids*
    - – When nutrients are used to yield energy, the energy is measured in kilocalories (kcal), or calories, per gram of nutrient
    - – Adults require approximately 2,000 kcal daily
  - • All major nutrients must be digested in the GI tract by enzymes that hydrolyze (split) large units into smaller ones; then these smaller units are absorbed from the small intestine and transported to the liver through the portal venous system

---

Key pancreatic secretions

- ● Trypsin
- ● Chymotrypsin
- ● Carboxypeptidase
- ● Ribonuclease
- ● Deoxyribonuclease
- ● Amylase
- ● Lipase
- ● Cholesterol esterase

Types of cells in the endocrine pancreas

- ● Alpha cells: secrete glucagon
- ● Beta cells: secrete insulin
- ● Delta cells: secrete somatostatin

Key facts about nutrient digestion and absorption

- ● The body requires a continual supply of water and nutrients
- ● Virtually all nutrients come from digested food

- The body also needs vitamins (biologically active organic compounds essential to normal metabolism and growth and development); vitamins may be water-soluble or fat-soluble
    – Water-soluble vitamins include the B complex and C vitamins
    – Fat-soluble vitamins include vitamins A, D, E, and K
- The body also needs minerals—inorganic substances required for enzyme metabolism, membrane transfer of essential compounds, maintenance of acid-base balance and osmotic pressure, nerve impulse transmission, muscle contractility, and growth
    – Major minerals include calcium, chloride, magnesium, phosphorus, potassium, sodium, and sulfur
    – Trace minerals include chromium, cobalt, copper, fluorine, iodine, iron, manganese, molybdenum, selenium, and zinc

● **Carbohydrate digestion and absorption**
- Enzymes break down complex carbohydrates into hexoses by hydrolyzing the glycoside bonds; hydrolysis restores the water molecules that were released when the bonds were formed
- Salivary amylase begins breaking down starch into disaccharides in the oral cavity; pancreatic amylase continues this process in the small intestine
- Intestinal mucosal disaccharidases break down disaccharides into monosaccharides
    – Lactase splits lactose to glucose and galactose
    – Sucrase splits sucrose into glucose and fructose
- Monosaccharides (such as glucose, fructose, and galactose) are absorbed through the intestinal mucosa by diffusion and active transport; they're transported to the liver through the portal venous system
    – Enzymes in the liver convert fructose and galactose to glucose
    – Ribonucleases and deoxyribonucleases break down nucleotides from deoxyribonucleic acid and ribonucleic acid into pentoses and nitrogen-containing compounds (nitrogen bases), which are absorbed through the intestinal mucosa like glucose

● **Protein digestion and absorption**
- Enzymes digest proteins by hydrolyzing peptide bonds
    – These bonds link the amino acids that make up the protein chains
    – This process restores water molecules that were released when the peptide bonds were formed
- Gastric pepsin breaks proteins into polypeptides
- Pancreatic trypsin, chymotrypsin, and carboxypeptidase convert polypeptides to peptides
- Intestinal mucosal peptidases break peptides into their constituent amino acids

---

Key facts about carbohydrate digestion and absorption

- Salivary amylase breaks down starch into disaccharides
- Pancreatic amylase continues the process
- Intestinal mucosal disaccharidases break down disaccharides into monosaccharides
- Monosaccharides are absorbed through intestinal mucosa

Key facts about protein digestion and absorption

- Gastric pepsin breaks proteins into polypeptides
- Pancreatic enzymes convert polypeptides to peptides
- Intestinal mucosal peptidases break peptides into amino acids
- Amino acids are absorbed through intestinal mucosa

   – These amino acids are absorbed through the intestinal mucosa by active transport mechanisms
   – Then they're carried through the portal venous system to the liver, which converts amino acids not needed for protein synthesis into glucose

● **Lipid digestion and absorption**
   • Bile from the liver emulsifies fats and other lipids into small droplets for more efficient digestion and eventual absorption in the small intestine
   • Pancreatic lipase breaks fats and phospholipids into a mixture of glycerol, short- and long-chain fatty acids, and monoglycerides (fats composed of one molecule of a fatty acid and one molecule of glycerol); these substances are transported to the liver via the portal venous system
      – Lipase hydrolyzes the bonds between glycerol and fatty acids
      – This process restores water molecules that were released when the bonds were formed
   • Glycerol diffuses directly through the mucosa
   • Short-chain fatty acids diffuse into the intestinal epithelial cells and are transported to the liver via the portal venous system
   • Long-chain fatty acids and monoglycerides in the intestine dissolve in the bile salt micelles
      – They diffuse from the micelles into the intestinal epithelial cells
      – In the endothelial cells, lipase breaks down absorbed monoglycerides into glycerol and fatty acids
   • Fatty acids and glycerol are recombined to form fats in the smooth endoplasmic reticulum of epithelial cells
   • Triglycerides (fats), along with a small amount of cholesterol and phospholipid, are coated with a thin layer of protein to form lipoprotein particles called *chylomicrons*
      – Chylomicrons collect in the intestinal lacteals (lymphatic vessels) and are transported through lymphatic channels
      – Then chylomicrons enter the circulation through the thoracic duct and are distributed to body cells
         · In the cells, fats are extracted from the chylomicrons and broken down into fatty acids and glycerol by enzymes
         · They're absorbed and recombined in fat cells to reform triglycerides (fat) for storage and later use

CARBOHYDRATE METABOLISM

● **Key concepts**
   • *Metabolism* is the transformation of substances into energy or materials that the body can use or store; it consists of two processes

---

Key facts about lipid digestion and absorption

● Pancreatic lipase breaks down fats into glycerol, short- and long-chain fatty acids, and monoglycerides
● Glycerol diffuses directly through mucosa
● Short-chain fatty acids diffuse into intestinal epithelial cells
● Long-chain fatty acids and monoglycerides dissolve in bile salt micelles

Key facts about carbohydrate metabolism

● Metabolism consists of anabolism and catabolism
● All ingested carbohydrates are converted to glucose
● Glucose that isn't used immediately is stored as glycogen or converted to lipids

– *Anabolism* is the synthesis of simple substances into complex ones

– *Catabolism* is the breakdown of complex substances into simpler ones or into energy

- All ingested carbohydrates are converted to glucose, the body's main energy source
- Glucose that isn't needed for immediate energy requirements is stored as glycogen or converted to lipids
- Energy from glucose catabolism is generated in three phases: glycolysis, the citric acid cycle (also called *Krebs cycle* or *tricarboxylic acid cycle*), and the electron transport system

– Glycolysis, which occurs in the cell cytoplasm, doesn't require oxygen

– The citric acid cycle and electron transport system, which occur in mitochondria, require oxygen (see *The glucose pathway*)

● Glycolysis

- During glycolysis, enzymes break down the six-carbon glucose molecule into two three-carbon pyruvic acid (pyruvate) molecules; this process yields energy in the form of adenosine triphosphate (ATP)
- If the oxygen supply to the tissues is inadequate, pyruvic acid is reduced by cytoplasmic enzymes to lactic acid by the addition of two hydrogen atoms
- When adequate oxygen becomes available, lactic acid is oxidized back to pyruvic acid

● Citric acid cycle (Krebs cycle)

- The Krebs cycle is a pathway by which a molecule of acetyl coenzyme A (acetyl CoA) is oxidized enzymatically to yield energy
- In this phase of carbohydrate metabolism, pyruvic acid releases a carbon dioxide molecule and is converted in the mitochondria to a two-carbon acetyl fragment, which combines with coenzyme A (a complex organic compound) to form acetyl CoA
- Then the two-carbon acetyl fragments of acetyl CoA enter the citric acid cycle by combining with the four-carbon compound oxaloacetic acid to form citric acid, a six-carbon compound; in this process, the coenzyme A molecule is detached from the acetyl group and becomes available to form more acetyl CoA molecules
- Enzymes then convert citric acid into intermediate compounds and eventually convert it back into oxaloacetic acid, which is available to repeat the cycle
- Each turn of the Krebs cycle releases hydrogen atoms, which are picked up by the coenzymes nicotinamide adenine dinucleotide

---

Key facts about glycolysis

- Involves the breakdown of a glucose molecule, yielding ATP
- If oxygen is scarce, lactic acid is produced
- When oxygen becomes available, lactic acid is oxidized back to pyruvic acid

Key facts about the Krebs cycle

- The second phase of glucose catabolism
- Involves the enzymatic oxidation of acetyl CoA to yield energy

GO WITH THE FLOW

The glucose pathway

Glucose catabolism generates energy in three phases: glycolysis, the citric acid cycle (Krebs cycle), and the electron transport system The flowchart below summarizes the first two phases.

GLYCOLYSIS

Glycolysis, the first phase, breaks apart one molecule of glucose to form two molecules of pyruvate, which yields energy in the form of adenosine triphosphate and acetyl coenzyme A (CoA).

KREBS CYCLE

The second phase, the Krebs cycle, continues carbohydrate metabolism. Fragments of acetyl CoA join to oxaloacetic acid to form citric acid. The CoA molecule breaks off from the acetyl group and may form more acetyl CoA molecules. Citric acid is first converted into intermediate compounds and then back into oxaloacetic acid. The citric acid cycle also liberates carbon dioxide.

ELECTRON TRANSPORT SYSTEM

In the third phase of glucose catabolism, molecules on the inner mitochondrial membrane attract electrons from hydrogen atoms and carry them through oxidation-reduction reactions in the mitochondria. The hydrogen ions produced in the citric acid cycle then combine with oxygen to form water.

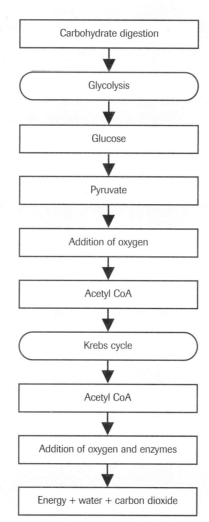

Carbohydrate digestion → Glycolysis → Glucose → Pyruvate → Addition of oxygen → Acetyl CoA → Krebs cycle → Acetyl CoA → Addition of oxygen and enzymes → Energy + water + carbon dioxide

(NAD) and flavin adenine dinucleotide (FAD); it also liberates carbon dioxide and generates energy

● **Electron transport system**
 • In the electron transport system, carrier molecules on the inner mitochondrial membrane pick up electrons from hydrogen atoms

Key facts about the electron transport system

• Third phase of glucose catabolism
• Involves oxidation-reduction reactions in mitochondria
• Reactions release energy and generate ATP

carried by NAD and FAD (each hydrogen atom consists of a hydrogen ion and an electron)
- Carrier molecules transport the electrons through a series of enzyme-catalyzed oxidation-reduction reactions in the mitochondria
    - During *oxidation,* a chemical compound loses electrons after combining with oxygen
    - During *reduction,* a compound gains electrons
- These reactions release the energy contained in electrons and generate ATP
- After passing through the electron transport system, hydrogen ions produced in the Krebs cycle combine with oxygen to form water

● **Role of the liver and muscle cells**
- The liver plays an essential role in regulating blood glucose levels
    - When the amount of glucose exceeds immediate needs, hormones stimulate the liver to convert glucose into glycogen or lipids
        · Glycogen is formed through *glycogenesis*
        · Lipids are formed through *lipogenesis*
    - When the blood glucose level is inadequate, the liver can form glucose by two processes
        · The liver can break down glycogen to glucose through *glycogenolysis*
        · It can also synthesize glucose from amino acids through *gluconeogenesis*
- Muscle cells can convert glucose to glycogen for storage, but they lack enzymes to convert glycogen back to glucose when needed
    - During vigorous muscular activity, when oxygen demand exceeds supply, muscle cells break down glycogen to yield lactic acid and energy
        · Lactic acid accumulates in muscles, and muscle glycogen is depleted
        · Some lactic acid diffuses from muscle cells; it's transported to the liver and reconverted to glycogen
        · Then the liver converts the newly formed glycogen to glucose, which is transported through the bloodstream to the muscles and reformed into glycogen
    - When muscular exertion ceases, part of the accumulated lactic acid is reconverted to pyruvic acid and then oxidized completely to yield energy by means of the Krebs cycle and electron transport system

PROTEIN METABOLISM

Key concepts

- Proteins are absorbed as amino acids; they're transported by the portal venous system to the liver and then throughout the body by blood
- Absorbed amino acids mix with other amino acids in the body's amino acid pool; these other amino acids may be produced by protein breakdown or synthesized in the body from other substances such as keto acids
- Amino acids can't be stored; they're converted to protein or glucose or are catabolized to provide energy
- For these changes to occur, amino acids must be transformed by deamination or transamination
  - In *deamination,* an amino group is removed and the amino residue is excreted as urea
  - In *transamination,* an amino group is exchanged for a keto group in a keto acid, through the action of transaminase enzymes; the process converts the amino acid to a keto acid and the original keto acid to an amino acid

Amino acid synthesis

- Body proteins are synthesized from 20 different amino acids selected from the body's amino acid pool
- The body can synthesize 12 amino acids from carbohydrates, fats, or other amino acids; they're called *nonessential amino acids*
- The body can't synthesize the other eight amino acids and must obtain them through dietary intake; they're called *essential amino acids*

Amino acid conversion

- Amino acids that aren't used for protein synthesis can be converted to keto acids and metabolized by the citric acid cycle and electron transport system to yield energy
  - Some keto acids can enter the Krebs cycle directly by combining with one of the intermediate compounds in the cycle
  - Others must undergo one of two possible conversions
    - They may be converted to pyruvic acid and then to acetyl CoA, which combines with oxaloacetic acid to form citric acid
    - They may be converted directly to acetyl CoA, which combines with oxaloacetic acid to form citric acid
- Amino acids can be converted to other nutrients

Key facts about protein metabolism

- Proteins are absorbed as amino acids
- Amino acids can't be stored
- Amino acids are converted to protein or glucose or are catabolized for energy through deamination or transamination

Key facts about amino acid synthesis

- Twenty different amino acids are used to synthesize body proteins
- The body can synthesize 12 amino acids (nonessential amino acids)
- The body must obtain eight other amino acids through food (essential amino acids)

Key facts about amino acid conversion

- Amino acids that aren't used for protein synthesis can be converted to keto acids and metabolized to yield energy
- Amino acids can also be converted to other nutrients or converted to fat

– They can be converted to fats
  · Amino acids that aren't used for protein synthesis may be converted to pyruvic acid and then to acetyl CoA
  · Acetyl CoA fragments condense to form long-chain fatty acids; this process is the reverse of fatty acid breakdown
  · These fatty acids combine with glycerol to form fats
– Amino acids also can be converted to glucose
  · They're converted to pyruvic acid
  · Pyruvic acid then may be converted to glucose

LIPID METABOLISM

● **Key concepts**
  • Fats (lipids) are stored in adipose tissue within cells until required for energy
  • When required for energy, each fat molecule is hydrolyzed to glycerol and three molecules of fatty acids
  • Glycerol is converted to pyruvic acid and then to acetyl CoA, which enters the citric acid cycle to yield energy
  • Long-chain fatty acids are catabolized into two-carbon fragments, which combine with coenzyme A to form acetyl CoA fragments; the acetyl CoA then enters the Krebs cycle to yield energy

● **Ketone body formation**
  • The liver normally forms ketone bodies from acetyl CoA fragments, which are derived primarily from fatty acid catabolism
  • Acetyl CoA molecules yield three types of ketone bodies: acetoacetic acid, beta-hydroxybutyric acid, and acetone
    – Acetoacetic acid forms when two acetyl CoA molecules combine and coenzyme A is released from them
    – Beta-hydroxybutyric acid forms when hydrogen is added to the oxygen atom in the acetoacetic acid molecule; the designation *beta* refers to the location of the carbon atom that contains the hydroxyl group
  • Acetone forms when the carboxyl group of acetoacetic acid releases carbon dioxide
  • Muscle, brain, and other tissues oxidize ketone bodies for energy
  • Certain conditions may cause production of more ketone bodies than the body can oxidize for energy
    – Such conditions include fasting, starvation, and uncontrolled diabetes (in which the body can't break down glucose)
    – In all these conditions, the body must use fat, rather than glucose, as a primary energy source

　　　– The resulting excess of ketone bodies disturbs the body's normal acid-base balance and homeostatic mechanisms, leading to ketosis

● **Lipid formation from proteins and carbohydrates**
　• Excess amino acids can be converted to fat through keto acid–acetyl CoA conversion
　• Glucose may be converted to pyruvic acid and then to acetyl CoA, which is converted into fatty acids and then fat in the same way that amino acids are converted into fat

HORMONAL REGULATION OF METABOLISM

● **Key concepts**
　• Blood glucose levels must remain within a certain range for the body to maintain its normal functions
　• Various hormones are secreted in response to changes in blood glucose level
　• These hormones stimulate metabolic processes that return the blood glucose level to normal

● **Hormones that increase blood glucose level**
　• Glucagon, epinephrine, growth hormone (GH), cortisol, and thyroxine can increase the blood glucose level
　• Glucagon promotes glycogen breakdown to glucose (glycogenolysis), amino acid conversion to glucose (gluconeogenesis), and lipid breakdown (lipolysis), which liberates free fatty acids and glycerol that can be converted to glucose
　• Epinephrine promotes glycogenolysis, gluconeogenesis, and lipolysis
　• GH has multiple effects
　　– It promotes protein synthesis by facilitating amino acid entry into cells
　　– It causes fat lipolysis from adipose tissue and promotes the use of fat rather than carbohydrate as an energy source
　　– It suppresses carbohydrate use for energy, causing blood glucose to rise as a result of reduced glucose use
　　– It promotes conversion of liver glycogen to glucose, which also tends to increase blood glucose level
　• Cortisol promotes protein hydrolysis to amino acids, which can be converted to glucose through gluconeogenesis
　• Thyroxine usually raises the blood glucose level by promoting gluconeogenesis and lipolysis

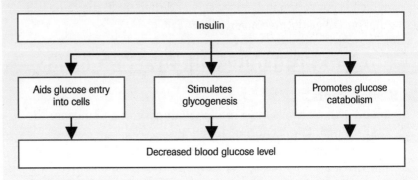

Insulin regulation of blood glucose levels

Unlike most hormones, insulin tends to decrease the blood glucose level. It does this by helping glucose to enter cells, thereby promoting glycogenesis and stimulating glucose catabolism.

Insulin

Aids glucose entry into cells	Stimulates glycogenesis	Promotes glucose catabolism

Decreased blood glucose level

TOP 9

Items to study for your next test on the gastrointestinal system

1. Structure and function of organs of the GI tract
2. Basic functions of the GI tract
3. Structure and function of accessory organs of the GI tract
4. Processes used in the digestion and absorption of food
5. Function of digestive enzymes
6. Ways in which energy is produced from glucose metabolism
7. Processes of protein and lipid metabolism
8. Hormones that affect blood glucose levels
9. Teaching tips for patients with irritable bowel syndrome

● **Hormones that decrease blood glucose level**
  • Insulin is the only hormone that substantially lowers the blood glucose level (see *Insulin regulation of blood glucose levels*)
  • Insulin promotes cell uptake and use of glucose as an energy source
  • It promotes glucose storage as glycogen (glycogenesis) and lipids (lipogenesis)

NCLEX CHECKS

It's never too soon to begin your NCLEX preparation. Now that you've reviewed this chapter, carefully read each of the following questions and choose the best answer. Then compare your responses with the correct answers.

1. Which hormone would the nurse give a client to reduce his blood glucose level?
  ☐ **1.** Glucagon
  ☐ **2.** Epinephrine
  ☐ **3.** Growth hormone
  ☐ **4.** Insulin

2. The nurse is teaching a client with liver disease about his disorder. Which statement made by the client indicates that he understands the teaching?

□ **1.** "The liver secretes gastrin to help in digestion."
□ **2.** "The liver stores vitamins A, C, and K."
□ **3.** "The liver produces bile, which breaks down fats in the small intestine."
□ **4.** "The liver activates such substances as drugs, antibiotics, and steroid hormones."

3. The nurse is assisting a client with his meal. The nurse understands that sight, smell, and anticipation of food stimulates gastric acid secretion during which phase of digestion?
□ **1.** Cephalic
□ **2.** Gastric
□ **3.** Glycolysis
□ **4.** Krebs cycle

4. Which explanation would the nurse give to a client with irritable bowel syndrome?
□ **1.** Abnormal gastric acid secretion exacerbates irritable bowel syndrome.
□ **2.** Excess cholesterol in the bile can precipitate an attack.
□ **3.** A blocked pancreatic duct causes constipation and diarrhea.
□ **4.** Abnormal peristalsis can promote exacerbations.

5. The nurse is preparing a client for a transverse colostomy. Identify the area where the colostomy will be located.

6. The nurse tells a client that bacteria in the large intestine synthesize which vitamins?
□ **1.** Vitamin A and vitamin C
□ **2.** Vitamin K and some B vitamins
□ **3.** Vitamin A and vitamin K
□ **4.** Some B vitamins and vitamin C

7. The nurse teaches a client that water-soluble vitamins aren't stored in the body and must be consumed daily in the diet. Which vitamins are water-soluble?
- [ ] **1.** Vitamin B_1 and vitamin C
- [ ] **2.** Vitamin A and vitamin D
- [ ] **3.** Vitamin B_6 and vitamin K
- [ ] **4.** Vitamin B_{12} and vitamin E

8. The nurse explains to a client who has been recently diagnosed with diabetes mellitus that insulin is secreted by which pancreatic cells?
- [ ] **1.** Alpha cells
- [ ] **2.** Beta cells
- [ ] **3.** Delta cells
- [ ] **4.** Endothelial cells

9. When teaching a client about the importance of minerals to maintain body functions, the nurse correctly identifies which minerals as major?
- [ ] **1.** Calcium, chloride, iron
- [ ] **2.** Chloride, magnesium, potassium
- [ ] **3.** Sodium, copper, fluorine
- [ ] **4.** Phosphorus, manganese, selenium

10. A diabetic client asks the nurse to explain what happens in carbohydrate metabolism. The nurse tells her that sucrose is split into glucose and fructose by which enzyme?
- [ ] **1.** Salivary amylase
- [ ] **2.** Pancreatic amylase
- [ ] **3.** Lactase
- [ ] **4.** Sucrase

ANSWERS AND RATIONALES

1. CORRECT ANSWER: 4
Insulin is the only hormone that substantially lowers the blood glucose level. Glucagon, epinephrine, growth hormone, cortisol, and thyroxine can all increase the blood glucose level.

2. CORRECT ANSWER: 3
The liver has digestive, metabolic, regulatory, and storage functions. Its chief digestive function is bile production, which emulsifies fat in the small intestine. Gastrin is produced in the stomach. The liver stores vitamins A, B_{12}, D, E, and K. The liver inactivates such substances as drugs, antibiotics, and steroid hormones.

3. CORRECT ANSWER: 1
Stimulation of gastric acid secretion occurs during two phases of digestion. In the cephalic phase, secretion is stimulated by the sight, smell, or anticipation of food. In the gastric phase, secretion is stimulated by gastrin, the GI hormone released in response to food in the stomach and duodenum. Glycolysis and the Krebs cycle are phases of glucose catabolism, not digestion.

4. CORRECT ANSWER: 4
In irritable bowel syndrome, abnormal peristalsis can lead to constipation, diarrhea, or both. Abnormal gastric acid secretion doesn't cause irritable bowel syndrome. Excess cholesterol in the bile may cause gall stones. A blocked pancreatic duct may cause pancreatitis.

5. CORRECT ANSWER:

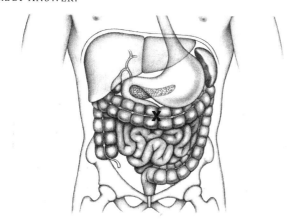

A transverse colostomy is located in the transverse colon.

6. CORRECT ANSWER: 2
Intestinal bacteria in the large intestine synthesize vitamin K and some B vitamins.

7. CORRECT ANSWER: 1
Water-soluble vitamins include the B-complex vitamins and vitamin C. Fat-soluble vitamins include vitamins A, D, E, and K.

8. CORRECT ANSWER: 2
The endocrine pancreas consists of three major cell types. The beta cells secrete insulin to lower blood glucose in response to increased blood glucose levels. Alpha cells secrete glucagon to increase blood glucose in response to decreased blood glucose levels. Delta cells secrete somatostatin, which inhibits glucagon and insulin secretion. Endothelial cells cover the body's surface, line body cavities, and form certain glands.

9. CORRECT ANSWER: 2

Major minerals include calcium, chloride, magnesium, phosphorus, potassium, sodium, and sulfur. Trace minerals include chromium, cobalt, copper, fluorine, iodine, iron, manganese, molybdenum, selenium, and zinc.

10. CORRECT ANSWER: 4

Sucrase splits sucrose into glucose and fructose. Salivary amylase begins breaking down starch into disaccharides in the oral cavity. Pancreatic amylase continues this process in the small intestine. Lactase hydrolyzes lactose to glucose and fructose.

16

Urinary system

LEARNING OBJECTIVES

After studying this chapter, you should be able to:

- Describe the structures and functions of the urinary system.
- Explain the process of urine production.
- Discuss hormonal regulation of urine volume and concentration.
- Describe the countercurrent mechanism of urine concentration.
- Understand renal regulation of blood pressure and volume.
- Discuss the voiding reflex and urine elimination.

CHAPTER OVERVIEW

Although metabolism of nutrients provides energy, it also creates toxic materials and excess essential materials. To maintain homeostasis, the body must eliminate both types of by-products. It does this through the urinary system as well as the lungs, skin, and GI tract. If these by-products aren't continually eliminated, they quickly build up to fatal levels. Because of the urinary system's vital contribution to homeostasis, the nurse must comprehend its basic structures and their functions. This chapter reviews major urinary structures (the kidneys, ureters, bladder, and urethra), urine production, hormonal regulation of urine volume and concentration, renal regulation of blood pressure and volume, and urine elimination.

Key facts about urinary system function

- Removes wastes
- Helps regulate acid-base balance
- Regulates fluid and electrolyte balance
- Assists in blood pressure control

Key urinary system structures

- Renal artery
- Renal vein
- Kidneys
- Inferior vena cava
- Abdominal aorta
- Ureters
- Bladder
- Urethra

MAJOR URINARY STRUCTURES

● Key concepts

- The urinary system is the organ system responsible for eliminating wastes from the body—primarily by producing, carrying, and storing urine
- Its major structures include the kidneys, ureters, bladder, and urethra (see *The urinary system*)

● Functions of the urinary system

- Urinary structures work together to help maintain homeostasis
  - They remove wastes from the body
  - They help govern acid-base balance by retaining and excreting hydrogen ions
  - They regulate fluid and electrolyte balance
  - They assist in blood pressure control
- The urinary system also works with the lungs, skin, and GI tract—all of which also excrete wastes—to maintain the body's overall fluid and chemical balance

The urinary system

This illustration shows the main structures of the urinary system.

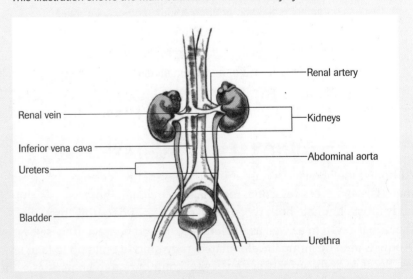

KIDNEYS

● **Key concepts**
- The kidneys are a pair of bean-shaped organs embedded in the dorsal part of the abdomen retroperitoneally, just behind the stomach and liver; the right kidney is situated slightly lower than the left
- Kidneys have several functions
  - They dispose of wastes and excess ions, in the form of urine
  - They filter blood, regulating its volume and chemical makeup
  - They maintain fluid, electrolyte, and acid-base balances
  - They produce several hormones and enzymes
  - They convert vitamin D to a more active form

● **Kidney structure**
- The kidney has an outer region, called the renal cortex; a middle region, called the renal medulla; and an inner region, called the renal pelvis (see *The kidneys,* page 308)
  - The *renal cortex* contains blood-filtering mechanisms
  - The *renal medulla* consists of eight to 12 triangular, striated wedges called *renal pyramids*
    · *Renal columns,* extensions of the renal cortex, jut inward among the renal pyramids
    · The *apices* (tips, or papillae) of the renal pyramids project into the *calyces* (cavities) of the renal pelvis
  - The funnel-shaped *renal pelvis* is an expansion of the upper end of the ureters
    · Urine is discharged at the apex of the renal pyramids into the calyces of the renal pelvis
    · From here, it flows into the ureters
- The kidneys are encased in three layers of supportive and protective tissue—an inner renal capsule, a middle adipose capsule, and an outer renal fascia
- The ureters, renal blood vessels, lymphatic vessels, and nerves enter or exit through the *hilus*—a notch on the inner, concave side of each kidney
- On top of each kidney is an adrenal (suprarenal) gland, which functions separately from the kidney

● **Nephron**
- The nephron is the structural and functional unit of the kidney; each kidney contains more than 1 million nephrons

Key regions of the kidneys
- Outer region is the renal cortex
- Middle region is the renal medulla
- Inner region is the renal pelvis
- Vessels and nerves exit through the hilus

Key characteristics of the nephron
- Structural and functional unit of the kidney
- Has a role in the reabsorption, secretion, and maintenance of osmolality of interstitial fluid

The kidneys

The kidneys are located in the lumbar area, with the right kidney situated slightly lower than the left to make room for the liver, which is just above it. The position of the kidneys shifts somewhat with changes in body position. Covering the kidneys are the true or fibrous capsule, perirenal fat, and renal fasciae.

BLOOD'S CLEANSING JOURNEY

The kidneys receive waste-filled blood from the renal artery, which branches off the abdominal aorta. After passing through a complicated network of smaller blood vessels and nephrons, the filtered blood returns to the circulation by way of the renal vein, which empties into the inferior vena cava.

CONTINUING THE CLEANUP

The kidneys excrete waste products that the nephrons remove from the blood; these excretions combine with other waste fluids (such as urea, creatinine, phosphates, and sulfates) to form urine. An action called *peristalsis* (the circular contraction and relaxation of a tube-shaped structure) passes the urine through the ureters and into the urinary bladder. When the bladder has filled, nerves in the bladder wall relax the sphincter. In conjunction with a voluntary stimulus, this relaxation causes urine to pass into the urethra for elimination from the body.

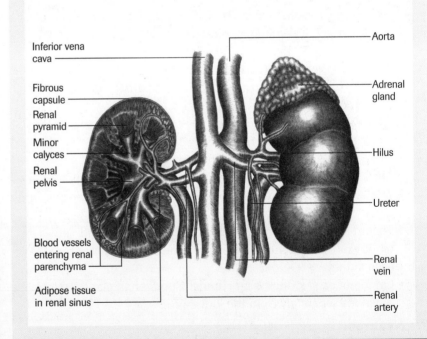

Inferior vena cava

Fibrous capsule

Renal pyramid

Minor calyces

Renal pelvis

Blood vessels entering renal parenchyma

Adipose tissue in renal sinus

Aorta

Adrenal gland

Hilus

Ureter

Renal vein

Renal artery

- Each nephron consists of a long tubule with a closed end, called the glomerular capsule, or Bowman's capsule (see *Internal structure of a nephron*)

Internal structure of a nephron

Within each nephron's glomerular capsule are a renal tubule and a glomerulus. The long tubule has three portions: the proximal convoluted tubule, loop of Henle, and distal convoluted tubule. This illustration shows a nephron and its blood supply.

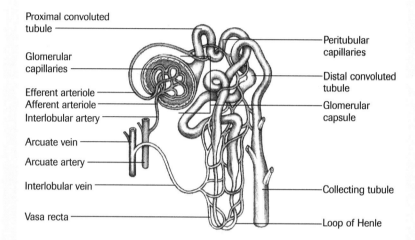

Proximal convoluted tubule

Glomerular capillaries

Efferent arteriole
Afferent arteriole
Interlobular artery

Arcuate vein

Arcuate artery

Interlobular vein

Vasa recta

Peritubular capillaries

Distal convoluted tubule

Glomerular capsule

Collecting tubule

Loop of Henle

Key nephron structures

- Proximal convoluted tubule
- Distal convoluted tubule
- Peritubular capillaries
- Glomerular capillaries
- Efferent arteriole
- Afferent arteriole
- Glomerular capsule
- Interlobular artery
- Interlobular vein
- Arcuate artery
- Arcuate vein
- Collecting tubule
- Vasa recta
- Loop of Henle

- Each glomerular capsule contains a renal tubule and a glomerulus, a structure consisting of a cluster of capillaries
  - The glomerular capsule and glomerulus make up the *renal corpuscle*
  - The renal corpuscle is the main filtration site; it's highly porous
- The long tubule of the nephron is divided into three portions
  - The *proximal convoluted tubule* is the first portion, nearest to the glomerular capsule
  - The *loop of Henle* is the second portion, just beyond the proximal tubule; it has an ascending and a descending limb
  - The *distal convoluted tubule* is the third portion, most distal to the glomerular capsule
- The distal end of the tubule joins the distal ends of adjacent nephrons to form a larger *collecting tubule*
- Reabsorption, secretion, and maintenance of an osmolality gradient within the interstitial fluid take place in different regions of the nephron
  - In the proximal tubule, certain solutes are reabsorbed from the glomerular filtrate back into the blood

– In the descending tubule of the loop of Henle, water is removed from the filtrate (by osmosis) and returned to the interstitial fluid

– In the ascending limb of the loop of Henle, salts (sodium and chloride) are removed to maintain osmolality

– In the distal tubule, potassium and hydrogen ions are secreted and reabsorbed

– Some urea diffuses out of the collecting tubule and some returns to the nephron; however, most urea enters the interstitial fluid

• The juxtaglomerular apparatus regulates blood flow through the glomerulus and regulates blood pressure by producing renin; it consists of juxtaglomerular cells and the macula densa

– *Juxtaglomerular cells* are specialized cells that contain renin granules; they're located in the wall of the afferent arteriole, where the tubule is in contact with the arteriole

– The *macula densa* is an area of compact, heavily nucleated cells in the distal convoluted tubule, where the tubule makes contact with the vascular pole of the glomerulus

● **Blood supply and innervation**

• Blood enters the kidney via large renal arteries, which branch from the abdominal aorta; these arteries deliver blood to the kidneys at a rate of about 1,200 ml/minute

– Each renal artery branches into five lobar (segmental) arteries

– Each lobar artery, in turn, branches into several interlobar arteries

– Each interlobar artery branches into arcuate arteries at the junction of the renal medulla and renal cortex

– Afferent arterioles deliver blood to the glomerulus

• Blood exits the kidneys via the arcuate, interlobar, lobar, and renal veins; from the glomeruli, efferent arterioles from the glomerular capsule form a capillary network (vasa recta) around the convoluted tubules and loop of Henle

• The renal plexus, a network of autonomic nerve fibers and ganglia, innervates the kidneys and ureters

URETERS

● **Key concepts**

• The two *ureters* are fibromuscular tubes that are extensions of the renal pelvis

– Each ureter remains behind the peritoneum as it descends to the level of the bladder

---

Key facts about blood supply and innervation of the kidneys

• Blood enters the kidneys through renal arteries
• Blood exits through the arcuate, interlobar, lobar, and renal veins
• The renal plexus innervates the kidneys and ureters

Key characteristics of the ureters

• Two fibromuscular tubes
• Extensions of the renal pelvis
• Collect and convey urine to the bladder

– Then it courses obliquely through the bladder wall before opening into the bladder
* The ureters collect urine as it forms in the kidneys; then they convey it to the bladder

● **Ureter structure**
* The walls of the ureters have three layers: the mucosa, the muscularis, and the fibrous coat
* As the bladder fills, pressure constricts the ureters at their point of entry into the bladder

BLADDER

● **Key concepts**
* The *bladder* is a freely movable, collapsible, muscular sac
* It's located retroperitoneally, just posterior to the symphysis pubis
    – In men, the bladder lies anterior to the rectum; its neck is surrounded by the prostate gland at the urethral junction
    – In women, the bladder is located anterior to the uterus
* The bladder stores urine until it's excreted; along with the urethra, it eliminates urine from the body
* Folds of peritoneum hold the bladder in place
* When empty, the bladder resembles a deflated balloon; as urine volume increases, it takes on a pear shape

● **Bladder structure**
* A small, triangular area called the *trigone* lies at the base of the bladder
    – The base of the trigone is formed by the openings of each ureter
    – The apex of the trigone is formed by the opening of the urethra
* The bladder wall has four layers
    – The innermost mucosa consists of transitional epithelium
    – The middle submucosa consists of connective tissue
    – The third layer is muscular; the detrusor muscle in this layer contracts to expel urine
    – The outermost layer consists of fibrous adventitia and parietal peritoneum

URETHRA

● **Key concepts**
* A thin, muscular tube extending from the floor of the bladder to the surface of the body, the *urethra* drains urine from the bladder, then expels it from the body
* The urethra has two sphincters

Key characteristics of the bladder
* Is a freely movable, collapsible, muscular sac
* Stores urine until it's excreted
* Held in place by folds of the peritoneum

Key characteristics of the urethra
* Drains urine from the bladder and out of the body
* Has an internal sphincter, composed of smooth muscle
* Has an external sphincter, composed of skeletal muscle
* Male urethra also serves as passageway for semen

Key facts about the male urethra

- Connects the bladder with the urethral meatus
- Is longer than the female urethra
- Has three regions (prostatic, membranous, and penile)
- Expels urine from the body
- Also serves as a passage for semen discharge

Key facts about the female urethra

- Connects the bladder with the urethral meatus
- Has three layers (mucous membrane, spongy tissue, muscle)
- Expels urine from the body

Key facts about urine production

- Glomeruli filter blood
- Filtrate flows into renal tubules
- Tubules reabsorb and secrete various substances and ultimately produce urine

– The *internal urethral sphincter* is located at the junction with the bladder; it's composed of smooth (involuntary) muscle
– The *external urethral sphincter* is located at the pelvic floor; it's composed of skeletal (voluntary) muscle

● **Male urethra**
- The male urethra is approximately 8″ (20 cm) long
- It passes vertically through the prostate gland, then extends through the urogenital diaphragm and the penis
- It includes three regions
  – The prostatic region connects to the bladder and passes through the prostate gland
  – The membranous region passes through the urogenital diaphragm
  – The penile region passes through the penis and terminates at the external urethral orifice
- Besides expelling urine from the body, the male urethra serves as a passageway for semen discharge

● **Female urethra**
- The female urethra is approximately 1″ to 1½″ (2.5 to 4 cm) long
- Embedded in the anterior wall of the vagina behind the symphysis pubis, it connects the bladder with an external opening (urethral orifice or meatus)
- It has three layers—an inner layer of mucous membrane, a middle layer of spongy tissue, and an outer layer of muscle
- Expels urine from the body

URINE PRODUCTION

● **Key concepts**
- The kidneys receive and filter a large volume of blood from the renal artery; tubular reabsorption and secretion converts glomerular filtrate into urine (see *Urine formation*)
- Within the nephrons, glomeruli filter the blood; then the filtrate flows through the renal tubule
- The tubules reabsorb and secrete various substances from the filtrate, changing its composition and concentration and ultimately producing urine
- The glomerular filtration rate (GFR) depends on glomerular capillary permeability, blood pressure, and effective filtration rate
- The juxtaglomerular apparatus regulates glomerular filtration pressure by varying the glomerular filtration volume
- Urine and the urinary system are normally sterile
  – When bacteria enter through the urethra, a urinary tract infection (UTI) can occur (see *Teaching a patient with a UTI,* page 314)

GO WITH THE FLOW

Urine formation

Urine formation occurs in three steps: glomerular filtration, tubular reabsorption, and tubular secretion.

Step 1: Filter

As blood flows into the glomerulus, filtration occurs. Active transport from the proximal convoluted tubules leads to reabsorption of sodium (Na^+) and glucose into nearby circulation. Osmosis then causes water (H_2O) reabsorption.

↓

Step 2: Reabsorb

In tubular reabsorption, a substance moves from the filtrate in the distal convoluted tubules to the peritubular capillaries. Active transport results in Na^+, potassium (K^+), and glucose reabsorption. The presence of antidiuretic hormone causes H_2O reabsorption.

↓

Step 3: Secrete

In tubular secretion, a substance moves from the peritubular capillaries into the tubular filtrate. Peritubular capillaries then secrete ammonia (NH_3) and hydrogen (H^+) into the distal tubules via active transport.

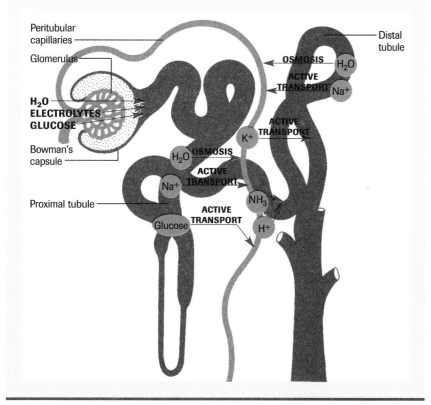

Key teaching topics for a patient with a UTI

- Explain risk factors, signs and symptoms, and complications
- Review diagnostic tests and antibiotic treatment
- Stress dietary guidelines and prevention techniques

Key facts about glomerular filtration rate

- Depends on glomerular capillary permeability, blood pressure, and effective filtration rate
- Stability is aided by the juxtaglomerular apparatus

TIME-OUT FOR TEACHING

Teaching a patient with a UTI

Make sure you teach a patient with a urinary tract infection (UTI):
- signs and symptoms of infection, such as burning on urination, fever, increased frequency, and cloudy or bloody urine
- risk factors for UTIs
- complications of UTIs (such as renal failure)
- diagnostic tests to anticipate (such as urinalysis)
- treatment recommendations (such as antibiotic therapy)
- the importance of taking the full course of antibiotics, if prescribed
- dietary guidelines, such as increased consumption of water and fruit juice (especially cranberry juice)
- prevention techniques, such as perineal hygiene measures, avoiding tub baths, and frequent bladder emptying.

- Lower UTIs (which include urethritis and cystitis) affect the urethra and bladder, respectively
- Upper UTIs (which include pyelonephritis) affect the kidneys

● Glomerular filtration

- Glomeruli filter about 125 ml of water and dissolved materials every minute from the blood as it flows through their capillary network
- GFR depends on three factors: permeability of the glomerular capillary walls, blood pressure, and effective filtration rate
  - A change in any of these factors can alter GFR significantly
  - For example, decreased cardiac output and blood pressure can reduce renal blood flow and GFR
- The juxtaglomerular apparatus helps maintain a stable GFR, despite wide variations in systemic arterial pressure
  - A change in the GFR causes a change in filtration volume and sodium concentration of the filtrate
  - The macula densa detects this change as the fluid flows into the distal convoluted tubule; it conveys the information to the juxtaglomerular cells in the walls of the adjacent afferent arterioles, controlling blood flow into the glomerulus
  - In response, the juxtaglomerular cells constrict or dilate the afferent arterioles and possibly the efferent arterioles to maintain a stable GFR by controlling rennin release
  - The changes in the glomerular filtration pressure (regulated by the juxtaglomerular apparatus) adjust the GFR of each nephron based on the character (volume and sodium concentration) of the glomerular filtrate

● **Tubular reabsorption and secretion**
  • As the filtrate passes through, the renal tubule selectively reabsorbs and secretes substances required by the body; reabsorption and secretion between tubular filtrate and peritubular blood occur via active and passive transport mechanisms
    – Such substances as sodium, potassium, glucose, calcium, some phosphates, and amino acids undergo active transport, which requires energy
    – Such substances as urea, water, chloride, some bicarbonates, and some phosphates undergo passive transport, which doesn't require energy
  • Waste products and other unwanted substances are reabsorbed incompletely or not at all
  • Most reabsorption occurs in the proximal convoluted tubule, which reabsorbs such substances as water, glucose, amino acids, sodium ions, chloride ions, and other electrolytes; the tubule also secretes hydrogen ions, foreign substances, and creatinine
  • The proximal tubule also reabsorbs small amounts of protein that filter through the glomerular capillaries; the protein molecules are engulfed via pinocytosis, broken down by intracellular enzymes into amino acids, and reabsorbed
  • The loop of Henle primarily reabsorbs sodium and chloride ions; it secretes sodium chloride
  • The distal convoluted tubule reabsorbs sodium, chloride, and bicarbonate ions and water; it secretes such substances as hydrogen and ammonium ions, which help maintain the normal hydrogen ion concentration (pH) of body fluids
  • The distal tubule also secretes potassium ions in exchange for sodium ions, which are reabsorbed from the filtrate; this exchange is controlled by the adrenal cortical hormone aldosterone
    – Potassium and hydrogen ions compete for secretion
    – Increased hydrogen ion secretion reduces potassium excretion; decreased hydrogen ion secretion increases potassium excretion
  • The collecting tubule can reabsorb or secrete sodium, potassium, hydrogen, and ammonium ions depending on the body's requirements; it also reabsorbs some water in the filtrate and secretes urea
  • Because of reabsorption in the renal tubule and collecting tubule, only about 1% of the original filtrate volume is excreted as urine

---

Key characteristics of the proximal convoluted tubule

● Reabsorbs water, glucose, amino acids, sodium ions, chloride ions
● Secretes hydrogen ions, foreign substances, creatinine

Key characteristics of the loop of Henle

● Reabsorbs sodium and chloride ions
● Secretes sodium chloride

Key characteristics of the distal convoluted tubule

● Reabsorbs sodium, chloride, and bicarbonate ions and water
● Secretes hydrogen and ammonium ions; exchanges potassium ions for sodium ions

Key characteristics of the collecting tubule

● Reabsorbs or secretes sodium, potassium, hydrogen, and ammonium ions
● Reabsorbs some water
● Secretes urea

Key facts about aldosterone's role in urine regulation

- Acts in the ascending limb of the loop of Henle and distal tubule
- Promotes sodium reabsorption and potassium secretion
- Secretion depends on sodium and potassium concentration in body fluids

Key facts about ADH's role in urine regulation

- Allows collecting tubules to absorb more water from filtrate, which concentrates urine
- Depends on osmoreceptors in the hypothalamus to respond to osmotic pressure changes in blood and body fluids
- When body fluids are concentrated, osmotic pressure rises and ADH is released
- When body fluids are dilute, osmotic pressure falls and ADH isn't released

URINE VOLUME AND CONCENTRATION REGULATION

● **Key concepts**
- The hormones aldosterone and antidiuretic hormone (ADH) regulate urine volume and concentration
- Aldosterone, a steroid hormone produced by the adrenal cortex, regulates the rate of sodium reabsorption from the tubules
- ADH, a posterior pituitary hormone, is released in response to the solute concentration of blood flowing through the hypothalamus; it regulates water reabsorption from the collecting tubules

● **Aldosterone**
- This hormone acts primarily in the ascending limb of the loop of Henle and the distal tubule (see *Aldosterone production*)
- It promotes sodium reabsorption and potassium secretion
- Because chloride ions are absorbed along with sodium, aldosterone indirectly promotes chloride reabsorption
- Aldosterone secretion depends primarily on the sodium and potassium concentration in body fluids
  - A decreased sodium concentration in body fluids stimulates aldosterone secretion; this increases sodium reabsorption, raising the sodium concentration in body fluids
  - An increased sodium concentration in body fluids reduces aldosterone secretion; this reduces sodium reabsorption, decreasing the sodium concentration in body fluids
  - An increased potassium concentration in body fluids also stimulates aldosterone secretion; this increases sodium reabsorption and potassium secretion by the tubules, raising the sodium concentration and lowering the potassium concentration in body fluids
  - A decreased potassium concentration in body fluids inhibits aldosterone release; this reduces potassium secretion, raising the potassium concentration in body fluids

● **ADH**
- ADH regulates water reabsorption from the collecting tubules
  - The hormone increases collecting tubule permeability, which allows tubules to absorb more water from filtrate; this makes urine more concentrated (see *Antidiuretic hormone regulation of urine,* page 318)
  - Without ADH, the collecting tubules are relatively impermeable to water; they reabsorb less water from the filtrate, and the urine remains dilute

GO WITH THE FLOW

Aldosterone production

Aldosterone (a hormone that helps regulate fluid balance) is released by the adrenal gland through the actions of the renin-angiotensin system.

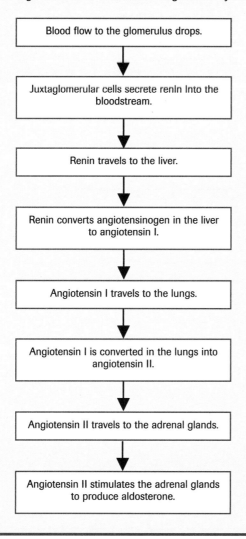

- Specialized cells in the hypothalamus, called *osmoreceptors*, regulate ADH release from the pituitary; these cells respond to osmotic pressure changes in blood and body fluids
- When body fluids are too concentrated (relatively low water and high solute content), osmotic pressure rises

GO WITH THE FLOW

Antidiuretic hormone regulation of urine

Antidiuretic hormone (ADH) regulates fluid balance in four steps.

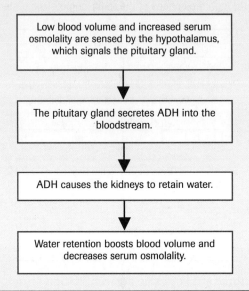

Low blood volume and increased serum osmolality are sensed by the hypothalamus, which signals the pituitary gland.

↓

The pituitary gland secretes ADH into the bloodstream.

↓

ADH causes the kidneys to retain water.

↓

Water retention boosts blood volume and decreases serum osmolality.

- Pressure change stimulates osmoreceptors, which cause ADH secretion
- ADH causes more water to be reabsorbed from the tubules, diluting body fluids and lowering osmotic pressure
• When body fluids are too dilute (relatively high water and low solute content), osmotic pressure decreases
  - ADH isn't released and water isn't reabsorbed from the tubules
  - Excess water is excreted in dilute urine
  - Water excretion increases the relative concentration of substances dissolved in blood, raising osmotic pressure toward normal

COUNTERCURRENT MECHANISM

● **Key concepts**
  • The kidneys can also adjust body fluid concentrations
    - When body fluids are too dilute, the kidneys eliminate excess water; this makes fluids more concentrated

- When body fluids are too concentrated, the kidneys conserve water by excreting more concentrated urine; this makes fluids more dilute
- The countercurrent mechanism allows the kidneys to concentrate urine
- Body fluid concentration is expressed in terms of fluid osmolarity, which is a measure of the osmotic pressure exerted by substances dissolved in the fluid
  - Upon leaving the glomerulus, filtrate normally has the same osmolarity as body fluids—about 300 mOsm/L
  - As filtrate passes along the renal tubule, its osmolarity changes in different parts of the nephron—from 1,200 mOsm/L in the descending limb of the loop of Henle to 70 mOsm/L in the collecting tubule
  - The osmolarity of interstitial fluids in the kidney varies from 300 mOsm/L in the cortex to 1,200 mOsm/L in the medulla near the renal papillae
- The kidneys' ability to excrete urine of variable osmolarity depends on the anatomic arrangement of the loop of Henle, vasa recta, and collecting tubules, which pass through the medulla to empty at the renal papillae
  - These three structures lie adjacent to one another in the medulla
  - They're surrounded by interstitial fluid
- The countercurrent mechanism concentrates urine
  - This mechanism is based on the theory of the countercurrent multiplication system
    · The system assumes the presence of two side-by-side tubes, each with a current flowing in opposite directions
    · It also assumes that the two tubes are joined at one end in a U shape
    · Because tubular material is transported osmotically from one tube to another across the membrane separating them, the concentration of material in the U joint is greater than that entering or leaving the tubes
  - This theory describes what occurs in the nephron
    · When the nephron is functioning normally, sodium is actively transported out of the solution in the proximal convoluted tubule, with water flowing passively
    · The solution that enters the descending limb is *isotonic* (able to bathe cells without extracting water)
    · At this point, however, sodium from extracellular fluid enters passively, so that when the solution in the limb reaches the

loop of Henle, it's highly concentrated and *hypertonic* (able to extract water from cells)

- When the solution enters the ascending limb, it flows along membranes that are impermeable to water but allow active transport of chlorine and passive flow of sodium
- When the solution enters the distal convoluted tubule, it's *hypotonic,* which allows additional sodium and chlorine to be pumped out actively, with water flowing passively
- When the solution enters the collecting tubule, the action of ADH makes the membrane permeable to water and urea; this leaves a hypertonic solution that enters the renal pelvis as urine

● Countercurrent mechanism function

- Glomerular filtrate flows through the proximal tubule, which reabsorbs water and dissolved substances in equal proportions; this reabsorption reduces the filtrate volume by 80% but doesn't change its osmolarity
- The filtrate flows into the descending limb of the loop of Henle, which is freely permeable to water and sodium chloride
- As filtrate passes down the descending limb, it's exposed to the high osmolarity of the interstitial fluid in the medulla
  - Water moves from the descending limb into the interstitial tissue by osmosis
  - Sodium chloride diffuses into the tubular filtrate from the interstitial tissue, where the sodium chloride concentration is much higher
  - As a result, tubular filtrate osmolarity increases as the fluid passes down the descending limb until its osmolarity is as high as that of the interstitial fluid in the medulla
- The filtrate moves into the ascending limb of the loop of Henle
  - This limb is relatively impermeable to water and possesses an aldosterone-regulated transport mechanism that pumps sodium out of the filtrate
  - Chloride moves out passively with sodium; water remains in the filtrate
  - As a result, tubular filtrate osmolarity falls as the filtrate moves through the ascending limb
- When the filtrate reaches the distal tubule, its osmolarity has fallen to 100 mOsm/L; it continues to fall to as low as 70 mOsm/L until it enters the collecting tubule
- ADH regulates the final urine concentration
  - If the body has insufficient water, ADH is secreted and collecting tubule permeability increases

Key facts about countercurrent mechanism function

- Reabsorption in the proximal tubule reduces the filtrate volume but doesn't change osmolarity
- Osmolarity of filtrate falls as it passes through the descending and ascending limbs of the loop of Henle
- Osmolarity continues to fall until it enters the collecting tubule
- ADH regulates final urine concentration

– This allows water to move out of the collecting tubule by osmosis into the hypertonic interstitial fluid, which produces concentrated urine for excretion
– If the body has excess water, ADH isn't excreted; the collecting tubules remain impermeable to water, which produces dilute urine for excretion

RENAL REGULATION OF BLOOD PRESSURE AND VOLUME

● **Key concepts**
  • Juxtaglomerular cells in the kidneys regulate blood pressure and blood volume by secreting renin
  • They secrete renin in response to decreased blood pressure, blood volume, or plasma sodium concentration

● **Regulation process**
  • Renin interacts with a blood protein called renin substrate to yield the polypeptide angiotensin I
  • Angiotensin I is converted to angiotensin II by enzymes in endothelial cells in the lungs and other tissues
  • Angiotensin II raises blood pressure by increasing vasoconstriction and stimulating the adrenal cortex to secrete aldosterone
  • Aldosterone increases sodium and water reabsorption in the renal tubule, which increases blood volume
  • The renin-angiotensin-aldosterone system is self-regulating
    – Blood pressure, blood volume, and sodium concentration rise in response to renin secretion
    – When these levels reach the normal range, the juxtaglomerular cells are no longer stimulated, causing renin secretion to fall
  • When the renin-angiotensin-aldosterone system functions improperly, hypertension can result

URINE ELIMINATION

● **Key concepts**
  • After urine is formed in the nephrons, it passes from the collecting tubules through the calyxes of the kidney to the renal pelvis
  • From the renal pelvis, urine is conveyed by the ureters to the bladder
    – Smooth-muscle contractions move urine down the ureter
    – These peristaltic contractions occur at a rate of about one to five per minute
  • The bladder stores urine until the voiding reflex is triggered; the bladder can hold 500 to 600 ml in an adult

---

Key facts about renal regulation of blood pressure and volume

• Juxtaglomerular cells secrete renin in response to decreased blood pressure, blood volume, or sodium concentration
• Renin stimulates production of angiotensin II
• Angiotensin II increases vasoconstriction and stimulates secretion of aldosterone
• Aldosterone increases sodium and water reabsorption, which increases blood pressure

Key facts about urine elimination

• Urine passes from the collecting tubules, through the calyxes, to the renal pelvis
• Urine then flows through the ureters to the bladder
• Urine passes from the bladder through the urethra and out of the body

- Urine elimination results from involuntary and voluntary processes
- Urine flows from the bladder through the urethra; it's expelled from the body through the external urethral opening

● **Voiding reflex**
- The voiding reflex is typically activated when the bladder contains 300 to 400 ml of urine
- As urine fills the bladder, it stretches the bladder walls, triggering the voiding reflex
- Stretch receptors in the bladder walls transmit sensory impulses to the spinal cord, which stimulates parasympathetic neurons
- The spine relays motor impulses that cause bladder wall contraction and relaxation of the external urethral sphincter; this leads to urination unless voluntary control is exerted
  - In neurogenic bladder, normal impulse transmission from the spinal cord to the bladder is interrupted or delayed
  - This leads to voiding problems, such as incontinence and incomplete bladder emptying
- Besides being transmitted to the spinal cord, sensory impulses from the bladder walls are sent to higher brain centers; they're interpreted as a sense of bladder fullness or the need to urinate
- The brain can inhibit or stimulate the voiding reflex
  - When urination must be delayed, the person inhibits the reflex by contracting the external sphincter, which is composed of striated muscle and is under voluntary control
  - When the opportunity to urinate becomes available, the person voluntarily contracts the abdominal muscles, which raises intra-abdominal pressure and helps expel urine from the bladder

NCLEX CHECKS

It's never too soon to begin your NCLEX preparation. Now that you've reviewed this chapter, carefully read each of the following questions and choose the best answer. Then compare your responses with the correct answers.

1. The nurse is helping a client with bladder retraining and explains that the voiding reflex is triggered when the bladder reaches which volume of urine?
- ☐ **1.** 100 to 200 ml
- ☐ **2.** 200 to 300 ml
- ☐ **3.** 300 to 400 ml
- ☐ **4.** 400 to 500 ml

2. A client has a low cardiac output and low blood pressure. Which change in the GFR should the nurse anticipate?

☐ **1.** The GFR will increase.
☐ **2.** The GFR will decrease.
☐ **3.** The GFR will remain unchanged.
☐ **4.** The GFR will become erratic.

3. The nurse explains to a client with diabetes insipidus that this disorder is characterized by ADH deficiency. Place the steps of ADH regulation, listed below, in chronological order to show how fluid balance is achieved. Use all the options.

1. The hypothalamus signals the pituitary gland.	
2. ADH causes the kidneys to retain water.	
3. The hypothalamus senses low blood volume and increased serum osmolality.	
4. The pituitary gland secretes ADH into the bloodstream.	
5. Water retention boosts blood volume and decreases serum osmolality.	

4. During a physical examination, the nurse palpates a client's kidneys. Which of the following best describes the location of the kidneys?
☐ **1.** Anterior to the stomach and liver
☐ **2.** Retroperitoneally, in the right and left lower abdominal quadrants
☐ **3.** Retroperitoneally, on either side of the thoracic vertebrae
☐ **4.** Posterior to the stomach and liver

5. While teaching a client with acute renal failure about his condition, the nurse realizes that the client understands basic kidney function when he identifies which structure as the functional unit of the kidney?
☐ **1.** Nephron
☐ **2.** Renal cortex
☐ **3.** Hilus
☐ **4.** Renal corpuscle

6. Which fact about aldosterone should the nurse keep in mind when interpreting the laboratory results of a client with impaired aldosterone secretion?

☐ **1.** Decreased potassium concentration in body fluids stimulates aldosterone release.

☐ **2.** Increased potassium concentration in body fluids reduces aldosterone secretion.

☐ **3.** Increased sodium concentration in body fluids stimulates aldosterone secretion.

☐ **4.** Decreased sodium concentration in body fluids stimulates aldosterone secretion.

7. A client with high blood pressure is scheduled to receive a loop diuretic. The nurse understands that the drug was prescribed because it acts on the loop of Henle to control the flow of water and electrolytes. However, what occurs in the nephron's distal tubule?

☐ **1.** Certain solutes are reabsorbed from the glomerular filtrate back into the blood.

☐ **2.** Water is removed from the filtrate and returned to the interstitial fluid.

☐ **3.** Potassium and hydrogen ions are secreted and reabsorbed.

☐ **4.** Sodium and chloride are removed to maintain osmolality.

8. When catheterizing the bladder of a male client, it's important for the nurse to keep in mind that the male urethra is approximately how many inches long?

☐ **1.** 1" to 1½" (2.5 to 4 cm)
☐ **2.** 4" (10 cm)
☐ **3.** 6" (15 cm)
☐ **4.** 8" (20 cm)

9. Which information should the nurse include in the teaching plan for a client with a UTI?

☐ **1.** Take antibiotics as prescribed.
☐ **2.** Limit fluid intake to reduce the need to urinate.
☐ **3.** Take tub baths while symptoms persist.
☐ **4.** Urinate at least every 3 to 4 hours.

10. The nurse would expect a healthy client to have a GFR of what value?

☐ **1.** 25 ml/minute
☐ **2.** 50 ml/minute
☐ **3.** 100 ml/minute
☐ **4.** 125 ml/minute

ANSWERS AND RATIONALES

1. CORRECT ANSWER: 3

The voiding reflex is typically triggered when the bladder contains 300 to 400 ml of urine.

2. CORRECT ANSWER: 2

GFR depends on three factors: permeability of the glomerular capillary walls, blood pressure, and effective filtration rate. A change in any of these factors significantly alters the GFR. For example, decreased cardiac output and blood pressure reduces renal blood flow, resulting in a decreased GFR.

3. CORRECT ANSWER:

> **3.** The hypothalamus senses low blood volume and increased serum osmolality.

> **1.** The hypothalamus signals the pituitary gland.

> **4.** The pituitary gland secretes ADH into the bloodstream.

> **2.** ADH causes the kidneys to retain water.

> **5.** Water retention boosts blood volume and decreases serum osmolality.

ADH normally regulates fluid balance in a set sequence. First, the hypothalamus senses low blood volume and increased serum osmolality. Then specialized cells in the hypothalamus, called *osmoreceptors,* send signals to the pituitary about changes in blood volume and serum osmolality. The pituitary then releases ADH, causing more water to be absorbed from the tubules of the kidney. This dilutes body fluids and lowers the osmotic pressure.

4. CORRECT ANSWER: 4

The kidneys lie retroperitoneally, on either side of the lumbar vertebrae, posterior to the stomach and liver, and in front of the muscles attached to the vertebral column.

5. CORRECT ANSWER: 1
The nephron is the basic structural and functional unit of the kidney. The renal cortex contains the blood-filtering mechanisms. The ureters, renal blood vessels, lymphatic vessels, and nerves enter or exit the kidney through the hilus, a notch on the inner, concave side of each kidney. The glomerular capsule and glomerulus make up the renal corpuscle.

6. CORRECT ANSWER: 4
A decreased sodium concentration in body fluids stimulates aldosterone secretion; this increases sodium reabsorption, raising the sodium concentration in body fluids. An increased sodium concentration in body fluids reduces aldosterone secretion; this reduces sodium reabsorption, decreasing the sodium concentration in body fluids. An increased potassium concentration in body fluids stimulates aldosterone secretion; this increases sodium reabsorption and potassium secretion by the tubules, raising the sodium concentration and lowering the potassium concentration in body fluids. A decreased potassium concentration in body fluids inhibits aldosterone release; this reduces potassium secretion, raising the potassium concentration in body fluids.

7. CORRECT ANSWER: 3
In the distal tubule, potassium and hydrogen ions are secreted and reabsorbed. In the proximal tubule, certain solutes are reabsorbed from the glomerular filtrate back into the blood. In the descending tubule of the loop of Henle, water is removed from the filtrate (by osmosis) and returned to the interstitial fluid. In the ascending loop of Henle, sodium and chloride are removed to maintain osmolality.

8. CORRECT ANSWER: 4
The male urethra is approximately 8" (20 cm) long. The female urethra is approximately 1" to 1½" (2.5 to 4 cm) long.

9. CORRECT ANSWER: 1
Antibiotics are usually ordered to eliminate the causative bacteria and should be taken for the full course of therapy, as prescribed. Fluids should be encouraged to flush the infection from the urinary tract. Tub baths should be avoided because they can irritate the urethral opening and may allow bacteria to enter the urinary tract. The client should be encouraged to void every 2 hours to empty the bladder.

10. CORRECT ANSWER: 4
The glomeruli filter about 125 ml of water and dissolved materials every minute from the blood as it flows through their capillary network.

17

Fluid, electrolyte, and acid-base balance

LEARNING OBJECTIVES

After studying this chapter, you should be able to:

- Identify the major fluid compartments and their contents.
- Describe fluid movement and balance in the body.
- Identify the major electrolytes and their mechanisms of balance.
- Differentiate between an acid and a base.
- Explain how the buffer systems, lungs, and kidneys maintain acid-base balance.

CHAPTER OVERVIEW

Fluid, electrolyte, and acid-base balance is essential to homeostasis, health, and well-being. However, numerous factors (such as illness, injury, surgery, and treatments) can disrupt this balance—in some cases, leading to potentially fatal changes in metabolic activity. Because most patients are at risk for a fluid, electrolyte, or acid-base imbalance, the nurse must have current, comprehensive knowledge of the substances and their regulatory mechanisms. This chapter reviews body fluids, fluid balance, electrolyte balance, acid-base balance, and mechanisms of acid-base balance.

Key facts about
body fluids

- More than 50% of an adult's body weight is water
- Proportion of body water varies inversely with body fat
- Women have lower percentage of water than men do

Key facts about body
fluid compartments

- Intracellular fluid compartment comprises 70% of body fluids
- Extracellular compartment includes intravascular and interstitial compartments
- ICF and ECF have different compositions

BODY FLUIDS

● Key concepts

- Homeostasis depends on a complex interrelationship among fluid, electrolyte, and acid-base metabolism
- More than 50% of the average adult's body weight consists of water
- The proportion of body water varies inversely with the body's fat content because fat contains no water
    - An obese individual has a lower percentage of water than a lean person
    - Most women have a lower percentage of water than men because their bodies normally have a higher percentage of body fat
- Body water contains dissolved substances (solutes) that are necessary for physiologic functioning
- Solutes include electrolytes, glucose, amino acids, and other nutrients
- Body fluid composition differs by compartment

● Body fluid compartments

- The intracellular fluid compartment consists of the fluid in the body's cells and comprises 70% of body fluids
- The extracellular fluid compartment is found in spaces between the cells and comprises 30% of body fluids
    - This includes the *intravascular compartment* and the *interstitial compartment*
    - The intravascular fluid consists of the fluid in blood plasma and the lymphatic system
    - The interstitial fluid consists of fluid distributed diffusely through the loose tissue surrounding the cells
    - Intravascular and interstitial fluids are separated by a capillary endothelium that's freely permeable to water, electrolytes, and other solutes; consequently, the composition of both types of extracellular fluids is similar
- The composition of intracellular fluid (ICF) differs from that of extracellular fluid (ECF)
    - ICF has higher concentrations of protein, potassium, magnesium, phosphate, and sulfate
    - ICF has lower concentrations of sodium, calcium, chloride, and bicarbonate
- Active transport helps maintain different concentrations of sodium and potassium in the ICF and ECF

Body fluid osmolarity
- When a semipermeable membrane separates two solutions of unequal solute concentration, water shifts by *osmosis* from the less concentrated solution to the more concentrated solution
- The ability of the more concentrated solution to attract water is called its *osmotic activity*
- The solution's osmotic activity depends on the number of particles dissolved in the solution
  - Osmotic activity is unrelated to the particles' molecular weight or valence
  - The same osmotic activity results from a solution that contains equal numbers of sodium ions, calcium ions, or glucose molecules
    - Sodium ions are monovalent (able to form only one ionic bond)
    - Calcium ions are divalent (able to form two ionic bonds)
    - Glucose molecules don't dissociate into ions
  - The osmotic pressure of a solution (pressure exerted by a solution on a semipermeable membrane) is usually measured in terms of *osmolarity*
    - A solution of 1 L of water that contains 1 gram molecular weight of a substance that doesn't dissociate in solution (such as glucose) has an osmolarity of 1 Osm/L
    - A solution of 1 L of water that contains 1 gram molecular weight of an electrolyte that dissociates into two ions (such as sodium chloride) has an osmolarity of 2 Osm/L
    - A solution of 1 L of water that contains 1 gram molecular weight of an electrolyte that dissociates into three ions (such as calcium chloride) has an osmolarity of 3 Osm/L
    - Because body fluids have low concentrations of dissolved particles, their osmolarity usually is expressed in milliosmols per liter (mOsm/L)

FLUID BALANCE

Key concepts
- Water is essential to normal physiologic functioning
- The body gains and loses water daily through fluid intake and output
- Water enters the body via the GI tract and leaves via the skin, lungs, GI tract, and urinary tract (see *How the body gains and loses fluids,* page 330)
- These gains and losses must be balanced to stabilize the body's water content and to permit proper physiologic functioning

How the body gains and loses fluids

Each day, the body takes in fluid from the GI tract (in foods, liquids, and water of oxidation) and loses fluids through the skin, lungs, intestines (stool), and urinary tract (urine). This illustration shows the primary sites involved in fluid gains and losses as well as the amount of normal daily fluid intake and output.

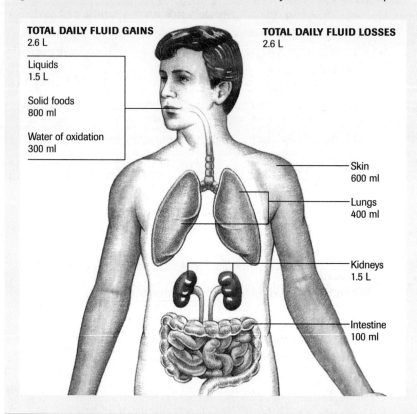

TOTAL DAILY FLUID GAINS
2.6 L

Liquids
1.5 L

Solid foods
800 ml

Water of oxidation
300 ml

TOTAL DAILY FLUID LOSSES
2.6 L

Skin
600 ml

Lungs
400 ml

Kidneys
1.5 L

Intestine
100 ml

- Two mechanisms help maintain fluid balance: thirst, which regulates water intake, and the *countercurrent mechanism*, which regulates urine concentration

● **Fluid intake**
- Water normally enters the body from the GI tract
- Each day, the body derives about 1,500 ml of water from consumed liquids
- The body also receives 700 ml from consumption of solid foods, which may contain up to 97% water
- Food oxidation in the body generates carbon dioxide and 250 ml of water (water of oxidation)

Fluid output

- Water leaves the body through the skin (in perspiration), lungs (in exhaled air), GI tract (in feces), and urinary tract (in urine)
- Each day, the body loses 800 ml of water through the skin and lungs
  - This amount of water loss may increase dramatically with strenuous exertion, predisposing the individual to dehydration
- Although the GI tract contents include large amounts of fluid, the colon normally absorbs almost all the water (the body loses only about 200 ml of water in feces)
- Urine excretion is the main route of water loss; output typically varies from 1,000 to 1,500 ml daily

Mechanisms of fluid balance

- Two mechanisms help maintain fluid balance: thirst and the countercurrent mechanism
- Thirst (conscious desire for water) primarily regulates fluid intake
  - Dehydration decreases the ECF volume, which increases its sodium concentration and osmolarity
  - When the sodium concentration reaches about 2 mEq/L above normal, it stimulates the neurons of the thirst center in the hypothalamus
  - When the brain directs motor neurons to satisfy thirst, a person usually drinks the proper amount of fluid to restore the ECF to normal
- Through the countercurrent mechanism, the kidneys can regulate fluid output by excreting urine of greater or lesser concentration
- Interruption or dysfunction of either the thirst or countercurrent mechanism can lead to a fluid imbalance

ELECTROLYTE BALANCE

Key concepts

- *Electrolytes* are substances that dissociate into *ions* (electrically charged particles) when dissolved in water
- Normal metabolism and function require sufficient quantities of each major electrolyte and proper balance among electrolytes
- Ions may be positively charged *cations* or negatively charged *anions*
- The ICF and ECF normally contain different concentrations of electrolytes
- Electrolyte balance is maintained by various mechanisms

Electrolytes

- Major cations include sodium, potassium, calcium, and magnesium
- Major anions include chloride, bicarbonate, and phosphate

Key facts about fluid output

- The body loses a large amount of water through the skin and lungs
- Amount of water lost increases dramatically with physical exertion
- Urine excretion is the main route of water loss

Key facts about fluid balance mechanisms

- Thirst helps regulate fluid balance by regulating input
- Countercurrent mechanism helps maintain fluid balance by regulating output

Key facts about electrolyte balance

- Electrolytes dissociate into ions when dissolved in water
- Positively charged ions are called *cations*
- Negatively charged ions are called *anions*

Key facts about electrolytes

- Cations and anions are normally balanced so body fluids are electrically neutral
- Ion concentration is referred to as the ion's equivalent weight
- ICF and ECF have different electrolyte compositions

Key facts about equivalent weight

- Equivalent weight refers to an ion's ability to combine with other ions
- It equals the ion's gram molecular weight divided by its chemical valence
- Ions with the same number of equivalents have equal combining powers

Key facts about electrolyte balance mechanisms

- Homeostasis depends on the interrelationship among water, electrolyte, and acid-base metabolism
- The kidneys regulate sodium, potassium, chloride, and phosphate
- Magnesium is regulated by aldosterone
- Calcium is regulated by parathyroid hormone

- Normally, the electrical charges of the cations and anions are balanced so that body fluids are electrically neutral
- Ion concentration is expressed in terms of the ion's *equivalent weight*
  - Equivalent weight refers to the ion's ability to combine with other ions
  - Equivalent weight equals the ion's gram molecular weight divided by its chemical valence
    - *Gram molecular weight* refers to the amount of a substance that has a weight in grams equal to its molecular weight
    - *Chemical valence* is the numerical expression of chemical-combining capacity
  - Ions with the same number of equivalents in a solution have equal combining powers; their concentrations are considered equal even though their gram molecular weights are different
  - In body fluids, ions exist in such low concentrations that they're usually expressed in milliequivalents per liter (mEq/L)
- The ICF and ECF normally have different electrolyte compositions because their cells are permeable to different substances
  - Sodium concentration in ICF is 10 mEq/L; in ECF, 136 to 146 mEq/L
  - Potassium concentration in ICF is 140 mEq/L; in ECF, 3.6 to 5 mEq/L
  - Calcium concentration in ICF is 10 mEq/L; in ECF, 4.5 to 5.8 mEq/L
  - Magnesium concentration in ICF is 40 mEq/L; in ECF, 1.6 to 2.2 mEq/L
  - Chloride concentration in ICF is 4 mEq/L; in ECF, 96 to 106 mEq/L
  - Bicarbonate concentration in ICF is 10 mEq/L; in ECF, 24 to 28 mEq/L
  - Phosphate concentration in ICF is 100 mEq/L; in ECF, 1 to 1.5 mEq/L

Mechanisms of electrolyte balance
- Homeostasis depends on a complex interrelationship among water, electrolyte, and acid-base metabolism
- Electrolytes profoundly affect water distribution, osmolarity, and acid-base balance
- The body uses various mechanisms to maintain electrolyte balance
  - Sodium is regulated chiefly by the kidneys through the action of aldosterone
    - Sodium is absorbed readily from food by the small intestine
    - It's excreted through the skin and kidneys

GO WITH THE FLOW

Osmotic regulation of sodium and water

This flowchart shows two compensatory mechanisms used to restore sodium and water balance.

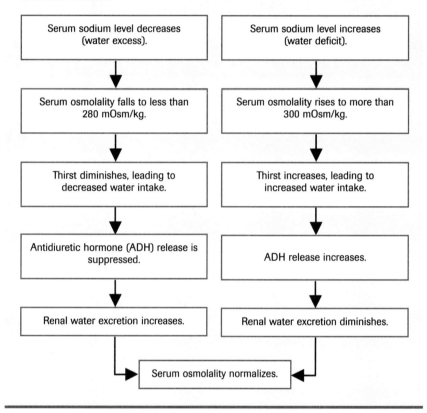

Serum sodium level decreases (water excess).	Serum sodium level increases (water deficit).
Serum osmolality falls to less than 280 mOsm/kg.	Serum osmolality rises to more than 300 mOsm/kg.
Thirst diminishes, leading to decreased water intake.	Thirst increases, leading to increased water intake.
Antidiuretic hormone (ADH) release is suppressed.	ADH release increases.
Renal water excretion increases.	Renal water excretion diminishes.

Serum osmolality normalizes.

- Sodium and water balances are closely interrelated (see *Osmotic regulation of sodium and water*)
- Potassium is also regulated by the kidneys through the action of aldosterone
  - Most of the body's potassium is absorbed from food in the GI tract
  - The amount of potassium excreted in urine normally equals dietary potassium intake
- Calcium in blood is in equilibrium with calcium salts in bone
  - Calcium is regulated primarily by parathyroid hormone
  - Parathyroid hormone controls both calcium uptake from the intestinal tract and calcium excretion by the kidneys
- Magnesium is regulated by aldosterone
  - Aldosterone controls renal reabsorption of magnesium

Key teaching topics for a patient with an electrolyte imbalance

- Describe possible causes and signs and symptoms
- Explain diagnostic tests and treatments
- Stress the need for avoiding foods and substances that contain the electrolyte
- Discuss the need for follow-up testing

TIME-OUT FOR TEACHING

Teaching a patient with an electrolyte imbalance

Make sure you teach a patient with an electrolyte imbalance:
- the type and possible causes of his specific imbalance
- signs and symptoms of the imbalance
- which diagnostic tests (such as serum electrolyte levels and electrocardiography) to anticipate
- which treatments (such as drugs, electrolyte replacement, and dietary supplementation) may be ordered
- the importance of avoiding or limiting foods and over-the-counter drugs that contain the electrolyte
- the need for medical follow-up, including diagnostic testing.

- Magnesium is absorbed from the GI tract and excreted in urine, breast milk, and saliva
 - Chloride is regulated by the kidneys; chloride ions move with sodium ions
 - Bicarbonate is regulated by the kidneys
   - The kidneys may excrete, absorb, or form bicarbonate
   - Bicarbonate plays an important role in regulating *acid-base balance*
 - Phosphate is regulated by the kidneys
   - It's absorbed well from food
   - It's incorporated with calcium in bone
   - It's regulated by parathyroid hormone along with calcium
- Interruption or dysfunction of any regulatory mechanism can lead to an electrolyte imbalance (see *Teaching a patient with an electrolyte imbalance*)

ACID-BASE BALANCE

● Key concepts
- Acid-base balance results in a stable hydrogen ion concentration in body fluids
- An *acid* is a substance that dissociates in water and releases hydrogen ions
  - A strong acid dissociates virtually completely, releasing a large number of hydrogen ions
  - A weak acid doesn't dissociate readily and releases fewer hydrogen ions
- A *base* is a substance that dissociates in water and releases ions that can combine with hydrogen ions such as hydroxyl ions
  - A strong base dissociates virtually completely, releasing a large number of ions

Key facts about acid-base balance

- An acid dissociates in water and releases hydrogen ions
- A base dissociates in water and releases ions that can combine with hydrogen ions
- The concentration of hydrogen ions determines whether it's acidic or basic

– A weak base doesn't dissociate readily and releases fewer ions
- The hydrogen ion concentration of a fluid determines whether it's acidic or basic (alkaline)
    – A neutral solution, such as pure water, dissociates only slightly
        · It contains 0.0000001 (one ten-millionth) gram molecular weight (mol) of hydrogen ions per liter
        · It contains the same amount of hydroxyl ions
    – This minute quantity may be expressed in exponential form as 10^{-7} g/L
    – More commonly, hydrogen ion concentration is expressed as pH
        · pH is the value of the exponent without the minus sign; for example, a neutral solution that contains 10^{-7} mols of hydrogen ions per liter has a pH of 7.0
        · An acidic solution contains more hydrogen ions; its pH is less than 7.0
        · An alkaline solution contains fewer hydrogen ions; its pH is greater than 7.0
    – Because pH is an exponential expression, a change of 1 pH unit represents a tenfold change in hydrogen ion concentration (for example, a solution with a pH of 6.0 has 10 times more hydrogen ions than one with a pH of 7.0)

Sources of hydrogen ions
- The human body is an acid-producing organism
- Protein catabolism produces several nonvolatile acids, such as sulfuric, phosphoric, and uric acid
- Fat oxidation produces acid ketone bodies (acetoacetic acid and beta-hydroxybutyric acid)
- Anaerobic glucose catabolism produces lactic acid
- Intracellular metabolism creates a large quantity of carbon dioxide as a by-product
    – Some of the carbon dioxide dissolves in body fluids to form carbonic acid
    – This makes intracellular fluids slightly more acidic than extracellular fluids

MECHANISMS OF ACID-BASE BALANCE

Key concepts
- Buffer systems and the lungs and kidneys maintain the blood pH within the narrow range of 7.38 to 7.42
    – These systems neutralize and eliminate acids as rapidly as they're formed
    – These actions help maintain acid-base balance

- The sodium bicarbonate–carbonic acid buffer system is the principal buffer in the ECF
- The lungs affect acid-base balance by excreting carbon dioxide and regulating the carbonic acid content of the blood
- The kidneys regulate acid-base balance by allowing tubular filtrate reabsorption of bicarbonate and by forming bicarbonate
- Interruption or dysfunction of a buffer system or other regulatory mechanism can lead to an acid-base imbalance

● **Buffer systems**
- Buffer systems minimize pH changes caused by excess acids or bases
- A buffer system consists of a weak acid and a salt of that acid, or a weak base and its salt
- The buffer system reduces the effect of a sudden change in hydrogen ion concentration by converting a strong acid or base (which normally would dissociate completely) into a weak acid or base (which releases a smaller number of free hydrogen or hydroxyl ions)
- The pH of any buffer system depends on the ratio of the two components in the buffer and not on their absolute amounts
- The *sodium bicarbonate–carbonic acid buffer system* is the principal buffer in ECF
  – This system works better in vivo than in vitro
    · If acid were added continuously to a fixed amount of bicarbonate–carbonic acid buffer in a beaker, eventually all of the sodium bicarbonate would be consumed by neutralizing the acid
    · The buffer would lose its effectiveness because it would no longer contain bicarbonate
  – In the body, this buffer system maintains its efficiency for two reasons
    · Both components of the buffer are replenished continually
    · The concentration of both components is regulated physiologically—sodium bicarbonate by the kidneys and carbonic acid by the lungs
  – In the sodium bicarbonate–carbonic acid buffer system, the normal ratio of the components (20 parts sodium bicarbonate to 1 part carbonic acid) maintains a pH of 7.4
    · A change in the 20:1 ratio causes a corresponding change in the pH of the buffer and the body fluids it regulates
    · This relationship can be visualized in terms of a board on a fulcrum

- Normally, one end of the board is weighted by 20 parts sodium bicarbonate and the other end is weighted by 1 part carbonic acid
- The fulcrum is positioned so the board balances at a pH of 7.4
- Changes in the ratio of sodium bicarbonate to carbonic acid will unbalance the board and shift the system to a higher or lower pH
- The *phosphate buffer system* also helps maintain normal pH, especially in ECF
    - The phosphate buffer uses sodium dihydrogen phosphate as the acidic component and sodium monohydrogen phosphate as the alkaline component
    - This buffer system is especially important in neutralizing hydrogen ions secreted by the renal tubules
- The *protein buffer system* helps maintain normal pH; in this system, intracellular proteins function as buffers by absorbing hydrogen ions generated by the body's metabolic processes

● **Lungs**
- The lungs excrete carbon dioxide (CO_2) and regulate the carbonic acid (H_2CO_3) content of the blood
    - Carbonic acid is derived from the carbon dioxide and water (H_2O) released as a by-product of cellular metabolic activity
    - Carbon dioxide is soluble in blood plasma
        · Some of the dissolved gas reacts with water to form carbonic acid, a weak acid that partially dissociates to form hydrogen (H^+) and bicarbonate (HCO_3^-) ions
        · All three substances are in equilibrium: $CO_2 + H_2O \leftrightarrow H_2CO_3 \leftrightarrow H^+ + HCO_3^-$
    - Carbon dioxide dissolved in plasma is in equilibrium with the carbon dioxide in the pulmonary alveoli
        · The alveolar carbon dioxide concentration is expressed as a partial pressure (PCO_2)
        · Consequently, an equilibrium exists between alveolar PCO_2 and the various forms of carbon dioxide in the plasma: $PCO_2 \leftrightarrow CO_2 + H_2O \leftrightarrow H_2CO_3 \leftrightarrow H^+ + HCO_3^-$
- The carbon dioxide content of alveolar air and the alveolar PCO_2 vary with the rate and depth of respirations
- A change in alveolar PCO_2 causes a corresponding change in the amount of carbonic acid formed by dissolved carbon dioxide
- These changes stimulate the respiratory center to alter the respiratory rate and depth (see *Respiratory regulation of blood pH*, page 338)

Key facts about the lungs and acid–base balance

- The lungs excrete carbon dioxide and regulate carbonic acid content of blood
- Carbon dioxide, carbonic acid, and water are in equilibrium
- The carbon dioxide content of alveolar air and the alveolar PCO_2 vary with the rate and depth of respirations

Respiratory regulation of blood pH

A rise in the carbon dioxide (CO_2) content of arterial blood or a decrease in blood pH stimulates the respiratory center, causing hyperventilation. As a result, less CO_2 and, therefore, less carbonic acid and fewer hydrogen ions remain in the blood. Consequently, blood pH increases, possibly reaching a normal level.

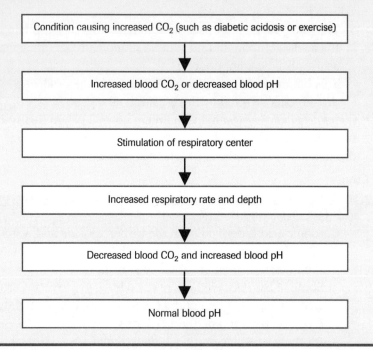

Key facts about respiratory regulation of blood pH

- A rise in alveolar PCO_2 increases the blood concentration of carbon dioxide and carbonic acid
- This stimulates the respiratory center to increase the rate and depth of respirations
- In turn, alveolar PCO_2 declines, which leads to a decline in the carbonic acid and carbon dioxide concentrations in blood

Key facts about the kidneys and acid-base balance

- The kidneys excrete waste products
- The kidneys regulate bicarbonate concentration by reabsorption of bicarbonate as well as by forming additional bicarbonate

– A rise in alveolar PCO_2 increases the blood concentration of carbon dioxide and carbonic acid
  · This stimulates the respiratory center to increase the rate and depth of respirations
  · In turn, alveolar PCO_2 declines
  · This leads to a corresponding decrease in the carbonic acid and carbon dioxide concentrations in blood
– A decrease in the rate and depth of respirations has an opposite effect
  · Alveolar PCO_2 becomes elevated
  · This leads to a corresponding increase in the carbon dioxide and carbonic acid concentrations in blood

● **Kidneys**
- The kidneys excrete various acid waste products
- They regulate the bicarbonate concentration in the blood in two ways

– They allow bicarbonate reabsorption from tubular filtrate
– They can form additional bicarbonate to replace that used in buffering acids

• Bicarbonate recovery and formation in the kidneys depend on hydrogen ion secretion by the renal tubules in exchange for sodium ions, which simultaneously are reabsorbed from the tubular filtrate into the circulation

• The renal tubules secrete hydrogen ions
– Under the influence of the enzyme carbonic anhydrase, tubular epithelial cells form carbonic acid from carbon dioxide and water
– This carbonic acid rapidly dissociates into hydrogen and bicarbonate ions
– The hydrogen ions enter the tubular filtrate in exchange for sodium ions
– The bicarbonate ions enter the bloodstream along with sodium ions that have been absorbed from the filtrate

• Bicarbonate is reabsorbed from tubular filtrate
– Each hydrogen ion secreted into tubular filtrate (in exchange for a sodium ion) combines with a bicarbonate ion
  · This forms carbonic acid
  · Carbonic acid rapidly dissociates into carbon dioxide and water
– The carbon dioxide diffuses into the tubular epithelial cell, where it can combine with more water to form more carbonic acid
– The leftover water molecule in the tubular filtrate is excreted in urine
– As each hydrogen ion moves into tubular filtrate to combine with a bicarbonate ion there, a bicarbonate ion in the tubular epithelial cell diffuses into the circulation
– This process is called *bicarbonate reabsorption,* even though the bicarbonate ion that enters the circulation isn't the same one as in the tubular filtrate

• To form more bicarbonate, the kidneys must secrete additional hydrogen ions in exchange for sodium ions
– The renal tubules can't continue to secrete hydrogen ions unless the excess ions can be combined with other substances in the filtrate and excreted
– Excess hydrogen ions in the filtrate may combine with ammonia (produced by the renal tubules) or with phosphate salts (present in tubular filtrate)
  · Ammonia is formed in the tubular epithelial cells by removal of the amino groups from glutamine (an amino acid deriva-

Key factors affecting bicarbonate recovery and formation in the kidneys

• Renal tubules secrete hydrogen ions
• The hydrogen ions enter filtrate in exchange for sodium ions
• Bicarbonate is reabsorbed from tubular filtrate
• The kidneys must secrete additional hydrogen ions in exchange for sodium ions to form more bicarbonate

tive) and from amino acids that are delivered from the circulation to the tubular epithelial cells

- Ammonia diffuses into the filtrate and combines with the secreted hydrogen ions to form ammonium ions (NH_4^+), which are excreted in urine with chloride and other anions
- Each ammonia molecule secreted eliminates one hydrogen ion in the filtrate
- Simultaneously, sodium ions that have been absorbed from the filtrate and exchanged for hydrogen ions enter the circulation
- The bicarbonate formed in tubular epithelial cells also enters the circulation

• Some secreted hydrogen ions combine with sodium dihydrogen phosphate, a disodium phosphate salt in the tubular filtrate

- Each secreted hydrogen ion that combines with the disodium salt converts it to the monosodium salt sodium monohydrogen phosphate
- This reaction releases a sodium ion, which is absorbed into the circulation along with a newly formed bicarbonate ion

• Two factors affect the rate of bicarbonate formation by the renal tubular epithelial cells: the amount of dissolved carbon dioxide in the plasma and the potassium content of the tubular cells

– If the amount of carbon dioxide in the plasma increases, the renal tubular cells form more bicarbonate

• Increased plasma carbon dioxide promotes increased carbonic acid formation by the renal tubular cells
• Carbonic acid partially dissociates, yielding more hydrogen ions for excretion into the tubular filtrate and additional bicarbonate ions for entry into the circulation
• This raises the plasma bicarbonate level and decreases the plasma level of dissolved carbon dioxide toward normal

– If the amount of carbon dioxide in the plasma decreases, the renal tubular cells form less carbonic acid

• Fewer hydrogen ions are formed and excreted
• This causes fewer bicarbonate ions to enter the circulation
• The plasma bicarbonate level falls correspondingly

– The potassium content of the renal tubular cells also regulates plasma bicarbonate concentration by influencing the rate at which the renal tubules secrete hydrogen ions

• Tubular cell potassium content and hydrogen ion secretion are interrelated
• The rates at which potassium and hydrogen ions are secreted vary inversely

Key factors affecting bicarbonate formation

- If plasma carbon dioxide levels increase, renal tubular cells form more bicarbonate and bicarbonate levels rise
- If plasma carbon dioxide levels decrease, renal tubular cells form less carbonic acid and bicarbonate levels fall
- If serum potassium levels fall, tubular epithelial cells secrete less potassium and more hydrogen, causing bicarbonate levels to rise
- When serum potassium levels rise, the tubules excrete more potassium and less hydrogen, causing bicarbonate levels to decline

- If tubular secretion of potassium ions falls, hydrogen ion secretion rises
- If tubular secretion of potassium ions increases, hydrogen ion secretion declines
- Each hydrogen ion secreted into the tubular filtrate is accompanied by the addition of a bicarbonate ion to the blood plasma
  - Therefore, the plasma bicarbonate content rises when tubular secretion of hydrogen ions increases
  - For example, if vomiting or diarrhea causes potassium depletion, then potassium secretion by the tubular epithelial cells falls and hydrogen ion secretion rises
  - When body potassium is depleted, more bicarbonate enters the circulation and the plasma bicarbonate level increases above normal
- The tubules excrete more potassium when the body contains excess potassium
  - When this occurs, fewer hydrogen ions are secreted and less bicarbonate is formed
  - As a result, the plasma bicarbonate concentration decreases

NCLEX CHECKS

It's never too soon to begin your NCLEX preparation. Now that you've reviewed this chapter, carefully read each of the following questions and choose the best answer. Then compare your responses with the correct answers.

1. The nurse is checking the pH of a client's gastric contents and obtains a pH of 4.0. Based on the pH, how would the nurse classify the client's gastric contents?
- ☐ **1.** Acidic
- ☐ **2.** Alkaline
- ☐ **3.** Neutral
- ☐ **4.** Basic

2. The nurse is counseling an obese female client about weight reduction. Which statement by the nurse is most appropriate?
- ☐ **1.** "Obese people have a higher percentage of water than lean people."
- ☐ **2.** "Obese people have a lower percentage of water than lean people."
- ☐ **3.** "Women tend to have a higher percentage of water than men."
- ☐ **4.** "Women have the same percentage of water as men."

TOP 8

Items to study for your next test on fluid, electrolyte, and acid-base balance

1. Characteristics of the ICF and ECF compartments and their contents
2. Major cations and anions
3. Mechanisms of electrolyte balance
4. Differences between acids and bases
5. How buffer systems maintain acid-base balance
6. Process of pulmonary and renal regulation of acid-base balance
7. Methods for maintaining fluid balance
8. Teaching tips for patients with an electrolyte balance

3. The nurse caring for a client with renal disease should keep in mind that ICF, when compared to ECF, has higher concentrations of which electrolytes?

- ☐ **1.** Potassium and sodium
- ☐ **2.** Calcium and sodium
- ☐ **3.** Calcium and phosphate
- ☐ **4.** Magnesium and potassium

4. To calculate a healthy client's fluid output, the nurse should know that fluid lost through the intestine normally totals what amount?

- ☐ **1.** 100 ml
- ☐ **2.** 400 ml
- ☐ **3.** 600 ml
- ☐ **4.** 1,500 ml

5. The nurse is completing an intake and output record for a client who has had 6 oz of apple juice, 10 oz of water, ½ cup of gelatin, and ½ cup of tea. His indwelling urinary catheter has drained 700 ml of urine. How many milliliters should the nurse document as intake?

_____

6. The nurse is caring for a client with an acid-base imbalance following a drug overdose. Nursing interventions focus on maintaining the blood pH within what range?

- ☐ **1.** 5.38 to 5.42
- ☐ **2.** 6.38 to 6.42
- ☐ **3.** 7.38 to 7.42
- ☐ **4.** 8.38 to 8.42

7. Which regulatory mechanism should the nurse keep in mind when developing a care plan for a client with an acid-base imbalance?

- ☐ **1.** The kidneys promote excretion of bicarbonate.
- ☐ **2.** The kidneys form carbonic acid.
- ☐ **3.** The lungs regulate the bicarbonate content of the blood.
- ☐ **4.** The lungs excrete carbon dioxide.

8. The nurse is assessing a client's serum electrolyte report. Which electrolyte is considered a major cation?

- ☐ **1.** Chloride
- ☐ **2.** Sodium
- ☐ **3.** Bicarbonate
- ☐ **4.** Phosphate

9. Which electrolytes would the nurse expect to be affected if a client has an aldosterone imbalance?

- ☐ **1.** Sodium, calcium, chloride
- ☐ **2.** Sodium, potassium, magnesium
- ☐ **3.** Magnesium, phosphate, bicarbonate
- ☐ **4.** Chloride, bicarbonate, potassium

10. Which instruction would the nurse give to a client with a high potassium level?

- ☐ **1.** "Eat foods high in potassium."
- ☐ **2.** "Use salt substitutes that contain potassium."
- ☐ **3.** "Anticipate the need for an electrocardiogram."
- ☐ **4.** "Continue with your current regimen; no medical follow-up is necessary."

ANSWERS AND RATIONALES

1. CORRECT ANSWER: 1

A solution with a pH of less than 7.0 contains more hydrogen ions and is considered acidic. A solution with a pH greater than 7.0 contains fewer hydrogen ions and is considered alkaline or basic. A neutral solution has a pH of 7.0.

2. CORRECT ANSWER: 2

The proportion of body water varies inversely with the body's fat content because fat contains no water. Therefore, an obese person has a lower percentage of water than a lean person. Most women have a lower percentage of water than men because their bodies normally have a higher percentage of body fat.

3. CORRECT ANSWER: 4

ICF has higher concentrations of magnesium, potassium, protein, phosphate, and sulfate, and lower concentrations of sodium, calcium, chloride, and bicarbonate.

4. CORRECT ANSWER: 1

Each day the body loses about 100 ml of fluid from the intestines through stool, 400 ml from the lungs, 600 ml through the skin, and 1,500 ml through the kidneys.

5. CORRECT ANSWER: 720

There are 30 ml in each ounce and 240 ml in each cup. The fluid intake for this client includes 6 oz (180 ml) of apple juice, 10 oz (300 ml) of water, ½ cup (120 ml) of gelatin, and ½ cup (120 ml) of tea for a total of 720 ml.

6. CORRECT ANSWER: 3

Buffer systems, lungs, and kidneys maintain the blood pH within the narrow range of 7.38 to 7.42.

7. CORRECT ANSWER: 4

The lungs affect acid-base balance by excreting carbon dioxide and regulating the carbonic acid content of the blood. The kidneys regulate acid-base balance by allowing tubular filtrate reabsorption of bicarbonate and by forming bicarbonate.

8. CORRECT ANSWER: 2

Major cations (positively charged) include sodium, potassium, calcium, and magnesium. Major anions (negatively charged) include chloride, bicarbonate, and phosphate.

9. CORRECT ANSWER: 2

Sodium, potassium, and magnesium are regulated by the kidneys through the action of aldosterone. Calcium is regulated primarily by parathyroid hormone, which controls calcium uptake from the intestinal tract and calcium excretion by the kidneys. Chloride is regulated by the kidneys; chloride ions move with sodium ions. Bicarbonate is regulated by the kidneys, which may excrete, absorb, or form bicarbonate. Phosphate is regulated by the kidneys and by the parathyroid along with calcium.

10. CORRECT ANSWER: 3

The client with a high serum potassium level should be prepared for diagnostic testing, such as electrocardiography and the monitoring of serum electrolytes. The client should also be instructed to avoid foods high in potassium as well as salt substitutes that contain potassium; both will further raise the serum potassium level. Medical follow-up is necessary, including diagnostic testing. The client should also be taught the causes of a high potassium level as well as which signs and symptoms to report.

18

Endocrine system

LEARNING OBJECTIVES

After studying this chapter, you should be able to:

- Describe the functions of hormones and their feedback mechanisms.
- Explain the structure, function, and hypothalamic control of the pituitary gland.
- Discuss the synthesis, secretion, and effects of thyroid hormones.
- Explain the relationship between parathyroid hormones and calcium metabolism.
- Compare the effects of the major hormones of the adrenal glands.
- Describe the endocrine and exocrine functions of the pancreas.

CHAPTER OVERVIEW

Endocrine glands are largely responsible for maintaining the homeostasis of about 50 billion cells. These glands secrete many hormones into the bloodstream, regulating the hundreds of chemical reactions involved in growth, maturation, reproduction, metabolism, and behavior. The complexity of endocrine function contributes to the number and diversity of endocrine disorders, which can challenge your health care skills. To meet these challenges, the nurse must be familiar with endocrine anatomy and physiology, including the functions of hormones and their effects on target cells. This chapter reviews the endocrine glands and hormones, with special focus on the pituitary gland, thyroid gland, parathyroid glands, adrenal glands, and pancreas.

GLANDS AND HORMONES

● **Key concepts**
- The endocrine system is composed of endocrine glands (which are located throughout the body) and other structures (see *Components of the endocrine system*)
  - The major endocrine glands include the *pituitary, thyroid, parathyroid,* and *adrenal glands; islets of Langerhans;* and the *ovaries* and *testes*
  - Other structures, such as the pineal and thymus glands, are considered minor endocrine glands
- *Endocrine glands* are ductless glands that release hormones directly into the blood or lymph
  - In contrast, *exocrine glands*—sweat glands, sebaceous glands, mucous glands, and digestive glands—secrete their products through one or more ducts into the body's cavities or onto its surface
  - Other tissues besides endocrine glands also produce hormones; these include the placenta and cell clusters in the walls of the GI tract and kidneys

● **Endocrine system function**
- The endocrine system and nervous system (sometimes collectively termed the *neuroendocrine system*) control all body functions
- The endocrine system exerts its control through hormones (chemical substances that regulate the activities of specific organs)
  - Hormones have several functions
    - They control reproduction and growth
    - They mobilize the body against stress
    - They maintain electrolyte, water, and nutrient balance
    - They regulate metabolism and energy balance
  - Once secreted by endocrine glands into the bloodstream, hormones travel to their target tissue
    - Specific hormone receptors within target cells or on their cell membranes determine the cell's responsiveness to a specific hormone
    - The number of hormone receptors in target cells varies with changes in circulating hormone levels
      - When hormone levels are above normal, the number of receptors decreases; this receptor decrease compensates for hormone excess by reducing target cell affinity for the hormone
      - When hormone levels are below normal, the number of receptors increases; this increase in receptors increases target cell affinity for the hormone

Components of the endocrine system

Endocrine glands secrete hormones directly into the bloodstream to regulate body function. This illustration shows the location of the major endocrine glands (except the gonads).

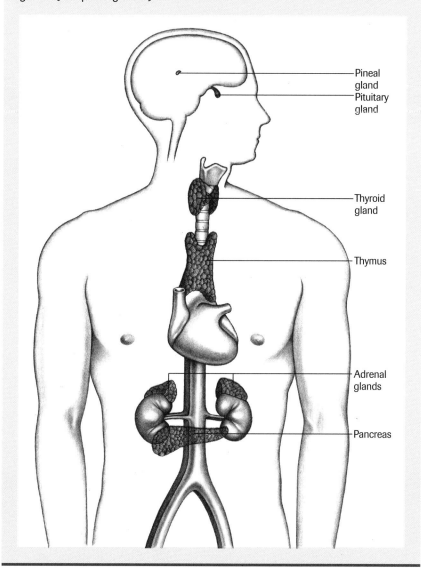

Pineal gland
Pituitary gland
Thyroid gland
Thymus
Adrenal glands
Pancreas

Key endocrine glands

- Pituitary
- Thyroid
- Parathyroid
- Adrenal
- Gonads
- Pineal
- Thymus

– Hormones alter the metabolism of specific cells in target tissue
– Hormones affect target tissue through one of two mechanisms
  · Acting directly, hormones activate deoxyribonucleic acid (DNA) in the cells of target tissue
  · In turn, DNA initiates synthesis of certain protein molecules, such as enzymes, that promote metabolic activity

• Acting indirectly, hormones produce one or more intracellular secondary messengers that mediate the response of target tissue
  - For example, an amino acid–based hormone produces cyclic adenosine monophosphate (cyclic AMP), an intracellular secondary messenger
  - Cyclic AMP, in turn, activates protein kinase enzymes within the cell

• Hormone output may be controlled directly or indirectly by feedback mechanisms
  – Output can be regulated *directly* by the hormone level produced by a gland
  – Output can be regulated *indirectly* by the level of a substance under hormonal control, such as glucose or sodium

• Usually, an elevated level of hormone or hormone-regulated substance suppresses further hormone output; this arrangement is called a *negative feedback mechanism*

• Less commonly, a rising hormone level stimulates hormone output; this arrangement is called a *positive feedback mechanism*, often within a negative process

● **Cyclic AMP and hormone function**

• Some hormones (steroid and thyroid hormones) can enter the cell and bind with intracellular hormone receptors to exert their effect

• Many hormones can't enter the target cell and must bind to receptors on the cell membrane; receptor binding to the cell membrane activates other enzymes to cause the desired effect in the cell
  – Receptor binding activates the enzyme adenylate cyclase, located on the inner surface of the cell membrane
  – This catalyzes the conversion of intracellular adenosine triphosphate into cyclic AMP; this conversion continues as long as the hormone acts on the cell membrane
  – Cyclic AMP activates certain intracellular enzymes in the target cells
  – The activated enzymes perform a specific function based on target cell characteristics; for example, enzymes cause glucose liberation from glycogen in liver cells or lipid synthesis in fat cells
  – Duration of cyclic AMP action is brief because the intracellular enzyme phosphodiesterase degrades cyclic AMP and converts it into the inactive form, AMP
  – Through this process, a hormone attached to the exterior of a cell can exert intracellular effects

---

Key facts about cyclic AMP and hormone function

- Many hormones bind to receptors on the cell membrane
- This activates the creation of cyclic AMP
- Cyclic AMP activates intracellular enzymes in the target cells, which activate other enzymes to cause the desired effect in the cell

PITUITARY GLAND

● **Key concepts**
- The *pituitary gland,* also called the *hypophysis,* is located at the base of the brain in the sella turcica of the sphenoid bone
- It receives chemical and nervous stimulation from the hypothalamus
- The pituitary gland has two main lobes—the anterior lobe (adenohypophysis) and the posterior lobe (neurohypophysis)

● **Pituitary gland structure**
- The pituitary gland is a small, pea-shaped gland connected to the hypothalamus by a narrow stalk
- It lies in a small depression at the base of the skull (sella turcica) just behind the optic chasm and optic nerves
- It has an anterior lobe and a posterior lobe
  - The lobes are connected by a small rudimentary intermediate lobe in the fetus; in adults, the cells are scattered throughout the anterior and posterior lobes
  - Releasing factors from the hypothalamus regulate hormone release from anterior lobe cells
  - After being synthesized in the hypothalamus, several hormones are transported by nerve axons to the posterior lobe cells, where they're stored
  - These hormones are released from the posterior lobe in response to nerve impulses transmitted from the hypothalamus down the pituitary stalk

● **Hypothalamic control**
- The hypothalamus, a portion of the diencephalon of the brain, activates, controls, and integrates various endocrine functions
- It produces releasing and inhibiting factors called *regulatory hormones*
  - These factors control the anterior pituitary
  - They enter the pituitary through portal venous pathways
- The hypothalamus also produces hormones that are stored in and secreted by the posterior pituitary
- A negative feedback mechanism controls the release of hypothalamic substances
  - Cells in the hypothalamus regulate the level of most pituitary hormones
  - These cells continually monitor the levels of circulating hormones produced by target glands such as the thyroid gland

Key characteristics of the pituitary gland
- Located in the base of the brain
- Receives chemical and nervous stimulation from the hypothalamus
- Has an anterior lobe and a posterior lobe

Key facts about hypothalamic control of the pituitary gland
- Produces regulatory hormones that control the anterior pituitary
- Produces hormones that are stored in and secreted by the posterior pituitary
- The release of substances is controlled by a negative feedback mechanism

- When the target gland hormone level declines, the hypothalamus produces releasing factors that are carried through the portal venous pathways to the pituitary
- The factors induce the release of tropic hormones that stimulate hormone production by the target gland
- The level of the hormone produced by the target gland rises until it reaches the upper range of normal
- The elevated hormone level then "shuts off" further release of releasing factors and tropic hormones
- The mechanism maintains a relatively steady hormone output from the target gland and prevents wide fluctuations in hormone levels that might disrupt normal body functions
- Higher cortical centers also can affect hypothalamic control of hormone release; for example, pituitary secretion may change in response to strong emotions, such as anxiety, anger, or fear (see *Mechanism of hypothalamic control*)

● **Anterior lobe hormones**
- The anterior lobe is composed of cords of epithelial cells that contain granules of stored hormone
- Five different cell types secrete six hormones
  - Somatotropes secrete *growth hormone* (GH), or somatotropin; GH stimulates bone and muscle growth
    - Hyposecretion of GH in children can lead to dwarfism (abnormal underdevelopment of the body)
    - Hypersecretion in children can result in gigantism
    - Hypersecretion in adults leads to acromegaly (chronic disease marked by elongation and enlargement of arm, leg, jaw, and nose bones)
  - Thyrotropes secrete *thyroid-stimulating hormone* (TSH), or thyrotropin; TSH stimulates the thyroid gland to release thyroid hormone
    - Hyposecretion of TSH in children results in cretinism (condition marked by hypothyroidism and arrested development)
    - Hyposecretion in adults causes myxedema (condition marked by slow speech, slow metabolism, hand and facial swelling, and coarse, edematous skin)
    - Hypersecretion causes Graves' disease (condition marked by hyperthyroidism and thyroid enlargement)
  - Corticotropes secrete *adrenocorticotropic hormone* (ACTH), or corticotropin; ACTH stimulates the adrenal cortex to release glucocorticoids and androgens
    - Hyposecretion of ACTH results in Addison's disease (disorder marked by increased pigmentation of skin and mucous

---

Key characteristics of anterior lobe hormones

● Five cell types secrete six hormones
● Somatotropes secrete GH
● Thyrotropes secrete TSH
● Corticotropes secrete ACTH
● Gonadotropes secrete FSH and LH
● Mammotropes secrete prolactin

GO WITH THE FLOW

Mechanism of hypothalamic control

Through a feedback mechanism, the hypothalamus regulates anterior pituitary hormones, which trigger hormone release by other endocrine glands, as illustrated below.

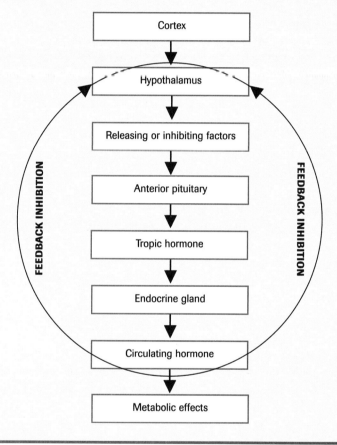

Hypothalamic control mechanism

- A feedback mechanism maintains steady hormone output to prevent wide fluctuations in levels
- Higher cortical centers can affect hypothalamic control of hormones
- Pituitary secretion may change in response to strong emotions

membranes, hypotension, nausea, anorexia and, in some cases, hypoglycemia)
- Hypersecretion results in Cushing's disease (disorder marked by fatigue, weakness, and adiposity of the face, neck, and trunk)
– Gonadotropes secrete follicle-stimulating hormone (FSH) and luteinizing hormone (LH)
- FSH stimulates ovarian follicle maturation and ovarian estrogen production in females and sperm production in males
   - Hyposecretion inhibits sexual maturation

- Hypersecretion results in precocious puberty
  - LH stimulates ovulation and ovarian production of progesterone in females and testicular production of testosterone in males
    - Hyposecretion results in primary or secondary hypogonadism, causing retarded growth and sexual development
    - Hypersecretion leads to hypergonadism, resulting in excessive growth and precocious puberty
  – Mammotropes secrete *prolactin;* this hormone stimulates the breast to produce milk
    - Hyposecretion results in poor milk secretion
    - Hypersecretion causes galactorrhea (persistent milk secretion) and cessation of menses in females and impotence in males
  – Melanocyte-stimulating hormone is secreted by the intermediate lobe and is responsible for pigmentation

● **Posterior lobe hormones**
  - The posterior lobe consists of a meshwork of nerve fibers and specialized cells called *pituicytes*
  - Bundles of nerve fibers in the pituitary stalk connect the posterior lobe to the hypothalamus; these structures aren't linked by the portal venous pathways
  - The posterior lobe secretes oxytocin and antidiuretic hormone (ADH)
    – *Oxytocin* stimulates uterine contractions and causes milk ejection from the breasts
      - Oxytocin stimulates contraction of the pregnant uterus
      - Milk ejection occurs when oxytocin stimulates contraction of specialized contractile cells surrounding the breast glands and ducts
        - Nipple stimulation from breast-feeding initiates nerve impulses
        - These impulses are transmitted to neurons in the hypothalamus, which send impulses to the posterior lobe and cause oxytocin release
    – *ADH* causes the cells of the renal and collecting tubules to become more permeable to water, altering urine concentration
      - Osmoreceptors in the hypothalamus regulate ADH secretion by responding to osmolarity variations in the extracellular fluid (ECF)
      - If ECF osmolarity rises above normal, hypothalamic neurons send impulses to the posterior lobe, stimulating ADH release
        - ADH triggers water retention

Key characteristics of posterior lobe hormones
- Oxytocin: stimulates uterine contractions and causes milk ejection from the breasts
- ADH: acts on the kidneys to alter urine concentration

- In turn, ECF becomes diluted, lowering its osmolarity
· If ECF osmolarity falls below normal, the hypothalamus reduces ADH output from the posterior lobe
  - Decline of ADH prevents reabsorption of excess water in the tubular filtrate, causing it to be excreted in the urine
  - This concentrates the ECF, increasing its osmolarity

THYROID GLAND

● **Key concepts**
  • One of the largest endocrine glands, the thyroid gland lies in the lower anterior neck
  • It's composed of spherical follicle cells that produce the hormones *thyroxine* (T_4) and *triiodothyronine* (T_3)
  • The thyroid gland secretes T_4, T_3, and *thyrocalcitonin*
  • The general term *thyroid hormone* refers to T_4 and T_3

● **Thyroid gland structure**
  • The thyroid gland is located in the anterior neck, overlying the inferior border of the larynx; it's fixed to the anterior surface of the upper trachea by loose connective tissue
  • It consists of two lateral lobes—one on either side of the trachea—connected by a narrow isthmus
  • The gland is composed of spherical thyroid follicles that contain colloid surrounded by a layer of cuboidal follicular cells; these cells synthesize the thyroid hormones T_4 and T_3
  • Parafollicular cells, located between the follicles, secrete the hormone thyrocalcitonin (also called *calcitonin*)

● **Thyroid hormones**
  • T_4 and T_3 are the major metabolic hormones of the body
  • They regulate metabolism by speeding cellular respiration
  • T_3 has several times the biologic activity of T_4
  • Thyrocalcitonin maintains the blood calcium level by inhibiting calcium release from bone
  • The calcium concentration of the fluid surrounding thyroid cells controls thyrocalcitonin secretion

● **Thyroid hormone synthesis**
  • Follicular cells actively concentrate iodine; they contain enzymes that can synthesize thyroid hormone from iodine and the amino acid tyrosine
  • Iodine circulates in the bloodstream as iodide ions
    – The thyroid gland takes up these ions and oxidizes them to iodine

Key characteristics of the thyroid gland

- Consists of two lobes, one on either side of the trachea
- Contains cuboidal follicular cells that secrete T_4 and T_3
- Contains parafollicular cells between the follicles that secrete thyrocalcitonin

Key characteristics of thyroid hormones

- T_4 and T_3 regulate metabolism by speeding cellular respiration
- Thyrocalcitonin inhibits calcium release from bone
- Follicular cells synthesize T_4 and T_3 from circulating iodide ions

Key facts about thyroid hormone synthesis

- Follicular cells concentrate iodine
- Iodine combines with amino acid tyrosine to yield thyroid hormone

Key facts about thyroid hormone secretion

- Pituitary TSH controls T_3 and T_4 output
- Most thyroid hormone is metabolically inactive and is bound to a plasma protein
- Only the unbound hormone is metabolically active

– Iodine combines with tyrosine to form monoiodotyrosine (MIT) and diiodotyrosine
– Condensation of MIT and diiodotyrosine molecules yields T_3 and T_4
- T_3 and T_4 combine with the large protein molecule thyroglobulin and form the colloid of the thyroid follicles

● Thyroid hormone secretion

- Pituitary TSH controls T_3 and T_4 output, which is regulated by a negative feedback mechanism
- Thyroid hormone stored as colloid must be released from thyroglobulin before it can be secreted
  – Thyroid follicular cells perform this function
  – These cells ingest colloid by pinocytosis
  – This causes T_3 and T_4 to split off and be secreted into the bloodstream
  – It also degrades thyroglobulin into its component amino acids, which become part of the amino acid pool
- Most of the thyroid hormone is metabolically inactive and circulates bound to a plasma protein called thyroidbinding globulin
- Only the small amount of free (unbound) hormone is metabolically active
- Most of the secreted hormone is T_4, but much of the T_4 is converted to T_3 in the tissues where it exerts its effect

● Metabolic effects of thyroid hormone

- Thyroid hormone controls the rate of metabolic processes
- It's required for normal growth and development and for development and maturation of the nervous system
- Thyroid hormone excess (hyperthyroidism) or deficiency (hypothyroidism) leads to a corresponding increase or decrease in metabolic processes (see *Teaching a patient with hypothyroidism*)

PARATHYROID GLANDS

Key characteristics of the parathyroid glands

- Located on the thyroid gland
- Secrete parathyroid hormone, which regulates calcium metabolism

● Key concepts

- The parathyroid glands are located on the thyroid gland; most people have four parathyroid glands
- These glands secrete *parathyroid hormone* (PTH, or parahormone), the principal regulator of calcium metabolism

● Parathyroid gland structure

- Four small parathyroid glands are embedded in the posterior surface of the thyroid gland
- Pea-sized, they're the smallest endocrine glands

TIME-OUT FOR TEACHING

Teaching a patient with hypothyroidism

Make sure you teach a patient with hypothyroidism:

- what hypothyroidism is and how it's caused
- signs and symptoms of hypothyroidism (such as fatigue, weight gain, cold intolerance, mental sluggishness, and dry, flaky, and "doughy" skin)
- possible complications of the disease

- diagnostic tests to anticipate (such as laboratory tests for blood levels of thyroid hormones)
- necessary activity restrictions
- dietary guidelines to ensure adequate nutrition
- the importance of lifelong thyroid hormone replacement therapy
- signs and symptoms of hyperthyroidism (such as heat intolerance, diaphoresis, tachycardia, and exophthalmos) in case of accidental thyroid hormone overdose.

● Parathyroid hormone

- The main function of PTH is to help control the calcium level in the blood
    - Blood calcium levels normally range from 8.5 to 10.5 mg/dl
    - An adequate calcium level is required for normal cardiac and skeletal muscle contraction, nerve impulse transmission, and blood coagulation
    - Hypocalcemia (too little calcium) greatly increases nerve and muscle excitability; it results from such disorders as burns, diarrhea, and vitamin D deficiency
    - Hypercalcemia (too much calcium) diminishes nerve and muscle excitability; it results from such disorders as hyperparathyroidism, vitamin D excess, prolonged immobilization, and renal or neoplastic disease
- PTH affects the kidneys by adjusting the rate at which calcium and magnesium ions are removed from urine
- It also increases the movement of phosphate ions from the blood to urine for excretion
- A reciprocal relationship exists between the calcium and phosphorus levels in the blood
    - A decreased calcium level tends to increase the phosphorus level
    - An increased calcium level tends to decrease the phosphorus level

- PTH, vitamin D, and thyrocalcitonin (from the thyroid gland) regulate the blood calcium level
  - PTH and vitamin D raise the blood calcium level
  - Thyrocalcitonin lowers the blood calcium level
- Because calcium in the blood is in equilibrium with calcium salts in bone, changes in the blood calcium level eventually cause changes in the amount of calcium salts in bone

● **Regulation of calcium metabolism**
- PTH helps regulate calcium metabolism
  - This hormone isn't stored but is synthesized and secreted continuously
  - The ionized calcium level in the blood regulates PTH output by a negative feedback mechanism
    · A decrease in the ionized calcium level causes increased PTH output, which raises the blood calcium level
    · An increase in the ionized calcium level suppresses PTH secretion, which reduces the blood calcium level
  - PTH has three sites of action—the skeletal system, intestines, and kidneys
    · Its main function is to mobilize calcium from bone by promoting bone matrix breakdown and liberating calcium, which diffuses into the blood and raises the blood calcium level
    · In the intestines, PTH increases calcium absorption, which tends to raise the blood calcium level
    · In the kidneys, PTH increases calcium reabsorption by the renal tubules and promotes phosphate excretion
      - Increased phosphate excretion in urine lowers the phosphate concentration in blood
      - Calcium and phosphate blood levels have a reciprocal relationship; therefore, the calcium level rises correspondingly
- Vitamin D also regulates calcium metabolism
  - This vitamin promotes calcium absorption from the intestines
  - Vitamin D is formed by a complex process from a cholesterol derivative in skin
    · Ultraviolet light in sunlight converts this sterol into an intermediate compound
    · The liver and kidneys further metabolize the intermediate compound into the active form of vitamin D
- Thyrocalcitonin acts as an antagonist to PTH
  - Thyrocalcitonin is secreted in response to an increased blood calcium level
  - It tends to lower the blood calcium level, primarily by inhibiting calcium mobilization from bone

Key facts about calcium metabolism regulation

- Decreased calcium levels increase PTH output; increased calcium levels decrease PTH output
- PTH acts on the skeletal system, intestines, and kidneys to increase calcium levels
- Vitamin D also regulates calcium metabolism
- Thyrocalcitonin is an antagonist to PTH

ADRENAL GLANDS

● **Key concepts**
  • The adrenal glands (also called *suprarenal glands*) are located on top of the kidneys
  • Each gland consists of an outer cortex, which is enclosed in a fibrous capsule, and an inner medulla
  • These two parts of the glands secrete different hormones
    – The adrenal cortex secretes three types of steroid hormones: glucocorticoids, mineralocorticoids, and sex hormones
    – The adrenal medulla produces two similar hormones: norepinephrine and epinephrine

● **Adrenal gland structure**
  • The two parts of the almond-shaped adrenal glands function as separate endocrine glands
    – The *adrenal cortex* forms the bulk of the gland
      · It has three zones, or cell layers
      · Although each zone primarily produces different hormones (called *corticosteroids*), all three zones produce the entire spectrum of corticosteroids
        - The zona glomerulosa, the outermost zone, secretes mineralocorticoids (such as aldosterone)
        - The zona fasciculata, the middle zone, secretes glucocorticoids (such as hydrocortisone, corticosterone, and cortisone)
        - The zona reticularis, the innermost layer, also secretes glucocorticoids and small amounts of gonadocorticoids (adrenal sex hormones); the principal gonadocorticoids are androgens (male sex hormones) and small amounts of estrogen and progesterone (female sex hormones)
    – The *adrenal medulla* forms the inner part of the adrenal gland
      · It functions as part of the sympathetic nervous system
      · The adrenal medulla's chromaffin cells secrete the catecholamines epinephrine (adrenaline) and norepinephrine (noradrenaline)

● **Glucocorticoids**
  • The major glucocorticoid is cortisol (hydrocortisone); others include corticosterone and cortisone
  • Cortisol and other glucocorticoids have similar actions
    – They raise the blood glucose level by decreasing glucose metabolism and by promoting glucose formation from protein and fat (gluconeogenesis)

– They promote protein breakdown into amino acids, some of which are converted by the liver into glucose; this depletes tissue proteins, which are converted to glucose
- Glucocorticoids are secreted in response to ACTH stimulation
- Their output is controlled by a negative feedback mechanism in which a low glucocorticoid level stimulates ACTH secretion and a high level suppresses it

● **Mineralocorticoids**
- Mineralocorticoids regulate electrolyte and water balance by promoting sodium ion absorption and potassium ion excretion by the renal tubule
- The major mineralocorticoid is aldosterone; its secretion is regulated by more than one mechanism
  – Although ACTH increases aldosterone secretion somewhat, the most potent stimulus is the renin-angiotensin-aldosterone system
  – This system responds to variations in blood volume, blood pressure, and blood sodium concentration; its effect is mediated by the juxtaglomerular apparatus of the kidneys

● **Sex hormones**
- Small amounts of estrogen, progesterone, and testosterone are produced by the adrenal glands of both sexes
- The amounts produced are minimal compared with the much larger quantities produced by the gonads
- The small amount of androgen produced by the adrenal glands appears to be responsible for the sex drive in women

● **Adrenal medulla hormones**
- The adrenal medulla produces the hormones norepinephrine and epinephrine from a precursor amino acid called tyrosine
- Both hormones belong to a class of compounds called *catecholamines*; epinephrine differs from norepinephrine only in the presence of a methyl group attached to the amino group in the molecule
- During synthesis, norepinephrine is formed first; then some of it is converted to epinephrine by the addition of the methyl group
- Both hormones are stored in the cytoplasmic granules of adrenal medulla cells; they're released into circulation in response to nerve impulses transmitted by preganglionic fibers of the sympathetic nervous system
- Epinephrine accounts for about 80% of the hormones produced by the adrenal medulla; norepinephrine accounts for roughly 20%

- Emotional stress, such as anger, fear, or anxiety, activates the sympathetic nervous system and causes the adrenal medulla to release these hormones
- The liberated catecholamines exert widespread effects that produce a physiologic response to stress—the fight-or-flight response
  - This response increases the heart rate and cardiac output and constricts the blood vessels, raising the blood pressure
  - It elevates the blood glucose level and mobilizes glycogen from the liver and free fatty acids from adipose tissue to provide glucose for energy
  - Other effects include tense muscles, dilated pupils, cold and clammy skin, and increased mental activity and nervous system response
- Small amounts of catecholamines are excreted unchanged in the urine, but most are inactivated by various enzymes and excreted in an inactive form
- Inactivation is accomplished in one of two ways
  - A methyl group can be added to one of the hydroxyl groups in the catecholamine ring, forming a compound called a *metanephrine*
  - The amino group can be removed, the terminal carbon oxidized to a carboxyl group, and a methyl group added to one of the hydroxyl groups attached to the ring; this produces vanillylmandelic acid

PANCREAS

● **Key concepts**
- The *pancreas* is a triangular organ located in the hypogastric area and left upper quadrant of the abdomen
- It has endocrine and exocrine functions
- Acinar cells make up most of the gland; they control the exocrine function of the pancreas, secreting pancreatic juice (an alkaline substance that contains digestive enzymes)
- Scattered among the acinar cells are clusters of endocrine cells called the *islets of Langerhans,* which secrete pancreatic hormones

● **Pancreas structure**
- The head and neck of the pancreas lie in the curve of the duodenum, its body stretches horizontally behind the stomach, and its tail reaches the spleen
- The islets of Langerhans are clusters of about 1 million hormone-secreting cells scattered throughout the pancreas; each islet is composed of three major cell types and three minor cell types

Key characteristics of the pancreas

- Has both exocrine and endocrine functions
- Acinar cells control exocrine functions
- The islets of Langerhans control endocrine function

- The major types are classified as alpha cells, beta cells, and gamma cells
- The minor types are classified as pancreatic polypeptide, D_1, and enterochromaffin cells
- Each cell type has a specific function
  - Alpha cells secrete glucagon, which raises the blood glucose level
  - Beta cells secrete insulin (the major islet hormone), which lowers the blood glucose level
  - Delta cells produce the hormone somatostatin, which suppresses insulin and glucagon release from the islets
  - Pancreatic polypeptide cells produce a hormone that stimulates GI enzyme secretion and inhibits intestinal motility
  - D_1 cells produce a hormone called *vasoactive intestinal polypeptide,* which increases the blood glucose level and stimulates GI secretions
  - Enterochromaffin cells synthesize serotonin
- Insulin is the islet cell hormone of major physiologic importance
  - Without sufficient insulin, diabetes mellitus develops

Glucagon

- *Glucagon* is a polypeptide that helps control carbohydrate metabolism
- The alpha cells secrete glucagon in response to hypoglycemia (decreased blood glucose level)
  - Glucagon increases the blood glucose level by working mainly in the liver, stimulating glycogenolysis (glycogen breakdown to glucose) and gluconeogenesis (glucose synthesis from noncarbohydrate materials)
  - This process rapidly liberates glucose, increasing the blood glucose level

Insulin synthesis and storage

- Within beta cells, insulin is synthesized by the endoplasmic reticulum and then transported to the Golgi apparatus
- Next, insulin is formed into secretory granules that accumulate in the cytoplasm of the beta cells and are eventually discharged into the circulation
- Insulin is synthesized as a large precursor peptide molecule called *proinsulin,* which is largely inactive
  - Chemical bonds join the two ends of the peptide chain
  - Each bond consists of a cross-bridge made of two sulfur atoms (disulfide bond); cross-linkage causes the chain to coil
- When proinsulin is being stored as secretory granules, a trypsin-like enzyme from Golgi apparatus membranes splits off the central

part of the proinsulin coil to yield the active enzyme insulin and the connecting peptide
- Insulin consists of two short peptide chains joined together by disulfide bonds
- Both cleavage parts are stored in the secretory granules and secreted together into the bloodstream

⬤ **Insulin secretion and action**
- Insulin secretion occurs in two phases
  - An initial outpouring results from the discharge of insulin stored in the cytoplasmic granules of the beta cells
  - A slower, more sustained release follows; this results from synthesis and release of additional insulin by beta cells
- The main stimulus for insulin secretion is blood glucose elevation, which occurs after eating
  - Digestion triggers the release of hormones and amino acids that also stimulate insulin release
  - Consequently, ingested glucose causes much more insulin to be secreted than does the same amount of intravenous glucose
- Several other hormones increase the blood glucose level, indirectly stimulating insulin secretion
  - Glucagon and catecholamines raise the blood glucose concentration by promoting conversion of liver glycogen into glucose
  - GH inhibits glucose use by the tissues; it promotes fat breakdown to yield free fatty acids, which are used instead of glucose for energy
  - Glucocorticoids raise the blood glucose level primarily by promoting protein breakdown into amino acids, which are converted into glucose by the liver
- Insulin's principal action is control of carbohydrate metabolism; it also influences protein and fat metabolism
- The chief sites of insulin action are liver cells and muscle and adipose tissue
  - Insulin promotes the entry of glucose into the cells and enhances the use of glucose as an energy source
  - It promotes the storage of glucose as glycogen in muscle and liver cells
  - In adipose tissue, insulin enhances the conversion of glucose to triglyceride and storage of the newly formed triglyceride within fat cells
  - Insulin also promotes the entry of amino acids into cells and stimulates protein synthesis

TOP 10

Items to study for your next test on the endocrine system

1. Characteristics of endocrine and exocrine glands
2. Details of the negative hormonal feedback mechanism
3. Process by which the hypothalamus controls the pituitary gland
4. Functions of the major pituitary hormones
5. Metabolic effects of thyroid hormones
6. Process by which parathyroid hormone regulates calcium metabolism
7. Comparison of mineralocorticoids and glucocorticoids
8. Details of the fight-or-flight response of adrenal hormones
9. Functions of pancreatic hormones
10. Teaching tips for patients with hypothyroidism

NCLEX CHECKS

It's never too soon to begin your NCLEX preparation. Now that you've reviewed this chapter, carefully read each of the following questions and choose the best answer. Then compare your responses with the correct answers.

1. In teaching a client with an endocrine disorder, the nurse explains that the endocrine system's chief function is to do what?
- ☐ **1.** Deliver nutrients to the body's cells
- ☐ **2.** Regulate and integrate the body's metabolic activities
- ☐ **3.** Eliminate waste products from the body
- ☐ **4.** Control body temperature and produce blood cells

2. A client is scheduled for surgical removal of a tumor in his pituitary gland. Which statement about the pituitary gland is true?
- ☐ **1.** It consists of three main lobes.
- ☐ **2.** It's regulated by the thalamus.
- ☐ **3.** It's located at the base of the skull.
- ☐ **4.** It's a large gland.

3. When teaching a client with myxedema about her disorder, the nurse knows that the client understands the etiology when she makes which statement?
- ☐ **1.** "It's caused by underproduction of prolactin."
- ☐ **2.** "It's caused by overproduction of follicle-stimulating hormone."
- ☐ **3.** "It's caused by too much growth hormone."
- ☐ **4.** "It's caused by too little thyroid-stimulating hormone."

4. A client is diagnosed with Addison's disease. What findings would the nurse expect to assess?
- ☐ **1.** Obesity, hypoglycemia, and weakness
- ☐ **2.** Pale skin, hypotension, and fatigue
- ☐ **3.** Hypotension, anorexia, and increased skin pigmentation
- ☐ **4.** Hyperglycemia, anorexia, and fatigue

5. A client has low parathyroid hormone levels. The nurse would expect which laboratory serum values to be abnormal?
- ☐ **1.** Calcium and phosphorus
- ☐ **2.** Chloride and glucose
- ☐ **3.** Sodium and potassium
- ☐ **4.** Magnesium and bicarbonate

6. A client is being treated for hyperthyroidism. Which signs and symptoms would the nurse expect to document?

☐ **1.** Weight gain, heat intolerance, and mental sluggishness
☐ **2.** Exophthalmos, tachycardia, and dry, flaky skin
☐ **3.** Fatigue, weight gain, and cold intolerance
☐ **4.** Heat intolerance, diaphoresis, and tachycardia

7. The nurse is teaching relaxation techniques to a client with a high level of anxiety and stress. Of the following signs and symptoms, which are commonly related to stress? Select all that apply.
☐ **1.** Tachycardia
☐ **2.** Dilated pupils
☐ **3.** Hypoglycemia
☐ **4.** Hot, dry skin
☐ **5.** Mental sluggishness
☐ **6.** Tense muscles

8. The nurse teaches a client about hormones related to his diabetic condition. Which hormone is secreted in response to hypoglycemia?
☐ **1.** Insulin
☐ **2.** Somatostatin
☐ **3.** Glucagon
☐ **4.** Aldosterone

9. Which finding would the nurse expect to observe in a child with hypersecretion of LH?
☐ **1.** Precocious puberty
☐ **2.** Growth retardation
☐ **3.** Lack of menses
☐ **4.** Persistent milk secretion

10. When palpating a client's thyroid gland, where would the nurse expect the gland to be located?
☐ **1.** In the anterior neck, over the inferior border of the larynx
☐ **2.** In the anterior neck, over the superior border of the larynx
☐ **3.** Fixed to the posterior surface of the upper trachea
☐ **4.** Fixed to the posterior surface of the lower trachea

ANSWERS AND RATIONALES

1. CORRECT ANSWER: 2
Along with the nervous system, the endocrine system regulates and integrates the body's metabolic activities. Through its hormones, the endocrine system also controls reproduction and growth; mobilizes the body against stress; maintains electrolyte, water, and nutrient balance; and regulates metabolism. Delivering nutrients to the body's cells, elimi-

nating bodily waste products, temperature control, and blood cell production aren't functions of the endocrine system.

2. CORRECT ANSWER: 3
The pituitary gland is a small, pea-sized gland located at the base of the skull. It's controlled by the hypothalamus and has two main lobes: the anterior lobe and the posterior lobe.

3. CORRECT ANSWER: 4
Hyposecretion of thyroid-stimulating hormone causes myxedema, which is characterized by slow speech, slow metabolism, hand and facial swelling, and coarse, edematous skin. Underproduction of prolactin results in poor milk secretion. Too much follicle-stimulating hormone leads to precocious puberty. Overproduction of growth hormone causes acromegaly.

4. CORRECT ANSWER: 3
Hyposecretion of adrenocorticotropin hormone results in Addison's disease, which is marked by hypotension, anorexia, increased skin pigmentation, hypoglycemia, nausea, and hypotension. Hypersecretion of the hormone results in Cushing's disease, which is characterized by fatigue, weakness, and adiposity of the face, neck, and trunk.

5. CORRECT ANSWER: 1
The main function of parathyroid hormone is to control the calcium level in the blood. A reciprocal relationship exists between calcium and phosphorus—a decreased calcium level increases the phosphorus level, and an increased calcium level tends to decrease the phosphorus level. Parathyroid hormone doesn't regulate chloride, glucose, sodium, potassium, magnesium, or bicarbonate.

6. CORRECT ANSWER: 4
Hyperthyroidism—an excess of thyroid hormone—is marked by heat intolerance, diaphoresis, tachycardia, exophthalmos, and a bruit or thrill over the thyroid gland. Hypothyroidism—a deficiency of thyroid hormone—is marked by fatigue, weight gain, mental sluggishness, and dry, flaky, and "doughy" skin.

7. CORRECT ANSWER: 1, 2, 6
Emotional stress activates the sympathetic nervous system, causing the adrenal medulla to release catecholamines. This leads to such signs and symptoms as increased heart rate (tachycardia), dilated pupils, tense muscles, vasoconstriction (causing increased blood pressure and cold, clammy skin), increased mental activity, and hyperglycemia.

8. CORRECT ANSWER: 3

The alpha cells of the pancreas secrete glucagon in response to hypoglycemia. The beta cells secrete insulin, which lowers the blood glucose level. The delta cells of the pancreas produce somatostatin, which suppresses insulin and glucagon release from the islets. Aldosterone is a mineralocorticoid secreted by the adrenal cortex that regulates water and electrolyte balance.

9. CORRECT ANSWER: 1

LH stimulates ovulation and ovarian production of progesterone in females and testicular production of testosterone in males. Hypersecretion of LH leads to hypergonadism, resulting in excessive growth and precocious puberty. Hyposecretion leads to retarded growth and sexual underdevelopment. Hypersecretion of prolactin causes persistent milk secretion (galactorrhea) and cessation of menses in females and impotence in males.

10. CORRECT ANSWER: 1

The thyroid gland is located in the anterior neck, overlying the inferior border of the larynx. It's fixed to the anterior surface of the upper trachea by loose connective tissue.

19

Reproductive system

LEARNING OBJECTIVES

After studying this chapter, you should be able to:

- Identify the structures and functions of the male reproductive system.
- Identify the structures and functions of the female reproductive system.
- Explain hormonal regulation of sexual development.
- Explain the hormones and events of the menstrual cycle.
- Describe the function and structure of the female breast.
- Understand the process of spermatogenesis and oogenesis.

CHAPTER OVERVIEW

Through reproduction, parents create new individuals and pass along their genetic information to them. In this way, the reproductive system is responsible for continuing the species. If every body system except the reproductive system were functioning perfectly, the individual could survive but the species couldn't. Because the reproductive system also has endocrine functions and is closely integrated with a person's self-concept, the nurse must understand its structures and functions. This chapter reviews both the male and female reproductive systems, with special focus on body structures, hormonal mechanisms, the reproductive process, and developmental considerations.

MALE REPRODUCTIVE SYSTEM

● **Key concepts**
  - Unlike other body systems, the human reproductive system is relatively inactive until puberty
  - Although male reproductive organs differ from those of their female counterparts, they have a common purpose: to produce offspring
  - The role of the male reproductive system is to produce gametes (spermatozoa) and transport them to the female reproductive tract for fertilization

● **Male reproductive structures**
  - Major structures include the penis, scrotum, testes, a duct system, and accessory organs (see *Structures of the male reproductive system*)
    - The *penis* is the copulatory organ
      · It's used to place spermatozoa in the female reproductive system

Structures of the male reproductive system

The male reproductive system includes the penis, the scrotum and its contents, the prostate gland, and the inguinal structures, as illustrated here.

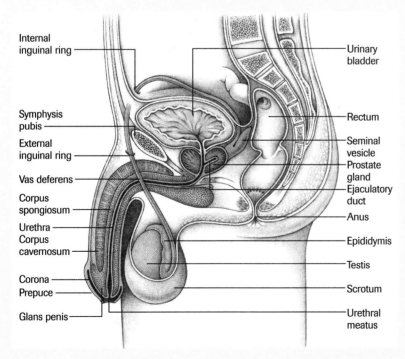

Internal inguinal ring — Urinary bladder — Symphysis pubis — Rectum — External inguinal ring — Seminal vesicle — Vas deferens — Prostate gland — Corpus spongiosum — Ejaculatory duct — Urethra — Anus — Corpus cavernosum — Epididymis — Corona — Testis — Prepuce — Scrotum — Glans penis — Urethral meatus

Major male reproductive structures

Penis
- Copulatory organ
- Includes the cavernous bodies corpora cavernosa and corpus spongiosum

Scrotum
- Covers and protects the testes
- Maintains the testes at the proper temperature

Testes
- Produce spermatozoa
- Produce testosterone

Duct system
- Moves spermatozoa to outside the body

Accessory glands
- Includes seminal vesicles, prostate gland, bulbourethral glands
- Secrete liquid portion of semen

- It consists of three cylinders of vascular erectile tissue called *cavernous bodies,* each encased by a layer of connective tissue
    - The upper (dorsolateral) two cylinders, the *corpora cavernosa,* are encased by dense fibrous tissue
    - The lower (midventral) cylinder, the *corpus spongiosum,* encloses the urethra
- Three pairs of superficial skeletal muscles attach to the bases of the cavernous bodies
- Contraction of these muscles compresses the urethra, which occurs during ejaculation and urination
– The *scrotum* is located posterior to the penis
- It covers and protects the testes and spermatic cords
- It maintains the testes at the proper temperature for spermatozoa production
– The *testes* (located in the scrotum) are the male gonads
- They produce spermatozoa in the *seminiferous tubules*
- They produce the hormone testosterone in *Leydig cells* (interstitial cells between the seminiferous tubules)
- Gonadotropic hormones regulate testicular functions
– The *duct system* moves spermatozoa from the testes to outside the body
- The rete testis and efferent ducts lie within each testis and drain into the epididymis, which is located on top of the testis
- The duct system continues as the vas deferens; the vas deferens extends to the prostate gland and joins the seminal vesicles to form the ejaculatory duct, which empties into the urethra
– The *accessory glands*—the seminal vesicles, prostate gland, and bulbourethral (Cowper's) glands—secrete the liquid portion of semen
- The seminal vesicles merge with the vas deferens and secrete a thick alkaline fluid that nourishes spermatozoa and enhances their motility
- The prostate gland, which surrounds the urethra and lies below the bladder, secretes a thin alkaline fluid that promotes sperm motility; this fluid is discharged into the urethra through small ducts that open near the orifices of the ejaculatory ducts
- Cowper's glands, which are located below the prostate, secrete a mucoid substance in response to sexual stimulation; this substance provides lubrication during intercourse
- The male reproductive system produces semen—a mixture of spermatozoa and various fluids

Hormonal regulation

- Two gonadotropic hormones regulate testicular function: *follicle-stimulating hormone* (FSH) and *luteinizing hormone* (LH)
  - The anterior pituitary gland releases FSH and LH
  - The hypothalamus controls FSH and LH secretion, which is continuous in males
  - A negative feedback mechanism controls FSH and LH output
    - Rising FSH and LH levels suppress further output of these hormones
    - As a result, gonadotropic hormone levels remain stable
- FSH has two functions
  - It promotes development and normal function of the seminiferous tubules
  - It also helps stimulate spermatozoa production
- Inhibin—a protein (polypeptide) hormone produced by specialized cells of the seminiferous tubules (called *Sertoli cells*)—suppresses FSH release
  - Inhibin levels rise with active spermatogenesis
  - Elevated inhibin levels suppress further FSH output, thereby preventing excessive spermatogenesis and maintaining normal sperm production
- LH promotes testosterone secretion from Leydig cells
  - Testosterone is responsible for sexual drive, development of secondary sex characteristics, and growth
  - Testosterone also promotes normal spermatogenesis in the seminiferous tubules
  - Rising testosterone levels suppress further LH output, thereby maintaining a stable testosterone level
- Spermatogenesis and testosterone production are separate functions

Spermatogenesis

- Spermatogenesis is the process of spermatozoa formation
- Precursor cells in the seminiferous tubules (called *spermatogonia*) contain 46 chromosomes
- Spermatogonia divide repeatedly by mitosis to form *primary spermatocytes*, which also contain 46 chromosomes
- Primary spermatocytes then undergo meiotic divisions in which the number of chromosomes in the cells is reduced by half
  - In the first meiotic division, each primary spermatocyte forms two *secondary spermatocytes* (each with 23 chromosomes)
  - In the second meiotic division, each secondary spermatocyte forms two *spermatids* (each with 23 chromosomes), which mature into spermatozoa (with 23 chromosomes)

- Spermatozoa are produced continuously in the testes and seminiferous tubules; the production process takes about 2 months
- LH and FSH are needed to maintain normal spermatogenesis
  - LH stimulates Leydig cells to secrete testosterone, which is required for spermatogenesis
  - FSH stimulates Sertoli cells in the seminiferous tubules to secrete androgen-binding protein
    - This protein binds with the secreted testosterone, maintaining a high hormone level at the site of spermatogenesis
    - Sertoli cells also provide nutrients to maturing spermatids, which attach themselves to these support cells

● **Spermatozoa structure and function**
- The spermatozoon is a tadpolelike structure that consists of three parts: head, middle piece, and tail
  - The head contains the chromosomes
    - It's partially covered by a thin membranelike structure called the *head cap,* or acrosome
    - The acrosome contains enzymes that allow the spermatozoon to penetrate and fertilize the ovum
  - The middle piece contains mitochondria with enzymes that provide the energy required to propel the spermatozoon
  - The tail propels the sperm by flagellated movement (to-and-fro motion)
- Spermatozoa discharged in semen must undergo activation via capacitation, which involves a structural change in the spermatozoon
  - Small perforations appear in the acrosome of the spermatozoon
  - These perforations allow the release of enzymes required for the spermatozoon to penetrate the ovum

● **Semen composition**
- Semen is a viscous secretion that consists of spermatozoa and secretions from the seminal vesicles and the prostate and Cowper's glands
  - Seminal vesicles and prostate secretions contribute most of the semen volume
  - The slightly alkaline secretions provide nutrients for spermatozoa and protect them from acidic vaginal secretions
  - Cowper's glands provide some lubricating fluid
- The average volume of ejaculated semen is about 3 ml (the volume normally varies from 2 to 5 ml, depending on the time interval between ejaculations)
- Normally, 1 ml of semen contains up to 100 million spermatozoa
- Although only one spermatozoon can enter the ovum to fertilize it, large numbers of spermatozoa are ejaculated

– This helps ensure that one survives to achieve fertilization
– A spermatozoa count under 20 million per ml of semen usually is associated with sterility

● **Male sexual response**
  • In men, sexual response consists of penile erection and semen discharge
  • The penile erectile tissue consists of three cylinders composed of a spongy meshwork of endothelium-lined blood sinuses that are supplied by many arterioles and drained by veins
  • The erectile tissue cylinders, surrounded by fibrous capsules, are called *cavernous bodies*
  • The arterioles that supply the erectile tissue of the cavernous bodies are normally contracted
    – Little blood flows into the cavernous bodies
    – The sinusoids remain collapsed
  • Sexual excitement causes reflex dilation of the arterioles
    – This results from parasympathetic nerve stimulation and concomitant inhibition of sympathetic nerves, which normally constrict arterioles
    – The cavernous bodies become engorged with blood, and the veins that drain them become compressed, causing the penis to become rigid
    – The penis returns to the flaccid state as a result of parasympathetic nerve inhibition and sympathetic nerve stimulation
      · This causes the arterioles to constrict again
      · Excess blood drains from the cavernous bodies
  • Semen discharge involves a two-phase spinal reflex, consisting of *emission* and *ejaculation*
  • Emission refers to semen movement into the urethra
    – Emission occurs when the sympathetic nervous system transmits efferent impulses from the lumbar spinal cord
    – These impulses cause rhythmic contractions of the muscles near the epididymis, vas deferens, seminal vesicles, and prostate gland to expel semen into the urethra
  • Ejaculation is the pulsatile expulsion of semen from the penis
    – It's associated with erotic sensations called *orgasm*
    – Ejaculation occurs when efferent impulses from the sacral portion of the spinal cord cause rhythmic contractions of the muscles around the base of the penis
    – This intermittently compresses the urethra, causing semen to be expelled from the penis in spurts
  • During emission and ejaculation, the sphincter muscle at the base of the bladder constricts, preventing semen reflux into the bladder

Key facts about male sexual response

● Consists of penile erection and semen discharge

Penile erection
● During sexual excitement, cavernous bodies become engorged with blood
● Penis becomes rigid

Semen discharge
● Involves two-phase spinal reflex
● Emission occurs when semen moves into urethra
● Ejaculation is the expulsion of semen from the penis

- The two-phase spinal reflex occurs when impulses from the penis and genital region, other skin areas, and cerebral cortex reach a critical level of intensity

● **Developmental considerations**
- Before *puberty,* trace amounts of sex hormones produced by the gonads are sufficient to suppress production of gonadotropin-releasing hormones by the hypothalamus
- At puberty, the hypothalamus matures and loses its extreme sensitivity to the inhibitory effect of low sex hormone levels
- Then the hypothalamus begins to release gonadotropin-releasing hormones, which cause the release of pituitary FSH and LH; these hormones then stimulate the gonads to release sex hormones (testosterone in men; estrogen and progesterone in women)
- Sex hormones induce sexual development and other body changes characteristic of sexual maturity; production of mature spermatozoa marks puberty in males
- With age, testosterone secretion slowly declines
  - This may lead to reduced sex drive
  - Spermatogenesis may also be somewhat reduced

FEMALE REPRODUCTIVE SYSTEM

● **Key concepts**
- The female reproductive system includes the ovaries, fallopian tubes, uterus, vagina, external genitalia, and mammary glands (see *Structures of the female reproductive system*)
- The role of the female reproductive system is to produce gametes (ova) and nurture a developing embryo
- The normal menstrual cycle prepares the endometrium to receive the fertilized ovum
- If fertilization doesn't occur, the prepared endometrium is discarded through menstruation and a new cycle starts

● **Structures**
- The female reproductive system includes external and internal genitalia and the mammary glands
- External genitalia, or *vulva,* include the mons pubis, labia majora, labia minora, clitoris, and vestibule
  - The *mons pubis* is a cushion of adipose and loose connective tissue over the symphysis pubis
  - The *labia majora* are twin folds of adipose and connective tissue that run from the mons pubis to the perineum
  - The *labia minora* are twin folds of connective tissue between the labia majora

Structures of the female reproductive system

The female reproductive system includes the vagina, cervix, uterus, fallopian tubes, ovaries, and other structures, as illustrated here.

VIEW OF EXTERNAL GENITALIA IN LITHOTOMY POSITION

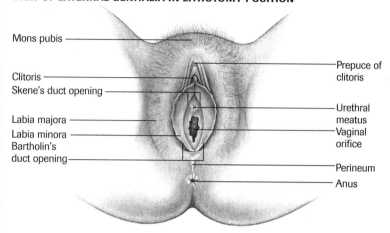

Mons pubis
Clitoris
Skene's duct opening
Labia majora
Labia minora
Bartholin's duct opening
Prepuce of clitoris
Urethral meatus
Vaginal orifice
Perineum
Anus

LATERAL VIEW OF INTERNAL GENITALIA

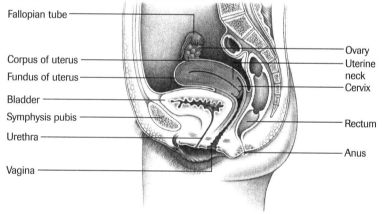

Fallopian tube
Corpus of uterus
Fundus of uterus
Bladder
Symphysis pubis
Urethra
Vagina
Ovary
Uterine neck
Cervix
Rectum
Anus

ANTERIOR CROSS-SECTIONAL VIEW OF INTERNAL GENITALIA

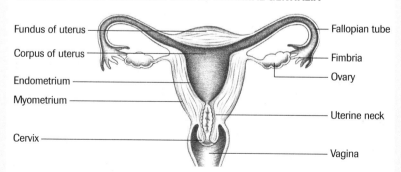

Fundus of uterus
Corpus of uterus
Endometrium
Myometrium
Cervix
Fallopian tube
Fimbria
Ovary
Uterine neck
Vagina

- – Similar to the penis, the *clitoris* is composed of erectile tissue; it's surrounded by mucosal folds (prepuce of the clitoris)
- – The *vestibule* is an oval-shaped structure surrounded by the clitoris and labia
  - · Several internal structures open into the vestibule, including the urethra, vagina, and ducts from Skene's and Bartholin's glands
  - · These structures secrete lubricating substances during intercourse
- Internal genitalia include the vagina, cervix, uterus, fallopian tubes, and ovaries
  - – The *vagina* is a fibromuscular tube that extends from the vestibule to the cervix
    - · It serves as a passageway for menstrual flow and as the receptacle for the penis during intercourse
    - · It also is the lower part of the birth canal
  - – The *cervix* is the narrow inferior portion of the uterus; it projects into the upper end of the vagina
  - – The *uterus,* a pear-shaped structure with a thick muscular wall, is designed to receive a fertilized ovum and support fetal development
    - · The organ is lined by a glandular mucous membrane (endometrium)
    - · It's held in position by bands of connective tissue called *ligaments*
  - – The *fallopian tubes* extend laterally from the upper corners of the uterus
    - · These tubes transport ova from the ovaries to the uterus
    - · The fringed (fimbriated) ends partially surround the adjacent ovaries
  - – The *ovaries* are the female gonads; they produce ova
- The *mammary glands,* located in the breasts, are specialized accessory glands that secrete milk
  - – Each mammary gland contains 15 to 25 lobes
  - – Lobes are separated by fibrous connective tissue and fat (see *The female breast*)
  - – Alveolar glands within the lobes produce milk during lactation
  - – Milk passes through excretory (lactiferous) ducts to the outside of the nipple

● **Menstrual cycle hormones**
- Pituitary and ovarian hormones induce cyclic changes in the endometrium that are responsible for the menstrual cycle (See *Events in the female reproductive cycle,* pages 376 and 377)

The female breast

The breasts are located on either side of the anterior chest wall over the greater pectoral and the anterior serratus muscles. Within the areola—the pigmented area in the center of the breast—lies the nipple. Erectile tissue in the nipple responds to cold, friction, and sexual stimulation.

SUPPORT AND SEPARATE

Each breast is composed of glandular, fibrous, and adipose tissue. Glandular tissue contains 15 to 20 lobes made up of clustered acini, tiny saclike duct terminals that secrete milk. Fibrous *Cooper's ligaments* support the breasts; adipose tissue surrounds each breast.

PRODUCE AND DRAIN

Acini draw the ingredients needed to produce milk from the blood in surrounding capillaries.

Sebaceous glands on the areolar surface, called *Montgomery's tubercles*, produce sebum, which lubricates the areolae and nipples during breast-feeding.

Key facts about the female breast

- Composed of glandular tissue separated by fibrous connective tissue and fat
- Each breast contains 15 to 25 lobes that secrete milk
- Sebaceous glands on areolar surface lubricate the nipples during breast-feeding

LATERAL CROSS SECTION

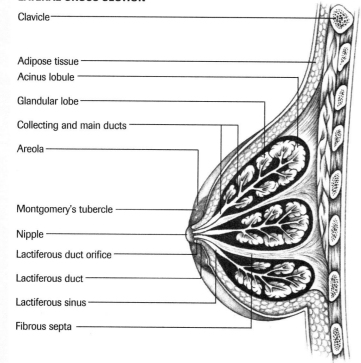

- Clavicle
- Adipose tissue
- Acinus lobule
- Glandular lobe
- Collecting and main ducts
- Areola
- Montgomery's tubercle
- Nipple
- Lactiferous duct orifice
- Lactiferous duct
- Lactiferous sinus
- Fibrous septa

- These hormones also produce less pronounced cyclic changes in the breasts, fallopian tubes, and cervical mucosa
- The pituitary hormones FSH and LH are secreted cyclically in women

Key events in the female reproductive cycle

- Cycle usually lasts 28 days
- Three major types of changes are ovulatory, hormonal, and endometrial
- Changes occur simultaneously
- Influential hormones include GnRH, FSH, LH, estrogen, and progesterone

Events in the female reproductive cycle

The female reproductive cycle usually lasts 28 days. During this cycle, three major types of changes occur simultaneously: ovulatory, hormonal, and endometrial (involving the lining [endometrium] of the uterus).

OVULATORY

- Ovulatory changes begin on the first day of the menstrual cycle.
- As the cycle begins, low estrogen and progesterone levels in the bloodstream stimulate the hypothalamus to secrete gonadotropin-stimulating hormone (GnRH). In turn, GnRH stimulates the anterior pituitary gland to secrete follicle-stimulating hormone (FSH) and luteinizing hormone (LH).
- Follicle development within the ovary (in the follicular phase) is spurred by increased levels of FSH and, to a lesser extent, LH.
- When the follicle matures, a spike in the LH level occurs, causing the follicle to rupture and release the ovum, thus initiating ovulation.
- After ovulation (in the luteal phase), the collapsed follicle forms the corpus luteum, which (if fertilization doesn't occur) degenerates.

HORMONAL

- During the follicular phase of the ovarian cycle, the increasing FSH and LH levels that stimulate follicle growth also stimulate increased secretion of estrogen.
- Estrogen secretion peaks just before ovulation. This peak sets in motion the spike in LH levels, which causes ovulation.

- After ovulation, estrogen levels decline rapidly. In the luteal phase of the ovarian cycle, the corpus luteum is formed and begins to release progesterone and estrogen.
- As the corpus luteum degenerates, levels of both of these ovarian hormones decline.

ENDOMETRIAL

- The endometrium is receptive to implantation of an embryo for only a short time in the reproductive cycle. Thus, it's no accident that the endometrium is most receptive about 7 days after the initiation of ovulation— just in time to receive a fertilized ovum.
- In the first 5 days of the reproductive cycle, the endometrium sheds its functional layer, leaving the basal layer (the deepest layer) intact. Menstrual flow consists of this detached layer and accompanying blood from the detachment process.
- The endometrium begins regenerating its functional layer at about day 6 (the proliferative phase), spurred by rising estrogen levels.
- After ovulation (about day 14), increased progesterone secretion stimulates conversion of the functional layer into a secretory mucosa (secretory phase), which is more receptive to implantation of the fertilized ovum.
- If implantation doesn't occur, the corpus luteum degenerates, progesterone levels drop, and the endometrium again sheds its functional layer.

– FSH stimulates the ovarian follicles to grow and secrete estrogen
– LH acts with FSH to promote follicle maturation
  · Under the influence of FSH and LH, a follicle develops and discharges its ovum; this action marks ovulation

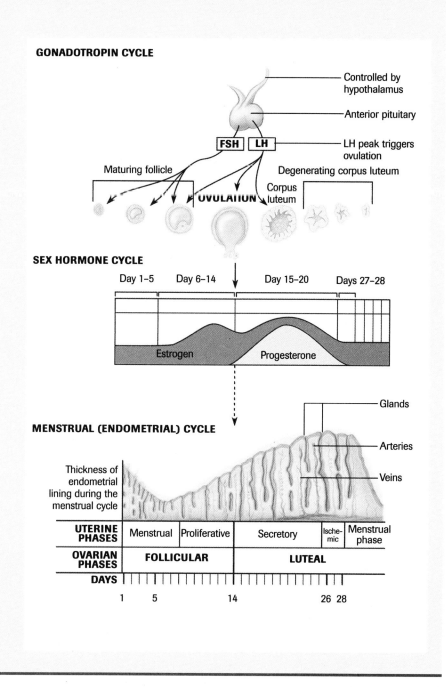

GONADOTROPIN CYCLE

Controlled by hypothalamus

Anterior pituitary

FSH   LH

LH peak triggers ovulation

Maturing follicle

Degenerating corpus luteum

OVULATION

Corpus luteum

SEX HORMONE CYCLE

Day 1–5   Day 6–14   Day 15–20   Days 27–28

Estrogen   Progesterone

MENSTRUAL (ENDOMETRIAL) CYCLE

Glands

Arteries

Veins

Thickness of endometrial lining during the menstrual cycle

UTERINE PHASES	Menstrual	Proliferative	Secretory	Ische-mic	Menstrual phase
OVARIAN PHASES	FOLLICULAR		LUTEAL		
DAYS					

1   5   14   26 28

- Then LH causes the ruptured follicle to change into a large convoluted yellow structure called the *corpus luteum,* which produces the steroid hormones estrogen and progesterone
- Under the influence of FSH and LH, the ovary secretes estrogen and progesterone

- The estrogen secreted by the ovaries exerts several effects
  - It induces sexual development at puberty, including proliferation of glandular tissue of the breasts
  - It stimulates endometrial growth during the first half (proliferative phase) of the menstrual cycle
  - It also stimulates the glandular epithelium of the cervix to secrete a thin, alkaline mucus that facilitates spermatozoa passage into the uterus and fallopian tubes
  - It causes general metabolic effects such as stimulation of bone growth
- Progesterone, secreted by the corpus luteum, produces several effects
  - It induces marked secretory activity in the endometrial glands during the second half (secretory phase) of the menstrual cycle, preparing the endometrium for implantation of the fertilized ovum
  - It increases cervical mucus thickness and viscosity, making it relatively resistant to spermatozoa penetration during the postovulatory phase
  - It causes breast development
- Pituitary (gonadotropic) and ovarian hormones have a reciprocal relationship
  - A high estrogen level inhibits FSH output, stabilizing the estrogen level
  - A high estrogen level also stimulates LH release, which increases progesterone output
  - A high progesterone level inhibits LH output

● Oogenesis

- *Oogenesis* is the process of ova formation
- Precursors of the ova, or *oogonia*, proliferate by mitosis in the fetal ovaries before birth; they form primary oocytes (with 46 chromosomes)
- Then a single layer of granulosa or follicular cells surrounds the oocytes, forming structures called *primary follicles*
  - Primary oocytes in the primary follicles enter the prophase of the first meiotic division during fetal development, but they don't continue to divide
  - A very large number of primary follicles form
    · A 5-month-old female fetus may have 7 million ova
    · By birth, only about 2 million ova remain
    · By puberty, about 300,000 to 400,000 remain
    · However, fewer than 500 ova are released in a lifetime
    · Only a few of those released are fertilized

Key facts about oogenesis

- A large number of primary follicles are present at birth
- The primary follicles remain inactive until puberty
- During each menstrual cycle, many follicles grow but one matures and is ovulated
- The oocyte completes its first meiotic division at ovulation
- The secondary oocyte doesn't complete its second meiotic division unless it's fertilized

- The primary follicles remain inactive until puberty, when cyclic ovulation begins under the influence of FSH and LH
- During each menstrual cycle, primary follicles begin to grow in the ovary, but normally only one matures and is ovulated
  - The granulosa cells around the follicles proliferate, and a layer of noncellular material called the *zona pellucida* is deposited on the surface of the oocyte
  - Fluid begins to accumulate in the layer of granulosa cells; a central fluid-filled cavity forms in the mature or graafian follicle
- About the time the oocyte is released at ovulation, it completes its first meiotic division, giving rise to two daughter cells—a secondary oocyte and the first polar body, which are of unequal size
  - The secondary oocyte contains half the chromosomes (23) and almost all the cytoplasm
  - The first polar body contains the remaining 23 chromosomes but almost no cytoplasm
- The newly formed secondary oocyte begins its second meiotic division, but it doesn't complete this division unless it's fertilized
  - Completion of the second division gives rise to a mature ovum and a second polar body, each containing 23 chromosomes
  - Whether fertilization occurs, the first polar body immediately undergoes a second meiotic division, giving rise to two additional haploid polar bodies (for a total of three), which degenerate
  - The ovum can survive for about 3 days after ovulation; however, it can only be fertilized successfully for about 36 hours after ovulation
- The ovum is swept into the fimbria of the fallopian tube by the beating of cilia that cover the tubal epithelium; it's then propelled down the fallopian tube by the cilia and by peristaltic contractions of smooth muscle in the wall of the tube
- Ova released late in a woman's reproductive life may have been arrested in prophase for up to 45 years before resuming meiosis at ovulation; this may explain the high incidence of congenital abnormalities related to abnormal chromosome separation in the offspring of older women

- **Menstrual cycle**
  - Customarily, the cycle begins on the first day of menstrual flow
  - Ovulation occurs around the middle of the cycle, dividing it into preovulatory (follicular) and postovulatory (luteal) phases
  - Menstrual cycle duration varies considerably among individuals; it may also vary somewhat from month to month in the same individual

Key facts about the menstrual cycle

- Ovulation occurs midcycle
- During preovulatory phase, FSH stimulates ovarian follicles to grow
- A surge of LH triggers ovulation
- In the postovulatory phase, the corpus luteum secretes estrogen and progesterone
- The corpus luteum degenerates if fertilization doesn't occur

- Variations usually result from differences in the preovulatory phase duration
- The duration of the postovulatory phase remains relatively constant, at about 14 days
- During the preovulatory phase, the pituitary gland begins to release FSH, which stimulates a group of ovarian follicles to grow
  - The first follicle to respond grows more rapidly and comes to full maturity
  - The other follicles undergo involution (atrophy)
- Soon after FSH output rises, LH output begins to increase; together FSH and LH promote estrogen secretion by the ovarian follicles
- The increasing estrogen output inhibits further FSH release and stimulates LH release
  - LH release eventually builds to a precipitous outpouring called the *LH surge,* which persists for about 24 hours
  - This surge leads to rupture of the follicle and ovulation
- The postovulatory phase is characterized by conversion of the ruptured follicle into a corpus luteum, which produces estrogen and progesterone
- The corpus luteum reaches maturity about 8 to 9 days after ovulation; then it begins to degenerate if pregnancy hasn't occurred
- Menstruation results from the decline in corpus luteum activity, which reduces estrogen and progesterone output
  - Eventually, the levels of these two hormones can't maintain the endometrium and the endometrium is shed, producing the menstrual flow
  - Menstruation lasts about 5 days; it's associated with an average total blood loss of 50 to 150 ml
  - Endometrial tissue occurring outside the uterine cavity leads to endometriosis, causing painful adhesions and infertility (see *Teaching a patient with endometriosis*)
- As estrogen and progesterone levels fall, their inhibitory effects on FSH and LH release also decline
- Eventually, when estrogen and progesterone have fallen to low levels, FSH and LH are released again and a new cycle begins

Female sexual response
- The physiologic effects of sexual excitement in women are similar to those in men
- The parasympathetic nervous system controls the dilation of arterioles that supply the erectile tissue in the clitoris and labia minora
  - During sexual excitement, nerve impulse transmission causes the tissues to become engorged with blood

TIME-OUT FOR TEACHING

Teaching a patient with endometriosis

Make sure you teach a patient with endometriosis:
- the disease process, including signs and symptoms (such as dysmenorrhea)
- possible complications (such as chronic pelvic pain and infertility)
- diagnostic tests (such as laparoscopy) that may be ordered
- prescribed treatments, including hormone therapy (androgens, progestins and hormonal contraceptives, and gonadotropin-releasing hormone agonists) and surgery (to rule out cancer or hysterectomy for women who aren't considering childbirth)
- the importance of an annual pelvic examination and Papanicolaou test
- methods to improve fertility (such as not postponing childbearing)
- the need to avoid minor gynecological procedures immediately before and during menstruation
- additional sources of information and support.

- Parasympathetic impulses also cause Skene's and Bartholin's glands to produce secretions that lubricate the vagina during intercourse
- Sensory input from nerve endings in the clitoris, labia, vaginal orifice, and perineal tissues is transmitted to the lumbar and sacral spinal cord
- When this input reaches a critical level, a spinal reflex response occurs, characterized by rhythmic contractions of the uterus and fallopian tubes; these contractions, together with rhythmic and pulsatile contractions of the skeletal muscles around the vagina, constitute the erotic sensations called *orgasm*
- Female sexual climax differs from male climax; it produces no secretions comparable to the ejaculate and isn't required to achieve fertilization

Developmental considerations
- The hypothalamus and pituitary gland perform the same actions to achieve puberty in females as in males; however, the release of pituitary FSH and LH stimulates the gonads to release estrogen and progesterone in females
- These sex hormones induce sexual development and other body changes characteristic of sexual maturity, including menarche in females

TOP 8

Items to study for your next test on the reproductive system

1. Structures and functions of the male and female reproductive systems
2. Male and female reproductive hormones
3. Events of the menstrual cycle
4. Process of spermatogenesis
5. Process of oogenesis
6. Male and female developmental considerations
7. Events occurring during male and female sexual response
8. Teaching tips for patients with endometriosis

- With age, women's ovarian follicles degenerate without producing mature egg cells
  - Mature egg cell production declines until about age 45, when few follicles remain
  - The ovaries no longer respond to FSH and LH stimulation and stop producing sex hormones
  - When the ovaries no longer can produce sufficient hormones to stimulate cyclic changes in the endometrium, menstruation ceases; this condition is called menopause
  - A woman is considered to have reached menopause after menses are absent for 1 year
  - Ovulation usually ceases 1 to 2 years before menopause

NCLEX CHECKS

It's never too soon to begin your NCLEX preparation. Now that you've reviewed this chapter, carefully read each of the following questions and choose the best answer. Then compare your responses with the correct answers.

1. While teaching a class on sexual health to adolescents, the nurse tells the students that the scrotum contains which structure?
- ☐ **1.** Testes
- ☐ **2.** Vas deferens
- ☐ **3.** Prostate gland
- ☐ **4.** Seminal vesicles

2. During a class on male reproduction, the nurse identifies which hormone as the principal regulator of male sexual drive?
- ☐ **1.** FSH
- ☐ **2.** LH
- ☐ **3.** Testosterone
- ☐ **4.** Inhibin

3. A couple is undergoing diagnostic testing for infertility. The nurse is aware that sterility is indicated by which value?
- ☐ **1.** 100,000,000 per ml of semen
- ☐ **2.** 80,000,000 per ml of semen
- ☐ **3.** 50,000,000 per ml of semen
- ☐ **4.** 10,000,000 per ml of semen

4. The nurse is caring for a client with menstrual irregularities and explains that the menstrual cycle is influenced by which hormones? Select all that apply.

☐ **1.** Testosterone
☐ **2.** LH
☐ **3.** Progesterone
☐ **4.** Gonadotropin-stimulating hormone
☐ **5.** Estrogen
☐ **6.** FSH

5. Which information should the nurse include in a teaching plan for a client with endometriosis?
☐ **1.** It's important to delay childbearing.
☐ **2.** It's important to avoid Papanicolaou tests.
☐ **3.** Infertility is a possible complication.
☐ **4.** Avoiding gynecologic procedures after menstruation is imperative.

6. The nurse discusses the reproductive cycle with a client who wants to become pregnant. Which hormone is responsible for ovulation?
☐ **1.** FSH
☐ **2.** LH
☐ **3.** Estrogen
☐ **4.** Progesterone

7. The nurse tells a client who's trying to become pregnant that the optimum time for fertilization is when?
☐ **1.** Just prior to ovulation
☐ **2.** On the day of ovulation
☐ **3.** Within 36 hours of ovulation
☐ **4.** Up to 72 hours after ovulation

8. The nurse is documenting the history of a client who thinks she may be pregnant and asks the client for the date of her last menstrual cycle. The nurse understands that the menstrual cycle begins on which day?
☐ **1.** The last day of menstrual flow
☐ **2.** The first day of menstrual flow
☐ **3.** The day ovulation occurs
☐ **4.** The day the corpus luteum reaches maturity

9. The nurse explains to a client who wants to become pregnant that fertilization occurs when?
☐ **1.** 2 to 3 days after the initiation of ovulation
☐ **2.** 4 to 6 days after the initiation of ovulation
☐ **3.** About 7 days after the initiation of ovulation
☐ **4.** Just before ovulation

10. The nurse discusses menopausal symptoms with a 47-year-old woman. When does menopause occur?

☐ **1.** When FSH and LH are no longer secreted
☐ **2.** When menses have been absent for 6 months
☐ **3.** When menses have been absent for 1 year
☐ **4.** When ovulation no longer occurs

ANSWERS AND RATIONALES

1. CORRECT ANSWER: 1
The testes are located in the scrotum. The vas deferens is a part of the duct system that moves spermatozoa from the testes to outside the body. The vas deferens extends to the prostate gland and joins the seminal vesicles to form the ejaculatory duct, which empties into the urethra.

2. CORRECT ANSWER: 3
Testosterone is responsible for sexual drive, development of secondary sex characteristics, and growth in males. FSH and LH regulate testicular function in males. Inhibin, a hormone secreted by Sertoli cells, inhibits the production of FSH by the pituitary.

3. CORRECT ANSWER: 4
Normally, 1 ml of semen contains up to 100,000,000 spermatozoa. A spermatozoa count under 20,000,000 per ml of semen is usually associated with sterility.

4. CORRECT ANSWER: 2, 3, 5, 6
The four hormones involved in the menstrual cycle are LH, progesterone, estrogen, and FSH. Testosterone is responsible for sexual drive and development of secondary sex characteristics in males. Gonadotropin-stimulating hormone is secreted by the hypothalamus and stimulates the anterior pituitary gland to secrete LH and FSH.

5. CORRECT ANSWER: 3
A woman with endometriosis should be taught that infertility is a possible complication of this disorder and, therefore, childbearing shouldn't be delayed. A pelvic examination and Papanicolaou test should be performed annually to detect complications and cancer. Minor gynecologic procedures should be avoided immediately before and during menstruation to reduce complications.

6. CORRECT ANSWER: 2
Estrogen secretion peaks just before ovulation, setting in motion the spike of LH levels that causes ovulation. After ovulation, estrogen levels decline rapidly. During the follicular phase of the ovarian cycle, the increasing FSH and LH levels stimulate follicle growth. In the luteal phase

of the ovarian cycle, the corpus luteum is formed and begins to release progesterone and estrogen.

7. CORRECT ANSWER: 3
The ovum can survive for about 3 days after ovulation; however, it can only be fertilized successfully for about 36 hours after ovulation.

8. CORRECT ANSWER: 2
The menstrual cycle begins on the first day of menstrual flow. Menstruation lasts about 5 days. Ovulation occurs approximately 14 days after the cycle starts. The corpus luteum reaches maturity about 8 to 9 days after ovulation.

9. CORRECT ANSWER: 3
The endometrium is receptive to implantation of an embryo for only a short time in the reproductive cycle, about 7 days after the initiation of ovulation.

10. CORRECT ANSWER: 3
A women reaches menopause when menses have been absent for 1 year. The pituitary gland still releases FSH and LH, but the ovaries no longer respond to these hormones. Ovulation usually ceases 1 to 2 years before menopause.

20

Reproduction and lactation

LEARNING OBJECTIVES

After studying this chapter, you should be able to:

● Describe the process of fertilization.

● Identify the changes that occur during pregnancy.

● Explain the events that occur in each stage of labor.

● Discuss postpartal adaptations that occur in the infant and mother.

● Understand the role of hormones in lactation.

CHAPTER OVERVIEW

Through the process of fertilization, a new being is formed. In order for fertilization to occur, a series of events that must be perfectly timed takes place. Following fertilization, the fetus develops in an amazing process that ends in delivery of a newborn. Changes occur in both the mother and newborn that allow the newborn to continue to develop and grow. The nurse must understand this complex series of events to provide optimal care. This chapter reviews fertilization, pregnancy, labor and postpartal adaptation, and lactation.

FERTILIZATION

- **Key concepts**
  - Fertilization is the union of a spermatozoon and an ovum (see *Fertilization*, page 388)
  - Fertilization occurs only when several basic prerequisites are met
    - Spermatozoa must be adequate in function and number
    - A mature ovum must be available and ready to be fertilized
    - Spermatozoa must be transported effectively through the female reproductive tract
  - Any structural or functional problem that interferes with these prerequisites can lead to infertility (see *Teaching a patient with infertility*, page 389)

- **Spermatozoa transport**
  - Spermatozoa move through the female reproductive tract by two mechanisms
    - Spermatozoa travel several millimeters per hour by flagellar propulsion
    - They're transported up into the uterus and fallopian tubes by rhythmic contractions of uterine muscles
  - Although several hundred million spermatozoa are deposited by a single ejaculation, many are destroyed by the acidity of vaginal secretions
  - Only the spermatozoa that enter the cervical canal, where they are protected by cervical mucus, can survive
  - The ease with which spermatozoa can penetrate cervical mucus is related to the menstrual cycle phase
    - Early in the cycle, spermatozoa have difficulty passing through the cervix because estrogen and progesterone levels cause the mucus to thicken
    - Midcycle, spermatozoa can pass readily through the cervix because the mucus is relatively thin
    - Later in the cycle, spermatozoa have difficulty passing through the cervix because the mucus is much thicker
  - After passing through the mucus, spermatozoa enter the uterus
    - Only spermatozoa (not seminal fluid) enter the uterus and fallopian tubes
    - Uterine contractions help spermatozoa ascend into the fallopian tubes
  - Spermatozoa can probably fertilize the ovum for up to 2 days after ejaculation, although they may survive for 3 to 4 days in the reproductive tract

Key facts about fertilization
- To occur, spermatozoa must be adequate in number and function
- A mature ovum must be available
- Spermatozoa must be transported effectively through the female reproductive tract

Key facts about spermatozoa transport
- All move by flagellar propulsion and uterine contractions
- Many are destroyed by vaginal secretions
- Only those reaching the cervical canal survive

Relationship between menstrual cycle and sperma survival
- Early in the cycle, cervical mucus is thick and impairs passage by spermatozoa
- Midcycle, mucus thins and spermatozoa can pass through readily
- Later in the cycle, mucus becomes much thicker and impairs passage

Steps in fertilization

- Spermatozoon approaches the ovum
- Spermatozoon penetrates the zona pellucida
- Ovum's second meiotic division occurs and it becomes impenetrable to other sperm
- Acrosome on sperm releases enzymes to aid penetration
- Upon penetration, sperm releases its nucleus into the ovum and its head fuses with the ovum's nucleus

GO WITH THE FLOW

Fertilization

Fertilization begins when a spermatozoon is activated upon contact with the ovum. Here's what happens.

1. The spermatozoon, which has a covering called the *acrosome,* approaches the ovum.

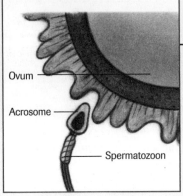

Ovum

Acrosome

Spermatozoon

2. The spermatozoon then penetrates the zona pellucida (the ovum's inner membrane). This triggers the ovum's second meiotic division (following meiosis), making the zona pellucida impenetrable to other spermatozoa.

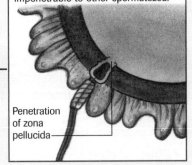

Penetration of zona pellucida

3. The acrosome develops small perforations through which it releases enzymes necessary for the sperm to penetrate the protective layers of the ovum before fertilization.

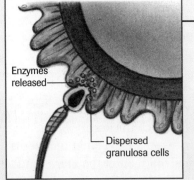

Enzymes released

Dispersed granulosa cells

4. After the spermatozoon penetrates the ovum, its nucleus is released into the ovum, its tail degenerates, and its head enlarges and fuses with the ovum's nucleus. This fusion provides the fertilized ovum, called a *zygote,* with 46 chromosomes.

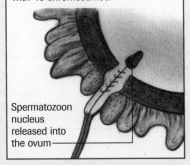

Spermatozoon nucleus released into the ovum

TIME-OUT FOR TEACHING

Teaching a patient with infertility

Make sure you teach a patient who's infertile:

- what infertility means and why it occurs (such as ovulatory dysfunction, structural abnormalities, or inadequate spermatozoa production)
- which diagnostic tests (such as semen analysis and laparoscopy) to anticipate
- recommended treatment options (such as fertility drugs that alter hormone levels)
- alternative techniques for becoming pregnant (such as in vitro fertilization and artificial insemination)
- surgical options to promote fertility (such as varicocelectomy and laparotomy)
- the benefits of psychological counseling and how to get help
- additional sources of information and support.

Ovum fertilization

- Fertilization normally occurs in the distal part of the fallopian tube
- The ovum remains viable for 24 to 36 hours, and spermatozoa remain viable for 48 hours or more; intercourse must occur around the time of ovulation for fertilization to occur
- Before a spermatozoon can penetrate the ovum, it must disperse the granulosa cells and penetrate the zona pellucida; enzymes in its acrosome allow this penetration
- After the spermatozoon has penetrated, the ovum completes its second meiotic division
- The zona pellucida then becomes impermeable to other spermatozoa
- The spermatozoon head fuses with the ovum nucleus, forming a cell nucleus with 46 chromosomes
- The fertilized ovum is called a *zygote*

PREGNANCY

Key concepts

- Pregnancy begins with fertilization and ends with childbirth; this time period (also called *gestation*) averages 38 weeks
  - Various structures develop as a result of pregnancy, such as the *decidua, amniotic sac and fluid, yolk sac,* and *placenta*
  - The zygote undergoes a complex sequence of *pre-embryonic, embryonic,* and *fetal development,* finally producing a full-term fetus

- Because the exact date of fertilization is usually unknown, the expected delivery date may be calculated from the beginning of the last menstrual period (LMP)
  - The length of gestation calculated from the LMP is 40 weeks—not 38 weeks—because the first day of the LMP occurs about 2 weeks before ovulation
  - Gestation length calculated from LMP may be expressed as 280 days, as 10 lunar (28-day) months, or as 9 calendar (31-day) months
- A 9-calendar-month gestation may be subdivided into three periods of 3 months, or *trimesters*
- Because the uterus grows throughout pregnancy, uterine size provides a rough estimate of the duration of pregnancy

● **Structural development**
- Pregnancy changes the usual development of the *corpus luteum*
  - Placental tissue secretes large amounts of human chorionic gonadotropin (HCG), which is similar to luteinizing hormone (LH) and follicle-stimulating hormone (FSH)
    · HCG prevents corpus luteum degeneration
    · It stimulates the corpus luteum to produce large amounts of estrogen and progesterone
  - During the first 3 months of pregnancy, the corpus luteum serves as the main source of estrogen and progesterone; these hormones are needed during pregnancy
  - Later in pregnancy, the placenta produces most of the hormones; although it persists, the corpus luteum is no longer needed to maintain the pregnancy
- The *decidua* covers the chorionic vesicle and eventually becomes part of the placenta
  - The decidua is the endometrial lining that has undergone the hormone-induced changes of pregnancy
  - It envelops the embryo and fetus during gestation
  - Decidual cells secrete three substances
    · The hormone prolactin promotes lactation
    · The hormone relaxin relaxes the connective tissue of the symphysis pubis and pelvic ligaments and facilitates cervical dilation
    · Prostaglandin mediates several physiologic functions
- The *amniotic sac* completely surrounds the developing embryo and fuses with the chorion, usually by 8 weeks' gestation
  - The fused amnion and chorion extend from the placental margins to form the fluid-filled amniotic sac
  - The amniotic sac gradually increases in size and ruptures at the time of delivery

- The amniotic sac and its fluid have two important functions
  - During gestation, they protect the fetus by creating a buoyant temperature-controlled environment
  - During childbirth, they form a fluid wedge that helps open the cervix
- Amniotic fluid source and volume vary with the gestational stage
  - Early in pregnancy, amniotic fluid is derived chiefly from maternal and fetal blood and from fluid from the fetal skin and respiratory tract
  - Later in pregnancy, fetal urine becomes the major source of amniotic fluid
  - Maternal and fetal blood filtration and fetal urine excretion continually add to the total amniotic fluid volume
- The *yolk sac* forms adjacent to the endoderm of the germ disc
  - Part of the yolk sac is incorporated in the developing embryo and forms the GI tract
  - Another part of the yolk sac gives rise to primitive germ cells, which migrate to the developing gonads and eventually form oocytes or spermatocytes
  - The yolk sac also forms blood cells during early embryonic development
  - The yolk sac never contains yolk and has no nutritive function; it eventually atrophies and disintegrates
- The *placenta* supplies nutrients to and removes wastes from the fetus from the 3rd month of pregnancy until childbirth
  - It's a flattened, disc-shaped structure that weighs about 18 ounces (500 grams) at delivery
  - The placenta forms from the chorion (and its chorionic villi) and the part of the decidua in which the villi are anchored
  - The umbilical cord connects the fetus to the placenta; the cord contains two arteries and one vein (see *The placenta,* page 392)
    - The arteries that carry blood from the fetus to the placenta follow a spiral course on the cord, divide on the placental surface, and send branches to the chorionic villi
    - Large veins on the placental surface collect blood returning from the villi; these veins join to form the single umbilical vein that enters the cord and returns blood to the fetus
  - The placenta has two circulatory systems
    - The *uteroplacental circulation* delivers oxygenated arterial blood from the maternal circulation to the intervillous spaces (large spaces between the chorionic villi in the placenta)

Key functions of the yolk sac

- Forms the GI tract in the embryo
- Gives rise to cells that migrate to developing gonads to form oocytes or spermatocytes
- Forms blood cells during early development

Key characteristics of the placenta

- Forms from the chorion and part of the villi
- Umbilical cord connects the fetus to the placenta
- Umbilical cord contains two arteries (to carry blood from the fetus to the placenta) and one vein (to collect blood from the villi and return it to the fetus)

The placenta

At term, the placenta (the spongy structure within the uterus from which the fetus derives nourishment) is flat, pancakelike, and round or oval. It measures 6" to 7¾" (15 to 20 cm) in diameter and ¾" to 1¼" (2 to 3 cm) in breadth at its thickest part. The maternal side is lobulated; the fetal side is shiny.

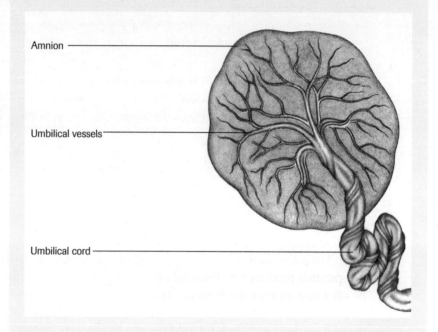

Amnion

Umbilical vessels

Umbilical cord

- Blood spurts into the intervillous spaces from many uterine arteries that penetrate the basal part of the placenta
- Blood leaves the intervillous spaces and flows back into the maternal circulation through veins that penetrate the basal part of the placenta near arteries
- The *fetoplacental circulation* delivers oxygen-depleted blood from the fetus to the chorionic villi
  - Blood travels to the chorionic villi by way of the two umbilical arteries
  - Oxygenated blood returns to the fetus by the single umbilical vein
- Although the maternal and fetal circulations exchange oxygen, nutrients, and wastes, fetal and maternal blood don't mix
- The placenta produces several peptide and steroid hormones
  - The peptide hormone *HCG* (detected as early as 9 days after fertilization) increases and peaks at about 10 weeks' gestation, and then gradually declines

- HCG stimulates the corpus luteum to produce the estrogen and progesterone needed to maintain pregnancy until the placenta takes over hormone production
- Highly sensitive pregnancy tests can detect HCG in blood and urine even before the first missed menstrual period
· The level of the peptide hormone *human placental lactogen* (HPL) rises progressively throughout pregnancy
  - HPL stimulates maternal protein and fat metabolism to ensure an adequate supply of amino acids, minerals, and fatty acids for the mother and fetus
  - It antagonizes the action of insulin, decreasing maternal glucose metabolism and making more glucose available to the fetus
  - It also stimulates breast growth in preparation for *lactation*
· The steroid hormone *estrogen* increases uterine muscle irritability and contractility
  - The placenta produces three different estrogens, which differ chiefly in the number of hydroxyl groups
  - The placenta lacks some of the enzymes needed to complete estrogen synthesis; it requires some precursor compounds produced by the fetal adrenal glands
  - Because neither the fetus nor the placenta can synthesize estrogens independently, estrogen production reflects the functional activity of the fetus and placenta
· The steroid hormone *progesterone* reduces uterine muscle irritability
  - The placenta synthesizes this hormone from maternal cholesterol
  - The fetus plays no part in progesterone synthesis

Pre-embryonic development
• The first period of prenatal development (pre-embryonic development) begins with ovum fertilization and lasts 2 weeks (see *Pre-embryonic development,* page 394)
• The zygote undergoes a series of mitotic divisions, or cleavage, as it passes through the fallopian tube
• The first cell division is completed about 30 hours after fertilization; subsequent divisions occur in rapid succession
• The zygote is converted into a ball of cells called a *morula,* which reaches the uterus about 3 days after fertilization
• Fluid accumulates in the center of the morula, forming a central cavity; the structure now is called a *blastocyst*
• Blastocyst cells differentiate in two ways

Key facts about hormones produced by the placenta
● Peptide hormone HCG peaks at 10 weeks' gestation and then declines
● HCG stimulates corpus luteum to produce estrogen and progesterone to maintain pregnancy until placenta takes over
● Peptide hormone HPL rises throughout pregnancy
● HPL stimulates maternal protein and fat metabolism and antagonizes action of insulin
● Steroid hormone estrogen increases uterine muscle irritability and contractility
● Steroid hormone progesterone reduces uterine muscle irritability

Key facts about pre-embryonic development
● First period of development begins with fertilization and lasts 2 weeks
● First cell division is completed 30 hours after fertilization
● Subsequent divisions occur in rapid succession

Key phases in pre-embryonic development

- Fertilized ovum
- Zygote: undergoes division in fallopian tube
- Morula: ball of cells arising from zygote; reaches uterus 3 days after fertilization
- Blastocyst: forms when fluid accumulates in the center of the morula, forming a central cavity
- Trophoblast: forms from the peripheral rim of the blastocyst; gives rise to fetal membranes and contributes to placenta formation
- Inner cell mass: cell cluster in the trophoblast that forms the embryo
- Germ disc: develops from the inner cell mass; differentiates into ectoderm, mesoderm, and endoderm
- Ectoderm: contributes to the formation of the amniotic sac and the yolk sac
- Chorionic sac: develops from connective tissue lining the blastocyst cavity
- Chorionic villi: extend from the chorion and anchor the chorionic vesicle to the endometrium

Pre-embryonic development

The pre-embryonic phase lasts from conception until around the end of the second week of development.

ZYGOTE FORMS

As the fertilized ovum advances through the fallopian tube toward the uterus, it undergoes mitotic division, forming daughter cells (initially called *blastomeres*), each containing the same number of chromosomes as the parent cell. The first cell division ends about 30 hours after fertilization; subsequent divisions occur rapidly.

The *zygote*, as it's now called, develops into a small mass of cells called a *morula*, which reaches the uterus at or around the third day after fertilization. Fluid that amasses in the center of the morula forms a central cavity.

The structure is now called a *blastocyst*. The blastocyst consists of a thin trophoblast layer (which includes the blastocyst cavity), and the inner cell mass. The trophoblast develops into fetal membranes and the placenta. The inner cell mass later forms the embryo (late blastocyst).

BLASTOCYST AND ENDOMETRIUM ATTACH

During the next phase, the blastocyst stays within the zona pellucida, unattached to the uterus. The zona pellucida degenerates and, by the end of the first week after fertilization, the blastocyst attaches to the endometrium. The part of the blastocyst adjacent to the inner cell mass is the first part to become attached.

The trophoblast, in contact with the endometrial lining, proliferates and invades the underlying endometrium by separating and dissolving endometrial cells.

During the next week, the invading blastocyst sinks below the endometrium's surface. The penetration site seals, restoring the continuity of the endometrial surface.

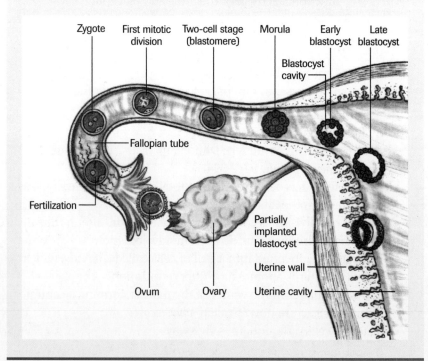

Zygote — First mitotic division — Two-cell stage (blastomere) — Morula — Early blastocyst — Late blastocyst — Blastocyst cavity — Fallopian tube — Fertilization — Ovum — Ovary — Partially implanted blastocyst — Uterine wall — Uterine cavity

- A peripheral rim of cells, called the *trophoblast,* develops; the trophoblast gives rise to the fetal membranes and contributes to placenta formation
  - A discrete cell cluster in the trophoblast, called the *inner cell mass,* eventually forms the embryo
- The blastocyst is enclosed in the zona pellucida and remains unattached to the uterus for several days
- The zona pellucida degenerates during the week after fertilization; this allows the blastocyst to attach to the endometrium and become implanted
- The inner cell mass becomes a flat structure, called the *germ disc*
- The germ disc differentiates into three germ layers: the *ectoderm, mesoderm,* and *endoderm* (see *Embryonic development,* page 396)
- A cleft appears between the ectoderm of the germ disc and the surrounding trophoblast, forming the amniotic sac
- The yolk sac forms on the opposite side of the germ disc
- A layer of connective tissue lines the enlarging blastocyst cavity and covers the amniotic and yolk sacs
  - At this point, the cavity contains the germ disc, amniotic sac, and yolk sac and is called the chorionic sac; its wall is called a *chorion*
  - The entire chorionic sac and embryo is called the *chorionic vesicle*
- Fingerlike columns of cells, called *chorionic villi,* extend from the chorion and anchor the chorionic vesicle to the endometrium (see *Development of the decidua and fetal membranes,* page 397)

● **Embryonic development**
- The embryonic period lasts from the fourth through the seventh week
- The developing zygote begins to assume a human shape and is called an *embryo*
- All the organ systems form during this period, making the embryo susceptible to injury by maternal drug use and other factors such as radiation
- Each germ layer forms specific tissues and structures
  - Ectoderm primarily forms the external covering of the embryo and the structures that will have contact with the environment
  - Mesoderm forms the circulatory system, muscles, supporting tissues, and most of the urinary and reproductive systems
  - Endoderm forms the internal linings of the embryo, such as the epithelial lining of the pharynx and respiratory and GI tracts

● **Fetal development**
- The fetal period extends from the eighth week until birth
- The fetus becomes larger and heavier as it matures, but it experiences no major changes in its basic structure

Key facts about embryonic development
- Lasts from fourth through seventh week
- The zygote assumes human shape and is called an *embryo*
- All organ systems form during this period

Key facts about fetal development
- Lasts from eighth week until birth
- The fetus grows larger and heavier but maintains basic structure
- Head is disproportionately large compared to rest of body
- Body lacks subcutaneous fat

Key facts about germ layers

- Ectoderm: outermost layer
- Mesoderm: middle layer
- Endoderm: innermost layer

Embryonic development

Each of the three germ layers—ectoderm, mesoderm, and endoderm—forms specific tissues and organs in the developing embryo.

ECTODERM

The ectoderm (outermost layer) develops into:
- the epidermis
- the nervous system
- the pituitary gland
- tooth enamel
- salivary glands
- optic lenses
- the lining of the lower portion of the anal canal
- hair.

MESODERM

The mesoderm (middle layer) develops into:
- connective and supporting tissue
- blood and the vascular system
- musculature
- teeth (except enamel)
- the mesothelial lining of the pericardial, pleural, and peritoneal cavities
- kidneys and ureters.

ENDODERM

The endoderm (innermost layer) becomes the epithelial lining of the:
- pharynx and trachea
- auditory canal
- alimentary canal
- liver
- pancreas
- bladder and urethra
- prostate.

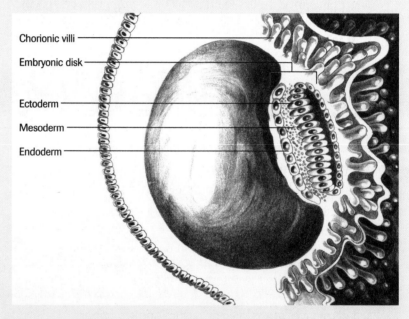

Chorionic villi

Embryonic disk

Ectoderm

Mesoderm

Endoderm

- The fetus displays two unusual features during early development
  - The head is disproportionately large compared to the rest of the body; this condition changes after birth as the infant grows
  - The body lacks subcutaneous fat; it fills out shortly before birth, when fat begins to accumulate

Development of the decidua and fetal membranes

Specialized tissues support, protect, and nurture the embryo and fetus throughout its development. Among these tissues, the decidua and fetal membranes begin to develop shortly after conception.

NESTING PLACE

During pregnancy, the endometrial lining is called the *decidua*. It provides a nesting place for the developing ovum and has some endocrine functions.

Based primarily on its position relative to the embryo (see illustration), the decidua may be known as the *decidua basalis,* which lies beneath the chorionic vesicle, the *decidua capsularis,* which stretches over the vesicle, or the *decidua parietalis,* which lines the rest of the endometrial cavity.

NETWORK OF BLOOD VESSELS

The chorion is a membrane that forms the outer wall of the blastocyst. Vascular projections, called *chorionic villi,* arise from its periphery. As the chorionic vesicle enlarges, villi arising from the superficial portion of the chorion, called the *chorion laeve,* atrophy, leaving this surface smooth. Villi arising from the deeper part of the chorion, called the *chorion frondosum,* proliferate, projecting into the large blood vessels within the decidua basalis through which the maternal blood flows.

Blood vessels form within the villi as they grow and connect with blood vessels that form in the chorion, in the body stalk, and within the body of the embryo. Blood begins to flow through this developing network of vessels as soon as the embryo's heart starts to beat.

ABOUT 4 WEEKS

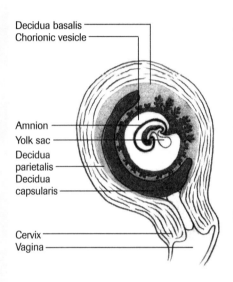

Decidua basalis
Chorionic vesicle
Amnion
Yolk sac
Decidua parietalis
Decidua capsularis
Cervix
Vagina

ABOUT 16 WEEKS

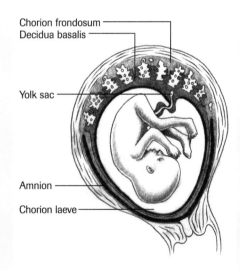

Chorion frondosum
Decidua basalis
Yolk sac
Amnion
Chorion laeve

Key characteristics of the decidua

- Decidua is the endometrial lining
- Decidua basalis: lies beneath the chorionic vesicle
- Decidua capsularis: stretches over the vesicle
- Decidua parietalis: lines the rest of the endometrial cavity

Key characteristics of fetal membranes

- Chorion: membrane forming the outer wall of the blastocyst
- Chorionic villi: vascular projections arising from the periphery of the chorion
- Chorion laeve: villi arising from the superficial portion of the chorion; atrophy as the chorionic vesicle enlarges
- Chorion frondosum: villi arising from the deeper part of the chorion; proliferate as the vesicle enlarges

LABOR AND POSTPARTAL ADAPTATION

Key facts about labor

- Labor begins when uterine contractions become strong and regular
- Contractions serve to expel the fetus from the uterus

Key factors contributing to the onset of labor

- Oxytocin receptors on uterine muscle fibers increase in number during pregnancy
- Stretching of uterus triggers secretion of oxytocin
- Fetus secretes cortisol, which diffuses into maternal circulation; this increases oxytocin and estrogen secretion and decreases progesterone secretion
- Decreasing progesterone leads to prostaglandin formation, which stimulates uterine contractions

Key factors contributing to maintenance of labor

- Cervical dilation stimulates the central nervous system to trigger increased oxytocin secretion
- As oxytocin stimulates uterine contractions, the cervix dilates further, which triggers the release of more oxytocin
- Oxytocin may also stimulate postaglandins formation, which enhances contractions

● **Key concepts**
- Childbirth (parturition, or delivery of the fetus) is accomplished through labor, the process in which the fetus is expelled from the uterus by uterine contractions
  – Weak uterine contractions occur irregularly throughout pregnancy
  – When labor begins, uterine contractions become strong and regular
  – Voluntary bearing-down efforts eventually supplement the contractions and lead to expulsion of the fetus and placenta
- Usually, the head of the fetus occupies the lowest part of the uterus; in this cephalic presentation, the fetus is delivered headfirst
- Childbirth is divided into three stages for descriptive purposes
- The duration of each stage varies with uterine size, maternal age, and the number of previous pregnancies
- After childbirth, the infant and mother undergo adaptation

● **Onset and maintenance of labor**
- Several factors contribute to the onset of labor
  – The number of oxytocin receptors on uterine muscle fibers increases progressively during pregnancy
    · These receptors reach a peak just before onset of labor
    · This increase causes the uterus to become more sensitive to the effects of oxytocin
  – The uterus stretches as the pregnancy progresses, initiating nerve impulses that stimulate oxytocin secretion from the posterior pituitary lobe
  – The fetus may also play a role in initiating labor
    · Near term, the fetal pituitary increases secretion of adrenocorticotropic hormone (ACTH)
    · This causes the fetal adrenal glands to secrete more cortisol, which diffuses into the maternal circulation through the placenta
    · Cortisol increases oxytocin and estrogen secretion and decreases progesterone secretion
    · These changes in hormone secretion increase uterine muscle irritability and make the uterus more sensitive to oxytocin stimulation
  – Prostaglandins may also play a role in initiating labor
    · Decreasing progesterone leads to conversion of esterified arachidonic acid into a nonesterified form
    · The nonesterified arachidonic acid biosynthesizes to form prostaglandins, which stimulate uterine contractions

- – Because postterm delivery carries an increased risk of fetal brain damage or death, labor induction or cesarean delivery may be needed if labor is delayed more than 2 weeks after the due date
- • After labor begins, several factors maintain it
    - – Cervical dilation causes nerve impulse transmission to the central nervous system, which increases oxytocin secretion from the pituitary gland
    - – Increased oxytocin secretion serves as a positive feedback mechanism
        - · Oxytocin stimulates more uterine contractions, which further dilate the cervix
        - · In turn, cervical dilation causes the pituitary to secrete more oxytocin
    - – Oxytocin may also stimulate prostaglandin formation by the decidua; prostaglandins diffuse into the uterine myometrium and enhance contractions

● Stages of labor

- • The first stage of labor is characterized by cervical effacement (thinning) and dilation; the fetus begins to descend (see *Cervical effacement and dilation,* page 400)
    - – Before labor begins, the cervix isn't dilated; by the end of the first stage, the cervix is dilated fully
    - – Uterine muscles contract actively while the cervix and the lower part of the uterus thin and dilate
    - – The amniotic sac and fluid function as a hydrostatic wedge to help dilate the cervix
    - – First stage typically lasts from 6 to 24 hours in primiparous women; it's much shorter in multiparous women
- • Second stage covers the time between full cervical dilation and expulsion of the fetus
    - – Uterine contractions increase in frequency and intensity, and the amniotic sac ruptures
    - – As the flexed head of the fetus enters the pelvis, pelvic muscles force the head to rotate anteriorly and force the back of the head (occiput) under the symphysis pubis
    - – Uterine contractions force the flexed head deeper into the pelvis
    - – Resistance of the pelvic floor gradually forces the head into extension
        - · As the head presses against the pelvic floor, the vulvar tissues stretch and the anus dilates
        - · At this stage, the vulvovaginal orifice may be enlarged surgically by a small incision, called an *episiotomy*
    - – As the head is delivered, the face passes over the perineum, and maternal tissues retract under the chin

Key characteristics of the first stage of labor

- • Uterine muscles contract while the cervix and lower uterus thin and dilate
- • The amniotic sac and fluid act as a wedge to help dilate the cervix
- • The cervix is fully dilated at the end of first stage
- • First stage lasts from 6 to 24 hours in primiparous women but is much shorter in multiparous women

Key characteristics of the second stage of labor

- • Uterine contractions increase in frequency and intensity
- • The amniotic sac ruptures
- • The head of the fetus enters the pelvis
- • Vulvar tissues stretch and the anus dilates
- • The head is delivered, followed by the shoulders and the rest of the fetus
- • This stage averages 45 minutes in primiparous women; it's shorter in multiparous women

Cervical effacement and dilation

THINNING WALLS

Cervical effacement is the progressive shortening of the vaginal portion of the cervix and the thinning of its walls during labor as it's stretched by the fetus. Effacement is described as a percentage, ranging from 0% (noneffaced and thick) to 100% (fully effaced and paper thin).

BIGGER EXIT

Cervical dilation refers to progressive enlargement of the cervical os to allow the fetus to pass from the uterus into the vagina. Dilation ranges from less than 1 cm to about 10 cm (full dilation).

NO EFFACEMENT OR DILATION

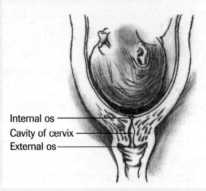

Internal os
Cavity of cervix
External os

EARLY EFFACEMENT AND DILATION

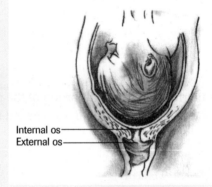

Internal os
External os

COMPLETE EFFACEMENT AND DILATION

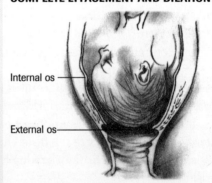

Internal os

External os

- The head, which had been rotated anteriorly during fetal descent, rotates back to its former position after passing through the vulvovaginal orifice
- Usually, the head undergoes lateral (external) rotation as the anterior shoulder rotates forward to pass under the pubic arch
- Delivery of the shoulders and the rest of the fetus follows shortly afterward
- This stage averages about 45 minutes in primiparous women; it may be much shorter in multiparous women
• Third stage of labor begins immediately after childbirth and ends with expulsion of the placenta
  - After delivery of the neonate, the uterus continues to contract intermittently and reduces in size
  - The area of placental attachment also is reduced correspondingly; because the bulky placenta can't decrease in size, it separates from the uterus
  - Blood seeps into the area of placental separation
  - As the uterus continues to contract, retroplacental blood is compressed and acts as a fluid wedge, cleaving the placenta from the uterus
  - Usually, the edges of the placenta are the last to separate from the uterine wall; the midportion of the placenta, covered by the fetal membrane, commonly is expelled first
  - This stage averages about 10 minutes in primiparous and multiparous women

Infant adjustment after birth
• The respiratory system undergoes changes after birth
  - The fetus depends on the mother to provide oxygen and remove carbon dioxide
  - At delivery, the oxygen supply from the mother ceases
    · This causes the infant's carbon dioxide level to increase, stimulating the respiratory center in the brain
    · In response, the brain causes the respiratory muscles to contract, allowing the infant to draw its first breath
• The cardiovascular system also makes several adjustments after birth
  - At birth, flaps of heart tissue fold together, closing the foramen ovale in the fetal heart and diverting blood to the lungs for the first time
  - When the infant's lungs start to function, heart muscle contractions close the ductus arteriosus
    · Closure normally becomes permanent about 3 months after birth
    · Incomplete closure results in patent ductus arteriosus

Key characteristics of the third stage of labor
- After childbirth, the uterus continues to contract and reduce in size
- The area of placental attachment reduces, causing the placenta to separate from the uterus
- Blood seeps into the area of separation, acting as a wedge to cleave the placenta from the uterus
- This stage averages 10 minutes

Key facts about infant adjustment after birth
- As oxygen supply from the mother ceases, the infant's carbon dioxide level rises
- This stimulates the respiratory center in the brain
- Respiratory muscles contract and the infant draws its first breath
- At the same time, flaps of heart tissue close the foramen ovale and heart muscle contractions close the ductus arteriosus
- The liver undergoes changes to regulate bile pigment production

Key facts about maternal adjustment after birth

- Uterus decreases in size in 2 weeks after childbirth
- The stretched tissues of the pelvis and vulva return to their former state more slowly
- The cervix becomes less elastic and returns to prepregnancy firmness
- Postpartal discharge persists for several weeks
- The reproductive tract requires 6 weeks to return to its former condition

Key facts about lactation

- As progesterone and estrogen levels fall after childbirth, the effects of prolactin are no longer inhibited
- Prolactin causes mammary glands to secrete milk
- Nipple stimulation triggers prolactin release
- Milk production continues as long as the nipples are stimulated
- Breast-feeding stimulates oxytocin, which causes milk ejection

- The liver must undergo changes at birth to regulate bile pigment production; this may lead to physiologic jaundice a few days after birth

● **Maternal adjustment after birth**
- After childbirth, the reproductive tract requires about 6 weeks to return to its former condition
  - This period is called the *puerperium,* or postpartal period
  - During this time, the uterus rapidly decreases in size; most of the involution occurs in the first 2 weeks after delivery
  - The stretched tissues of the pelvis and vulva return to their former state more slowly
  - The cervix becomes less elastic and returns to its prepregnancy firmness
- Postpartal vaginal discharge (lochia) persists for several weeks after childbirth
  - *Lochia rubra* (bloody discharge) occurs from 1 to 4 days postpartum
  - *Lochia serosa* (pink-brown, serous discharge) occurs from 5 to 7 days postpartum
  - *Lochia alba* (white, brown, or colorless discharge) occurs from 1 to 3 weeks postpartum

LACTATION

● **Key concepts**
- Milk production by the breasts, called *lactation,* is regulated by the interactions of four hormones
  - Estrogen and progesterone are produced by the ovaries and placenta; they stimulate proliferation of breast tissue
  - Prolactin and oxytocin are produced by the pituitary and decidua
    · Prolactin causes milk secretion after the breasts have been stimulated by estrogen and progesterone
    · Oxytocin causes contraction of specialized cells, which help expel milk during breast-feeding
- Breast-feeding stimulates prolactin secretion; the resulting high prolactin level causes changes in the mother's menstrual cycle

● **Hormonal initiation of lactation**
- Progesterone and estrogen levels fall sharply after childbirth when the placenta is expelled
- Because estrogen and progesterone no longer inhibit the effects of prolactin on milk production, the mammary glands begin to secrete milk

- Prolactin secretion also decreases after delivery unless the nipples are stimulated by breast-feeding
    - Sensory impulses from the nipples are transmitted to the hypothalamus; this stimulates prolactin release from the anterior pituitary lobe
    - Milk production continues as long as the nipples are stimulated regularly by breast-feeding; if breast-feeding is discontinued, the stimulus for prolactin release is removed and milk production stops
- Breast-feeding also stimulates oxytocin
    - Sensory impulses from the nipples are transmitted to the hypothalamus; this causes oxytocin release from the posterior pituitary lobe
    - Oxytocin causes contraction of the myoepithelial cells surrounding the breast lobules
    - This contraction causes *milk ejection* (expulsion of breast milk from the secretory lobules into larger ducts); the breast-feeding infant readily obtains milk from these ducts

● **Effects of breast-feeding on the menstrual cycle**
- The high prolactin level in a postpartal woman inhibits FSH and LH release
- If a woman doesn't breast-feed her infant, prolactin output soon declines and FSH and LH production by the pituitary is no longer inhibited
    - Cyclic release of FSH and LH soon follows
    - Normal menstrual cycles commonly resume about 6 weeks after delivery or a few weeks after discontinuation of breast-feeding
- If the woman breast-feeds her infant, the menstrual cycle doesn't resume because prolactin inhibits the cyclic release of FSH and LH necessary for ovulation; consequently, a breast-feeding woman has some protection from pregnancy
- The amount of prolactin released in response to breast-feeding gradually decreases
    - The inhibitory effect of prolactin on FSH and LH release also declines
    - As a result, ovulation and the menstrual cycle may resume; pregnancy may occur after this, even though the woman continues breast-feeding

Key facts about the effects of breast-feeding on the menstrual cycle

- High prolactin levels inhibit FSH and LH release, which prohibits ovulation
- If a woman breast-feeds, the menstrual cycle doesn't resume
- If breast-feeding doesn't occur, prolactin output declines, FSH and LH release follows, and the menstrual cycle resume after 6 weeks
- The amount of prolactin released in response to breast-feeding gradually decreases, making ovulation possible

TOP 10

Items to study for your next test on reproduction and lactation

1. Prerequisites necessary for fertilization to occur
2. The process of fertilization
3. Structural and hormonal changes occurring during pregnancy
4. The stages of embryonic and fetal development
5. The stages of labor
6. The processes of maternal and neonatal adaptation
7. Hormonal regulation of lactation
8. The effects of lactation on the menstrual cycle
9. Methods used to calculate the expected delivery date
10. Teaching tips for patients with infertility

NCLEX CHECKS

It's never too soon to begin your NCLEX preparation. Now that you've reviewed this chapter, carefully read each of the following questions and choose the best answer. Then compare your responses with the correct answers.

1. A nurse in a fertility clinic tells a client that cervical mucus is relatively thin, allowing spermatozoa to pass easily through the cervix during which part of the menstrual cycle?

☐ **1.** Menses
☐ **2.** Early in the cycle
☐ **3.** Midcycle
☐ **4.** Late in the cycle

2. A nurse knows that a client is in the second stage of labor when what occurs?

☐ **1.** Uterine contractions begin.
☐ **2.** The baby is delivered.
☐ **3.** The placenta is delivered.
☐ **4.** The cervix is fully dilated.

3. During a client's 1-week home visit, the visiting nurse documents the following on the chart below.

LOCHIA	
Date	10/7/06
Time	1400
Color	Pink
Odor	Normal
Consistency	No clots
Amount	1 pad/24 hr

What's the best term for the lochia described?

☐ **1.** Thrombic
☐ **2.** Alba
☐ **3.** Serosa
☐ **4.** Rubra

4. During a discussion about pre-embryonic development, the nurse correctly identifies which structure as the precursor to the placenta?

☐ **1.** Trophoblast
☐ **2.** Blastomere
☐ **3.** Zygote
☐ **4.** Morula

5. A nurse explains to a client that one purpose of the amniotic sac and its fluid is:

☐ **1.** to secrete estrogen and progesterone.
☐ **2.** to provide a steady temperature for the fetus.
☐ **3.** to supply nutrients to and remove wastes from the mother.
☐ **4.** to secrete prolactin and relaxin.

6. A nurse is assessing the umbilical cord following delivery. Which of the following would the nurse expect to see?

☐ **1.** Two arteries and one vein
☐ **2.** One artery and one vein
☐ **3.** Two arteries and two veins
☐ **4.** One artery and two veins

7. A nurse is assessing a client who thinks she may be pregnant. The nurse tells the client that HCG can be detected in the blood how soon in the pregnancy?

☐ **1.** As soon as fertilization occurs
☐ **2.** When implantation occurs
☐ **3.** As early as 9 days after fertilization
☐ **4.** At the time of the first missed period

8. After seeing her 12-week-old fetus on ultrasound, a client asks the nurse why the head of the fetus is so large. Which response by the nurse is most appropriate?

☐ **1.** "This is normal at this stage of fetal development."
☐ **2.** "There's probably something wrong with the fetus."
☐ **3.** "I'll tell the practitioner about your concerns."
☐ **4.** "Your baby will probably have a large head."

9. A nurse assesses a client in labor and determines that the fetus is in a cephalic presentation. The nurse would expect which body part to present first?

☐ **1.** Buttocks
☐ **2.** Foot
☐ **3.** Shoulder
☐ **4.** Head

10. Which type of vaginal discharge would the nurse expect to assess in a client who is 2 weeks' postpartum?

☐ **1.** No vaginal discharge
☐ **2.** Lochia rubra
☐ **3.** Lochia serosa
☐ **4.** Lochia alba

ANSWERS AND RATIONALES

1. CORRECT ANSWER: 3
Spermatozoa can pass readily through the cervix during the middle of the menstrual cycle, when mucus is relatively thin. Earlier in the menstrual cycle, spermatozoa have difficulty passing through the cervix because estrogen and progesterone levels cause the mucus to thicken. Later in the cycle, spermatozoa also have difficulty passing through the cervix because the mucus is much thicker. During menses, blood, mucus, and endometrial cells are discharged from the uterus as estrogen and progesterone levels fall to their lowest levels, reducing the likelihood of pregnancy.

2. CORRECT ANSWER: 4
The first stage of labor is characterized by cervical effacement and dilation. The second stage of labor begins when the cervix is fully dilated and ends with expulsion of the fetus. The third stage of labor begins immediately after childbirth and ends with expulsion of the placenta.

3. CORRECT ANSWER: 3
Lochia serosa is a pink or brownish discharge that occurs 4 to 10 days postpartum. Lochia alba is a creamy white or colorless discharge that occurs 10 to 14 days postpartum and may continue for up to 6 weeks. Lochia rubra is a red discharge that occurs 1 to 3 days postpartum. Lochia thrombic isn't a valid term.

4. CORRECT ANSWER: 1
The trophoblast develops into fetal membranes and the placenta. As the fertilized ovum advances through the fallopian tube toward the uterus, it undergoes mitotic division, forming daughter cells, called *blastomeres*. The zygote is the fertilized ovum, which develops into a small mass of cells called a *morula*.

5. CORRECT ANSWER: 2
The amniotic sac and its fluid protect the fetus by providing a buoyant, temperature-controlled environment. During the first 3 months of pregnancy, the corpus luteum is the main source of estrogen and progesterone. The placenta supplies nutrients to and removes wastes from the fetus. The decidua is the endometrial lining that has undergone the hormone-induced changes of pregnancy and secretes prolactin, relaxin, and prostaglandin.

6. CORRECT ANSWER: 1
The umbilical cord, which connects the fetus to the placenta, contains two arteries and one vein.

7. CORRECT ANSWER: 3
HCG can be detected in maternal blood as early as 9 days after fertilization, even before the first missed menstrual period.

8. CORRECT ANSWER: 1
During early development, the head of the fetus is disproportionately large compared to the rest of the fetus's body. This condition changes after birth as the infant grows.

9. CORRECT ANSWER: 4
Usually, the head of the fetus occupies the lowest part of the uterus. In this cephalic presentation, the head of the fetus is delivered first.

10. CORRECT ANSWER: 4
Lochia alba (white, brown, or colorless discharge) occurs from 1 to 3 weeks postpartum. Lochia rubra (bloody discharge) occurs from 1 to 4 days postpartum. Lochia serosa (pink-brown, serous discharge) occurs from 5 to 7 days postpartum. Vaginal discharge normally persists for several weeks after childbirth.

Glossary
Selected references
Index

Glossary

abdomen: area of the body between the diaphragm and pelvis

abduct: to move away from the midline of the body; the opposite of *adduct*

accommodation: adjustment of the eye's lens to change the focal length and bring images into sharp focus

acetabulum: hip joint socket into which the head of the femur fits

acetylcholine: neurotransmitter released at the synapses

acid: substance with excess hydrogen ions and a pH of less than 7.0

acid-base balance: stable concentration of hydrogen ions in body fluids

acinar cells: secretory cells surrounding a cavity such as those in the acinar glands of the pancreas

acromion: bony projection of the scapula

actin: contractile protein in muscle fibers

action potential: sudden change in electrical charge along a cell membrane

active transport: movement of a substance across a cell membrane by a chemical activity that allows the cell to admit larger molecules than would otherwise be able to enter; this transport mechanism requires energy

adduct: to move toward the midline of the body; the opposite of *abduct*

adenoids: paired lymphoid structures located in the nasopharynx

adrenal gland: one of two secretory organs that lie atop the kidneys; consists of a medulla and a cortex

afferent neuron: nerve cell that conveys impulses from the periphery to the central nervous system; the opposite of *efferent neuron*

agglutination: clumping of cells or microorganisms

air conduction: sound wave transmission through the tympanic membrane and auditory ossicles

albumin: protein in blood plasma

alimentary canal: GI tract; continuous tube open at both ends, extending through the ventral cavities from the mouth to the anus; functions in food digestion and absorption and waste elimination

all-or-none response: response that governs muscle fiber contractions in a motor unit; a nerve impulse strong enough to stimulate contraction causes all the fibers to contract

alpha cells: glucagon-secreting cells in the pancreatic islets

alveolus: small saclike dilation of the terminal bronchioles in the lung

ampulla: saclike dilation of a tube or duct

anabolism: synthesis of simple substances into complex ones, constructive part of metabolism

anaerobic metabolism: energy-releasing process that doesn't require oxygen in which glycogen and glucose are broken down into lactic acid

angiotensin: substance formed in the blood by the action of enzymes released from the kidneys

anterior: front or ventral; the opposite of *posterior* or *dorsal,* toward or near the head

antibody: immunoglobulin produced by the body in response to exposure to a specific foreign substance (antigen)

antigen: foreign substance that causes antibody formation when introduced into the body

anus: distal end or outlet of the rectum

aorta: main trunk of the systemic arterial circulation, originating from the left ventricle and eventually branching into the two common iliac arteries

apices: pointed extremities of conical structures such as the apices of the renal pyramids

aponeurosis: broad flat sheet of connective tissue that attaches muscle to bone or soft tissue

appendicular skeleton: division of the skeleton consisting of the pectoral and pelvic girdles and the upper and lower limbs

arachnoid: delicate middle membrane of the meninges

arcuate arteries: arc-shaped arteries that branch from the interlobar arteries

areola: pigmented ring around the nipple

arrectores pilorum: tiny smooth muscles of the skin, which are attached to hair follicles, that contract, causing the hair to stand erect (goose bumps)

arteriole: small branch of an artery

artery: vessel that carries blood away from the heart

arthrosis: joint or articulation

articulation: joint; point of junction of two or more bones

atom: unit of matter that contains a nucleus and electrons and makes up a chemical element

atrium: chamber or cavity

auricle: part of the ear that's attached to the head

axial skeleton: division of the skeleton consisting of the bones that form the longitudinal axis, including those of the skull, vertebral column, and bony thorax

axon: extension of a nerve cell that conveys impulses away from the cell body

base: substance with excess hydroxide ions and a pH greater than 7.0

basement membrane: extracellular, filamentous material composed mainly of collagen and found between the epidermis and dermis

beta cells: insulin-secreting cells in the pancreatic islets

binocular vision: vision that produces a three-dimensional image, which is necessary for normal depth perception

bladder: membranous sac that holds urine

bone: dense, hard connective tissue that composes the skeleton

bone conduction: sound wave transmission through the bones of the skull

bone marrow: soft tissue in the cancellous bone of the epiphyses; crucial for blood cell formation and maturation

bronchiole: small branch of the bronchus

bronchus: larger air passage of the lung

buccal: pertaining to the cheek

buffer system: system that minimizes pH changes caused by excess acids or bases (alkalies)

bursa: fluid-filled sac lined with a synovial membrane

calyces: cup-shaped organs or cavities such as those in the renal pelvis

capacitation: activation process for spermatozoa that allows ovum penetration; small perforations appear in the acrosome (head cap) of the spermatozoon, allowing enzyme release

capillary: microscopic blood vessel that links arterioles with venules

carbohydrate: organic compound that contains carbon, hydrogen, and oxygen in a specific arrangement

carbon dioxide: gaseous waste product of cell metabolism

cardiac cycle: events that occur during a single systole and diastole of the atria and ventricles; complete sequence of events in the heart from the beginning of one beat to the beginning of the next beat

cardiac output: amount of blood ejected per minute from a ventricle, which equals the stroke volume (volume of blood ejected from a ventricle at each contraction) multiplied by the heart rate in beats/minute

carpal: pertaining to the wrist

cartilage: connective supporting tissue occurring mainly in the joints, thorax, larynx, trachea, nose, and ear

catabolism: breakdown of complex substances into simpler ones or into energy

caudal: inferior, or toward the tail or lower part of the body

cecum: pouch located at the proximal end of the large intestine

celiac: pertaining to the abdomen

central nervous system: one of the two main divisions of the nervous system; consists of the brain and spinal cord

cerebellum: portion of the brain situated in the posterior cranial fossa behind the brain stem; coordinates voluntary muscular activity

cerebrospinal fluid: plasmalike fluid composed of secretions of the ventricles of the brain that fills the ventricles and surrounds the brain and spinal cord

cerebrum: largest and uppermost section of the brain, divided into hemispheres

chemotaxis: movement toward or away from a chemical stimulus

choroid plexus: any of the masses of capillaries in the ventricles of the brain that produce cerebrospinal fluid

chyme: mixture of partially digested food, water, and digestive juices

cilia: small, hairlike projections on the outer surfaces of some cells

citric acid cycle: metabolic pathway by which a molecule of acetyl-CoA is oxidized enzymatically to yield energy; also known as the *Krebs cycle*

coagulation: blood clotting

cochlea: spiral tube that makes up a portion of the inner ear

colon: part of the large intestine that extends from the cecum to the rectum

common bile duct: duct that receives bile from the hepatic and cystic ducts and transports it to the duodenum

complement system: collection of about 20 proteins in blood and tissue fluids that, when activated, augments the effects of antibodies

concentration gradient: differences in the concentration of the molecules on each side of a cell membrane

conditioned reflex: reflex that can be learned as a result of past associations; for example, salivation induced by the sight or smell of specific foods

condyle: rounded projection at the end of a bone

contralateral: on the opposite side; the opposite of *ipsilateral*

convergence: eye alignment so that the image of a newer object falls at corresponding points of both retinas, allowing depth perception

cornea: convex, transparent anterior portion of the eye

coronary: pertaining to the heart or its arteries

coronary sinus: enlarged vessel at the junction of the cardiac veins that empties blood into the right atrium

corpus luteum: the site of the ovum's expulsion; can produce estrogen and progesterone

cortex: outer part of an internal organ; the opposite of *medulla*

costal: pertaining to the ribs

countercurrent mechanism: process by which the kidneys concentrate urine

cranial: superior, or toward the head

cricoid: ring-shaped cartilage found in the larynx

cross bridges: structures formed by the binding of myosin filament heads to actin filaments; they pull actin filaments toward the center of the sarcomere, causing muscle contraction

cross over: mixing of genetic material in meiosis; during synapsis, chromatic segments of homologous chromosomes break off and interchange

cutaneous: pertaining to or affecting the skin

deamination: removal of the amino group-NH_2 from a compound

deep: farthest from the body surface

deltoid: shaped like a triangle (as in the deltoid muscle)

demarcate: limit or boundary

dendrite: branching process extending from the neuronal cell body that directs impulses toward the cell body

depolarization: change in resting membrane potential toward zero

dermis: skin layer beneath the epidermis

diaphragm: membrane that separates one part from another; the muscular partition separating the thorax and abdomen

diaphysis: shaft of a long bone

diarthrosis: freely movable joint

diastole: cardiac relaxation

diencephalon: part of the brain located between the cerebral hemisphere and the midbrain

diffusion: movement of dissolved particles (solute) across the cell membrane from one solution to a less concentrated one

digestion: breakdown of food into absorbable nutrients in the GI tract

distal: far from the point of origin or attachment; the opposite of *proximal*

diverticulum: outpouching from a tubular organ such as the intestine

dorsal: pertaining to the back or posterior; the opposite of *ventral* or *anterior*

duct: passage or canal

duodenum: shortest and widest portion of the small intestine extending from the pylorus to the jejunum

dura mater: outermost layer of the meninges

ear: organ of hearing

effector cells: cells capable of being stimulated to produce an effect

efferent neuron: nerve cell that conveys impulses from the central nervous system to the periphery; the opposite of *afferent neuron*

ejaculation: pulsatile expulsion of semen from the penis; associated with the erotic sensations called *orgasm*

ejection fraction: amount of blood ejected during each ventricular contraction in relation to the end-diastolic volume

electrolyte: substance that dissociates into ions when dissolved in water; can conduct an electrical current

electron: particle with a negative charge that orbits the nucleus in different electron shells

electron transport system: metabolic pathway that converts products of the citric acid cycle into energy

element: substance that can't be broken down into smaller substances

embryo: stage of fetal development through the eighth week of pregnancy

emission: semen movement into the urethra

end-diastolic volume: total blood volume in each ventricle before ventricular systole

endocardium: interior lining of the heart

endochondral bone formation: type of ossification in which a mass of cartilage forms, is invaded by osteoblasts, and is converted into bone

endocrine: pertaining to secretion into the blood or lymph rather than into a duct; the opposite of *exocrine*

end-systolic volume: blood volume that remains in a ventricle after systole

epidermis: outermost layer of the skin; lacking vessels

epiglottis: cartilaginous structure overhanging the larynx that guards against entry of food into the lung

epiphyses: ends of a long bone

epithelium: one of four main types of tissue

equilibrium: sense of balance

erythrocyte: red blood cell

erythropoiesis: process of red blood cell (erythrocyte) formation

esophagus: muscular canal that transports nutrients from the pharynx to the stomach

exocrine: pertaining to secretion into a duct; the opposite of *endocrine*

exocrine gland: gland that releases secretions through one or more ducts that open onto an internal or external body surface

expiratory reserve volume: amount of air that can be exhaled forcefully at the end of a normal tidal expiration (about 1,300 ml in the average adult)

extracellular fluid compartment: intravascular fluid (in blood plasma and lymph) and interstitial fluid (in loose tissue surrounding the cells)

eye: one of two organs of vision

facilitated diffusion: type of diffusion involving a carrier molecule in the cell membrane that picks up the diffusing substance on one side of the membrane and deposits it on the other side

fallopian tube: one of two ducts extending from the uterus to the ovary

fascia: fibrous membrane covering that supports and separates skeletal muscles

fasciculi: small bundles of muscle or nerve cells

fertilization: union of a spermatozoon and ovum

fetoplacental circulation: circulatory system that delivers oxygen-depleted blood from the fetus to the placenta by the umbilical arteries; it returns oxygenated blood to the fetus by the umbilical vein

fetus: term used to describe the unborn from the end of the eighth week of pregnancy until delivery

fibrinolysis: blood clot dissolution

fight-or-flight response: response to stimulation of the sympathetic nervous system that prepares an individual to cope with stress; also called *alarm response*

focal length: distance from a convex lens to its focal point

focal point: point behind a convex lens at which parallel light rays are brought into focus

fontanel: incompletely ossified area of a neonate's skull

foramen: small opening

fossa: hollow or cavity

functional areas: parts of the cerebral cortex related to specialized functions

fundus: base of a hollow organ; the part farthest from the organ's outlet

gallbladder: excretory sac lodged in the visceral surface of the liver's right lobe

gamete: sex cell (spermatozoon or ovum)

ganglion: cluster of nerve cell bodies found outside the central nervous system

gas exchange: process of respiration in which gases are transported between the air and capillaries in the lungs

genitalia: reproductive organs; may be external or internal

glabella: region above the root of the nose between the eyebrows

gland: organ or structure that secretes or excretes substances

glomerulus: compact cluster; kidney capillaries

gluconeogenesis: glucose synthesis from amino acids

glycogenolysis: glycogen breakdown into glucose

glycolysis: metabolic pathway that converts glucose to pyruvic or lactic acid and yields energy

gonad: sex gland in which reproductive cells form

gray matter: nervous tissue that appears gray from lack of myelinated fibers

heart: muscular, cone-shaped organ that pumps blood through the body

hematocrit: measurement of the volume of red blood cells packed by centrifuge, expressed as a percentage of the total blood volume

hematopoiesis: formation and development of blood cells from stem cells

hemoglobin: protein found in red blood cells that contains iron

hemostasis: arrest of bleeding by complex mechanisms that include vasoconstriction and coagulation

heterozygous: having different alleles at a given locus on homologous chromosomes

homeostasis: maintenance of a stable internal environment

homozygous: having identical alleles at a given locus on homologous chromosomes

hormone: substance secreted by an endocrine gland that triggers or regulates the activity of an organ or cell group

hyaline cartilage: flexible, semitransparent material composed of a basophilic, fibril-containing, interstitial substance with cavities containing chondrocytes; covers the articular surface of bones (also called *chondroid cartilage*)

hydrolysis: chemical reaction in which a chemical bond is broken and the atoms of a water molecule are added across the break; hydrogen is added to one side and the hydroxyl group to the other side

hydrostatic pressure: pressure that filters fluid from the blood through the capillary endothelium

hyoid: shaped like the letter U; the U-shaped bone at the base of the tongue

hypothalamus: structure in the diencephalon that secretes vasopressin and oxytocin

ileocecal valve: valve (sphincter muscle) located between the ileum of the small intestine and the cecum of the large intestine; permits only forward passage of intestinal contents

ileum: distal part of the small intestine extending from the jejunum to the cecum

immunity: ability to resist organisms or toxins that can damage tissues

incus: one of three bones in the middle ear

inferior: lower; the opposite of *superior*

inspiratory reserve volume: amount of air that can be inhaled forcefully at the end of a normal tidal inspiration (about 3,000 ml in the average adult)

integument: covering such as the skin and its derivatives

intestine: portion of the GI tract that extends from the stomach to the anus

intima: innermost structure

intracellular fluid compartment: fluid in the body's cells

intramembranous bone formation: type of ossification in which osteoblasts form bone without a preliminary cartilage mass

intrapleural pressure: pressure in the pleural cavity (space between the lung and the chest wall)

intrapulmonary pressure: air pressure in the lungs

involution: changes in the uterus occurring after childbirth in which the uterus shrinks in size

ion: charged particle formed when an electrolyte goes into a solution

ipsilateral: on the same side; the opposite of *contralateral*

jejunum: one of three portions of the small intestine; connects proximally with the duodenum and distally with the ileum

joint: fibrous, cartilaginous, or synovial connection between bones

kidney: one of two urinary organs on the dorsal part of the abdomen

labia: lips

lacrimal: pertaining to tears

lactation: milk production and secretion

larynx: voice organ; joins the pharynx and the trachea

lateral: pertaining to the side; the opposite of *medial*

leukocyte: white blood cell

ligament: band of white fibrous tissue that connects bones

lipids: organic compounds made of carbon, hydrogen, and water that's usually insoluble in water; fat

lipogenesis: lipid synthesis from glucose

liver: large gland in the right upper abdomen; divided into four lobes

lobe: defined portion of any organ, such as the liver or brain

lobule: small lobe

long bone: bone with a length that exceeds its width

lumbar: pertaining to the area of the back between the thorax and the pelvis

lungs: organs of respiration found in the chest's lateral cavities

lymph: watery fluid in lymphatic vessels

lymph node: small oval structure that filters lymph, fights infection, and aids hematopoiesis

lymphocyte: white blood cell; the body's immunologically competent cells

malleolus: projections at the distal ends of the tibia and fibula

malleus: tiny hammer-shaped bone in the middle ear

mammary: pertaining to the breast

manubrium: upper part of the sternum

mastication: the physical breaking up of food and mixing with saliva in the mouth, which is the first stage of digestion

matrix: extracellular substance secreted by connective tissue that determines the specialized function of the tissue; typically includes collagen, elastic, or reticular fibers and ground substances (material occupying intercellular spaces in fibrous connective tissue, cartilage, or bone)

meatus: opening or passageway

medial: pertaining to the middle; the opposite of *lateral*

mediastinum: middle portion of the thorax between the pleural sacs that contain the lungs

medulla: inner portion of an organ; the opposite of *cortex*

meiosis: special type of cell division in gametes in which the daughter cells receive half the number of chromosomes of the parent cells

membrane: thin layer or sheet

menarche: onset of menses

meninges: three connective tissue membranes that enclose the brain and spinal cord: the dura mater, arachnoid, and pia mater

menopause: cessation of menses, resulting from ovarian follicle depression; typically occurs around age 45

menstrual cycle: recurring cycle in which a layer of the endometrium is shed and then regrows, proliferates, and sheds again

metabolism: transformation of substances into energy or materials that the body can use or store; consists of the two processes anabolism and catabolism

metacarpals: bones of the hand located between the wrist and the fingers

metatarsals: bones of the foot located between the tarsal bones and the toes

milk ejection: expulsion of breast milk from the secretory lobules into larger ducts of the breast

mitochondria: cytoplasmic organelles that generate adenosine triphosphate

mitosis: type of cell division in which the parent cell produces identical daughter cells with chromosomes duplicated from the parent; it occurs in all human cells, except gametes

muscle: fibrous structure that contracts to initiate movement

myelin sheath: segmented, fatty wrapping around the axons of many nerve fibers

myocardium: thick, contractile layer of muscle cells that forms the heart wall

myofibril: threadlike contractile filaments found in skeletal muscle cells

myosin: contractile protein in muscle fibers; its interaction with actin is crucial to muscle contraction

Nägele's rule: method to determine the estimated date of delivery

nares: nostrils

negative feedback mechanism: mechanism in which an elevated level of a hormone or hormone-regulated substance suppresses further hormone output

nephron: structural and functional unit of the kidney

nerve: cordlike structure consisting of fibers that convey impulses from the central nervous system to the body

neurilemma: thin, membranous sheet composed of Schwann cells that surrounds the segmented myelin sheaths of peripheral nerve fibers

neuromuscular junction: motor endplate and the axon terminal associated with it

neuron: nerve cell

neutron: electrically neutral particle in an atom; mass nearly equal to that of the proton

neutrophil: white blood cell that removes and destroys bacteria, cellular debris, and solid particles

node: small mass of tissue; a swelling, knot, or protuberance that can be normal or pathologic

nucleic acid: organic compound made of nucleotides that contain pentose, a phosphate group, and a nitrogenous base

occiput: back of the head

olfactory: pertaining to the sense of smell

oogenesis: process of ova formation

ophthalmic: pertaining to the eye

opsonization: process by which phagocytosis increases

optic tracts: bundles of optic nerve fibers that connect the optic chiasma and the brain stem

orgasm: climax of sexual excitement usually accompanied by seminal fluid ejaculation in the male

osmolarity: measure of osmotic pressure exerted by a solution

osmosis: movement of water molecules across the membrane from a dilute solution (having a high concentration of water molecules) to a concentrated one (having a lower concentration of water molecules)

osmotic pressure: pressure exerted by a solution on a semipermeable membrane

ossicle: small bone, especially of the ear

osteoblast: mesodermal cell that participates in bone formation

osteoclast: large, multinucleated cell that reabsorbs the bone matrix

osteocyte: osteoblast embedded in the bone matrix

ovary: one of two female reproductive organs found on each side of the lower abdomen, next to the uterus

ovulation: ovum release from an ovarian follicle

oxidation: loss of electrons by a chemical compound

pacemaker: specialized cardiac tissue (specifically, the sinoatrial node) that generates impulses that spread to other regions of the heart; sets the contraction rate of the heart

pacinian corpuscles: encapsulated sensory nerve endings responsive to vibration and deep or heavy pressure found in sensitive skin, subcutaneous tissue, and other specialized areas, such as the pancreas, penis, clitoris, and nipple

pain: sensation of discomfort or suffering caused by pain receptor stimulation

palate: roof of the mouth

pancreas: secretory gland in the epigastric and hypogastric regions

parasympathetic: pertaining to the ocular, bulbar, and sacral divisions of the autonomic nervous system

parotid: located near the ear (as in the parotid gland)

partial pressure: pressure exerted by a single gas in a mixture of gases; designated by the letter "P" preceding the chemical symbol for the gas

passive transport: movement of small molecules across the cell membrane by diffusion; this transport mechanism requires no energy

patella: floating bone that forms the kneecap

pectoral: pertaining to the chest or breast

pelvis: funnel-shaped structure; lower part of the trunk

peptide: substance derived from two or more amino acids

pericardium: fibroserous sac that surrounds the heart and the origin of the great vessels

periosteum: fibrous membrane that covers bones except at joint surfaces

peripheral resistance: degree of impedance to blood flow, which may be increased by vasoconstriction

peristalsis: movement of tubular organ contents through wavelike, rhythmic muscular contractions

pH: measurement of the hydrogen ion concentration in body fluids; a pH of 7.0 is neutral, less than 7.0 is acidic, and greater than 7.0 is basic, or alkaline

phagocyte: cell that surrounds, engulfs, and digests harmful particles or cells

phagocytosis: process by which specialized cells engulf and dispose of organisms, other cells, and foreign particles

phalanx: one of the tapering bones that makes up the fingers and toes

pharynx: tubular passageway that extends from the base of the skull to the esophagus

phrenic: pertaining to the diaphragm

pia mater: innermost covering of the brain and spinal cord

pinocytosis: process in which specialized cells take in fluid

pituitary gland: gland attached to the hypothalamus that stores and secretes hormones

placenta: an organ of pregnancy that begins to develop in the third week; responsible for supplying nutrients and removing waste

plantar: pertaining to the sole

plasma: colorless, watery fluid portion of lymph and blood

platelet: small, disk-shaped blood cell necessary for coagulation

pleura: thin serous membrane that encloses the lung

plexus: network of nerves, lymphatic vessels, or veins

polarization: state of a nerve fiber not transmitting an impulse; the fiber exterior has a positive charge, the interior a negative charge

pons: portion of the brain that lies between the medulla and the mesencephalon

popliteal: pertaining to the back of the knee

posterior: back or dorsal; the opposite of *anterior* or *ventral*

process: prominence or projection (such as of bone)

pronate: to turn the palm downward; the opposite of *supinate*

prostate: male gland that surrounds the bladder neck and urethra

protein: organic compound made of carbon, hydrogen, oxygen, and nitrogen that contains amino acids

proton: particle with a positive electrical charge in an atom

proximal: situated nearest the center of the body; the opposite of *distal*

pseudostratified columnar epithelium: columnar epithelial tissue that appears to be (but isn't) multilayered

pupil: circular opening in the iris of the eye through which light passes

Purkinje fibers: modified cardiac muscle fibers that form part of the conduction system of the heart

pylorus: lower portion of the stomach through which stomach contents empty into the duodenum

receptor: molecular structure within or on the surface of a cell; sensory nerve terminal that responds to stimuli

reduction: gain of electrons by a chemical compound

referred pain: internal organ pain that's perceived as coming from the body surface at a site distant from the organ

reflex: involuntary action

reflex arc: chain of sensory, connecting, and motor neurons that produces a reflex when stimulated

refraction: bending of light rays as they pass from one medium to another of different density

refractive index: measurement of the refractive power of a medium; the greater the refractive index, the more the light rays are bent as they pass through the medium

refractory period: brief period after nerve impulse transmission during which the nerve fiber is unresponsive and can't transmit another impulse

renal: pertaining to the kidney

renal plexus: network of autonomic nerve fibers branching from the celiac plexus and accompanying the renal artery to the kidney; innervates the kidneys and ureters

renin-angiotensin-aldosterone mechanism: self-regulating mechanism that helps control blood pressure, blood volume, and sodium plasma concentration

residual volume: amount of air left after the lungs expel the expiratory reserve volume (about 1,200 ml in the average adult)

resorption: bone breakdown, which normally equals bone formation during adulthood

respiratory center: control center in the brain stem that regulates the rate and depth of respiration

resting membrane potential: voltage difference between the interior and exterior of a nerve fiber

retroperitoneally: behind the peritoneum or outside the peritoneal cavity

reuptake: absorption of a neurotransmitter into the synaptic vesicles of the axon terminals that originally released it

sagittal plane: vertical plane through the longitudinal axis of the trunk that divides the body into right and left regions

salt: substance that ionizes into anions and cations, but not into H^+ or OH^- ions

saltatory conduction: type of conduction in myelinated nerves in which the depolarization wave jumps between gaps in the myelin sheath rather than moving progressively along the fiber such as in unmyelinated nerves

sarcomere: smallest contractile unit of myofibrils in skeletal muscle

scrotum: skin pouch that houses the testes and parts of the spermatic cords

sebaceous gland: simple alveolar gland that secretes oil (sebum)

secretory coil: coiled secretory duct found in certain glands

semen: male reproductive fluid

serosa: serous membrane, such as the peritoneum, pleura, or pericardium

serum: watery fluid that remains after coagulating elements (clotting factors) have been removed from plasma

sexual response: penile erection and semen discharge (in men) or erection of the clitoris and labia minora without ejaculation of secretions (in women)

sinoatrial node: specialized cardiac tissue that sets the rate of cardiac contraction; also called the heart's *pacemaker*

sinus rhythm: normal cardiac rhythm, originating in the sinoatrial node

sodium-potassium pump: active transport mechanism that transports potassium ions through the cell membrane and simultaneously transports sodium ions out

spermatogenesis: process of spermatozoa formation

sphenoid: wedged-shaped bone at the base of the skull

spleen: highly vascular organ between the stomach and the diaphragm

stapes: tiny stirrup-shaped bone in the middle ear

Starling's law: the amount of cardiac muscle fiber stretching helps regulate stroke volume

sternum: long, flat bone that forms the middle portion of the thorax

stomach: major digestive organ located in the right upper abdomen

stratum germinativum: growth layer of the epidermis; collective term for the stratum basale and stratum spinosum

striated: marked with parallel lines such as striated (skeletal) muscle

stroke volume: volume of blood ejected from a single ventricle with each contraction

superficial: toward or at the body surface

superior: higher; the opposite of *inferior*

supinate: to turn the palm upward; the opposite of *pronate*

suture: fibrous joint in which the opposed surfaces are closely joined; an immovable articulation

symphysis: growing together; a type of cartilaginous joint in which fibrocartilage firmly connects opposing surfaces

synapse: point of contact between adjacent neurons

synovial fluid: viscid fluid that lubricates a joint

systole: contraction of the heart muscle

talus: anklebone

tarsus: instep

tendon: band of fibrous connective tissue that attaches a muscle to a bone

testis: one of two male gonads that produce semen

thyroid: secretory gland located at the front of the neck

tibia: shinbone

tidal volume: amount of air inhaled in one breath (about 500 ml in the average adult)

tongue: chief organ of taste found in the floor of the mouth

trachea: nearly cylindrical tube in the neck extending from the larynx to the bronchi that serves as a passageway for air

transamination: exchange of an amino group in an amino acid for a keto group in a keto acid through the action of transaminase enzymes

trimester: a 3-month period during pregnancy

tropic hormone: substance that stimulates hormone production by a target gland

tubercle: small, rounded process

tuberosity: elevation or protuberance; a broad, large process

turbinate: shaped like a cone or spiral; a bone located in the posterior nasopharynx

ureter: one of two thick-walled tubes that transport urine to the bladder

urethra: small tubular structure that drains urine from the bladder

uteroplacental circulation: circulatory system that delivers oxygenated arterial blood from the maternal circulation to the placenta by the uterine arteries; it returns blood to the maternal circulation by veins near the arteries

uterus: hollow, internal female reproductive organ in which the fertilized ovum is implanted and the fetus develops

uvula: tissue projection that hangs from the soft palate

vagina: sheath; the canal in the female extending from the vulva to the cervix

valve: structure that permits fluid to flow in only one direction

vein: vessel that carries blood to the heart

vena cava: one of two large veins that returns blood from the peripheral circulation to the right atrium

ventilation: process of respiration in which air moves in and out of the lungs

ventral: pertaining to the front or anterior; the opposite of *dorsal* or *posterior*

ventricle: small cavity, such as one of several in the brain or one of the two lower chambers of the heart

venule: small vessel that connects veins and capillary plexuses

vertebra: any of the 33 bones that make up the spinal column

viscera: internal organs

visceral peritoneum: serous membrane that covers the external surfaces of most abdominal organs; also called *perimetrium*

vital capacity: maximum amount of air that can be moved in and out of the lungs by maximum inspiration and maximum expiration (about 4,800 ml in the average adult)

vitreous: glasslike; referring to the body of the eye

voiding reflex: involuntary reflex that causes the urge to urinate when the bladder contains 300 to 400 ml of urine, which is under a high degree of voluntary control

white matter: nervous tissue that appears white from myelinated sheaths surrounding nerve fibers

xiphoid: sword-shaped; the lower portion of the sternum

zygote: fertilized ovum

Selected references

Anatomy & Physiology Made Incredibly Easy, 2nd ed. Philadelphia: Lippincott Williams & Wilkins, 2004.

Antevil, J.L., et al. *Anatomy Recall,* 2nd ed. Philadelphia: Lippincott Williams & Wilkins, 2005.

Atlas of Pathophysiology, 2nd ed. Philadelphia: Lippincott Williams & Wilkins, 2006.

Bartsch, T., and Goadsby, P.J. "Anatomy and Physiology of Pain Referral Patterns in Primary and Cervicogenic Headache Disorders," *Headache* 45(8):1100, September 2005.

Bray, R.C., et al. "Normal Ligament Structure, Physiology, and Function," *Sports Medicine & Arthroscopy Review* 13(3):127-35, September 2005.

Clemente, C. *Anatomy: A Regional Atlas of the Human Body,* 5th ed. Philadelphia: Lippincott Williams & Wilkins, 2006.

Clemente, C. *Clemente's Anatomy Dissector,* 2nd ed. Philadelphia: Lippincott Williams & Wilkins, 2006.

Farquhar, S., and Fantasia, L. "Pulmonary Anatomy and Physiology and the Effects of COPD," *Home Healthcare Nurse* 23(3):167-74, March 2005.

Gunstream, S.E. *Anatomy and Physiology Laboratory Textbook, Essentials Version,* 4th ed. New York: McGraw-Hill Book Co., 2007.

Hansel, D., and Dintzis, R. *Lippincott's Pocket Pathology.* Philadelphia: Lippincott Williams & Wilkins, 2005.

Le Vay, D. *Teach Yourself Human Anatomy and Physiology.* New York: McGraw-Hill Book Co., 2004.

Portable Pathophysiology. Philadelphia: Lippincott Williams & Wilkins, 2007.

Porth, C.M. *Pathophysiology: Concepts of Altered Health States,* 7th ed. Philadelphia: Lippincott Williams & Wilkins, 2004.

Ramsay, D.T., et al. "Anatomy of the Lactating Human Breast Redefined with Ultrasound Imaging," *Journal of Anatomy* 206(6):525-34, June 2005.

Robinson, A.G., et al. "Using Fresh Tissue Dissection to Teach Human Anatomy in the Clinical Years," *Academic Medicine. Special Theme: Administrative Issues in Medical Research* 79(7):711-16, July 2004.

Rubin, E., et al. *Rubin's Pathology Clinicopathologic Foundations of Medicine.* Philadelphia: Lippincott Williams & Wilkins, 2005.

Thibodeau, G.A., and Patton, K.T. *Anatomy and Physiology,* 6th ed. St. Louis: Mosby–Year Book, Inc., 2006.

Thibodeau, G.A., and Patton, K.T. *Anthony's Textbook of Anatomy & Physiology,* 18th ed. St. Louis: Mosby–Year Book, Inc., 2006.

Thibodeau, G.A., and Patton, K.T. *The Human Body in Health & Disease,* 4th ed. St. Louis: Mosby–Year Book, Inc., 2006.

Watson, R. *Anatomy and Physiology for Nurses,* 12th ed. Philadelphia: Elsevier, 2005.

Index

i refers to an illustration; t refers to a table.

i refers to an illustration; t refers to a table.

i refers to an illustration; t refers to a table.

---

i refers to an illustration; t refers to a table.

---

i refers to an illustration; t refers to a table.

---

i refers to an illustration; t refers to a table.

i refers to an illustration; t refers to a table.

---

i refers to an illustration; t refers to a table.

i refers to an illustration; t refers to a table.

i refers to an illustration; t refers to a table.

i refers to an illustration; t refers to a table.

i refers to an illustration; t refers to a table.

ABOUT THE CD-ROM

The enclosed CD-ROM is just one more reason why the *Straight A's* series is at the head of its class. The more than 250 additional NCLEX®-style questions contained on the CD provide you with another opportunity to review the material and gauge your knowledge. The program allows you to:

- take tests of varying lengths on subject areas of your choice
- learn the rationales for correct and incorrect answers
- print the results of your tests to measure progress over time.

Minimum system requirements

To operate the *Straight A's* CD-ROM, we recommend that you have the following minimum computer equipment:

- Windows XP-Home
- Pentium 4
- 256 MB RAM
- 10 MB of free hard-disk space
- SVGA monitor with High Color (16-bit)
- CD-ROM drive
- mouse.

Installation

Before installing the CD-ROM, make sure that your monitor is set to High Color (16-bit) and your display area is set to 800 × 600. If it isn't, consult your monitor's user's manual for instructions about changing the display settings. (The display settings are typically found in Start/Settings/Control Panel/Display/Settings tab.)

To run this program, you must install it onto the hard drive of your computer, following these three steps:

1. Start Windows XP-Home (minimum).
2. Place the CD in your CD-ROM drive. After a few moments, the install process will automatically begin. *Note:* If the install process doesn't automatically begin, click the Start menu and select Run. Type *D:\setup.exe* (where *D:* is the letter of your CD-ROM drive) and then click OK.
3. Follow the on-screen instructions for installation.

Technical support

For technical support, call toll-free 1-800-638-3030, Monday through Friday, 8:30 a.m. to 5 p.m. Eastern Time. You may also write to Lippincott Williams & Wilkins Technical Support, 351 W. Camden Street, Baltimore, MD 21201-2436, or e-mail us at *technicalsupport3@wolterskluwer.com.*